Y0-BGW-288

AN ATLAS OF DIAGNOSTIC AND THERAPEUTIC PROCEDURES FOR EMERGENCY PERSONNEL

To Mary Louise

AN ATLAS OF DIAGNOSTIC AND THERAPEUTIC PROCEDURES FOR EMERGENCY PERSONNEL

JAMES H. COSGRIFF, JR., M.D.
ATTENDING SURGEON
CHIEF OF TRAUMA SERVICE
SISTERS OF CHARITY HOSPITAL
ASSISTANT CLINICAL PROFESSOR OF SURGERY
STATE UNIVERSITY OF NEW YORK AT BUFFALO

with illustrations by
MELFORD D. DIEDRICK
DIRECTOR OF MEDICAL ILLUSTRATION
SCHOOL OF MEDICINE
STATE UNIVERSITY OF NEW YORK AT BUFFALO

J.B. LIPPINCOTT COMPANY
Philadelphia
New York / San Jose / Toronto

Copyright © 1978 by J. B. Lippincott Company

This book is fully protected by copyright and, with the exception of brief excerpts for review, no part of it may be reproduced in any form by print, photoprint, microfilm, or by any other means without the written permission of the publishers.

Distributed in Great Britain by
Blackwell Scientific Publications
London   Oxford   Edinburgh

ISBN 0-397-54213-5

Library of Congress Catalog Card Number 78-2943

Printed in the United States of America

2 4 6 8 9 7 5 3 1

Library of Congress Cataloging in Publication Data
Cosgriff, James H
    An atlas of diagnostic and therapeutic procedures for emergency personnel.

    Includes bibliographies and index.
    1. Medical emergencies—Atlases. 2. Diagnosis—Atlases. 3. Therapeutics—Atlases. I. Title.
RC86.7.C67   616'.025   78-2943
ISBN 0-397-54213-5

PREFACE

This Atlas is designed for all professional personnel who are actively engaged in direct patient care. It was written in response to a perceived need for a single reference guide which includes procedures commonly used in the diagnosis and treatment of the acutely ill or injured patient. With few exceptions, the methods described herein have been used personally by the author in the care of his own patients during the past 20 years.

Details of each procedure include indications for its use, specific equipment needs, important anatomical considerations and the step-by-step technique involved in performing it. Variations applying to pediatric patients are included. Approximately 70 procedures are described, ranging from the simple technique of venous puncture, to more complicated procedures such as pericardiocentesis, several methods of chest drainage, skeletal traction, single injection limb arteriography and others.

A comprehensive review of airway management technique and cardiopulmonary resuscitation is given. The Heimlich Maneuver, which admittedly may have little applicability in the hospital setting, but should be known to all health personnel, is presented in a detailed manner including an excellent illustration of the mechanism which makes the maneuver effective. The illustrations were designed and prepared by Melford D. Diedrich.

A detailed discussion of the principles of local anesthesia is among the contents with a number of specific nerve blocks useful in a variety of circumstances.

The procedures enumerated require no sophisticated gear. The equipment needed is readily available in any clinical setting. Thus it is hoped that readers will become familiar with each of the various techniques and be encouraged to include them in their armamentarium and utilize them in providing better patient care.

ACKNOWLEDGMENTS

The contents of this volume were derived from personal experience and discussion with numerous resident and attending physicians and emergency department and intensive care nurses whose recommendations were helpful to me in many ways.

I am particularly grateful to my good friends and colleagues, Doctor Ambrose A. Macie who prepared "Emergency Maternity Care" and Doctor Arthur J. Schaefer who performed the removal of a soft contact lens; Doctors Robert Dean, Anthony Federico, William Schemel and Joseph Serio who reviewed portions of the manuscript and provided much helpful advice.

Patricia Brady Pirrami, Karen Collins, Susan Schaefer Theeman, Carroll Becker and Joseph Pirrami, Jr. served as models or assisted with the illustrations, for which I am most appreciative.

Many thanks also to Anne Cohen who provided much help in securing needed references and to Sheila Fruehauf for her kind assistance.

Special appreciation must be expressed to my son, James, who endured long, tiring, sometimes painful hours of posing for many of the illustrations in this volume. His patience and high level of cooperation contributed significantly to ease this onerous task and to him I am most grateful.

Melford Diedrick, Director of Medical Illustration of The State University of New York at Buffalo gave freely of his time, knowledge and long experience to design and prepare the numerous illustrations required for this text. His patience in working with me in the interpretation of the manuscript and his insistence on accuracy and detail in the design of the illustrations has contributed enormously to whatever success this volume attains.

Dennis Atkinson, of The State University of New York at Buffalo, a talented medical photographer, spent many hours working on the details of photographing procedures and equipment. His availability at all times and his persistence in achieving the best from his work is deeply appreciated.

Geraldine Brady and Eleonore Barlog gave many hours to the arduous work of typing and retyping the manuscript and related correspondence. Their professional skills and willing assistance is gratefully acknowledged.

I am particularly indebted to David T. Miller, of J. B. Lippincott Co. whose encouragement and support has brought this endeavor to fruition. He reviewed each procedure with me and made many helpful suggestions, each of which has served to improve the volume. I look forward to working with him in future ventures.

Val Rementer, Head of Copy Editorial for Higher Education, J. B. Lippincott Co., rendered valuable assistance as my copy editor. Her flexibility and easy manner made the work of proof review much easier.

Lastly, I would be remiss indeed if I failed to acknowledge my many unnamed patients who have been the objects of my professional interest over the past 20 years and particularly those who allowed photographs to be taken during the course of their surgical procedure.

James H. Cosgriff, Jr., M.D.

CONTENTS

1
Airway management
1

2
Use of esophageal obturator airway
11

3
Endotracheal intubation
15

4
Needle cricothyrotomy
21

5
Tracheostomy
25

6
Heimlich maneuver
39

7
Single injection percutaneous femoral arteriogram
45

8
Single injection percutaneous axillary arteriogram
47

9
Vascular puncture techniques
53

10
Arterial puncture
59

11
Venipuncture
63

12
Venous cutdown
71

13
Injection of bicipital tendon sheaths
77

14
Aspiration of olecranon bursa
81

15
Aspiration of patellar bursa
83

16
Injection of radiohumeral bursa
85

17
Injection of subacromial bursa
87

18
Aspiration of ganglion
91

19
Cardiopulmonary resuscitation (CPR)
93

20
Temporary emergency transvenous pacemaker
111

21
Antishock suit
115

22
Central venous catheterization
121

23
Central venous catheter antecubital approach
125

24
Central venous catheter external jugular approach
127

25
Central venous catheter internal jugular approach
129

26
Central venous catheter subclavian approach
133

27
Eversion of upper eyelid
137

28
Removal of hard corneal (contact) lens
141

29
Removal of soft corneal (contact) lens
143

30
Drainage of felon
147

31
Drainage of subungual hematoma
149

32
Removal of finger ring
151

33
Removal of imbedded fish hook
155

34
Gastrointestinal tubes
157

35
Levin and Salem-sump tube
163

36
Cantor tube
167

37
Miller-Abbott tube
171

38
Blakemore-Sengstaken tube
175

39
Local anesthesia
179

40
Field block
185

41 Supraorbital nerve block 189

42 Infraorbital nerve block 193

43 Mental nerve block 197

44 Intercostal nerve block 201

45 Median nerve block 203

46 Radial nerve block 207

47 Ulnar nerve block 211

48 Digital nerve block 215

49 Lumbar puncture 219

50 Removal of foreign bodies in ear and nose 223

51 Anterior nasal packing 227

52 Posterior nasal packing
229

53 Indirect (mirror) laryngoscopy
233

54 Pericardiocentesis
237

55 Needle drainage of the pleural cavity
241

56 Thoracentesis
245

57 Closed thoracostomy
251

58 Peritoneal flank tap
259

59 Peritoneal four-quadrant tap
261

60 Peritoneal lavage
265

61 Cul-de-sac aspiration
269

62 Steinman pin insertion
271

63 Cervical traction
275

64
Cystography and stress cystography
279

65
Trocar suprapubic cystotomy
283

66
Urethral catheterization
287

67
Urethrogram
291

68
Emergency maternity care
295

69
Dental emergencies
309

Index
311

1 AIRWAY MANAGEMENT

Airway management is the ability to establish and maintain a patent airway and to allow for or provide adequate respiratory exchange. Emergency personnel should be well-practiced in this essential skill, since it has the highest priority in the treatment of the acutely ill or injured patient. Thousands of lives are lost annually because of failure to recognize and adequately treat airway difficulties.

ETIOLOGY

The common causes of airway problems may be classified as follows:
1. NEUROGENIC, which involves depression or failure of the respiratory center in the brain stem, may occur with a cerebrovascular accident, craniocerebral trauma, and drug overdose or secondary to injuries to the cervical spine and spinal cord.
2. OBSTRUCTIVE, resulting from retained secretions, vomitus, dentures, or other foreign bodies in the pharynx which prevent movement of air into the lungs.
3. PARENCHYMAL, which refers to loss of integrity of the air passages exemplified by penetrating wounds of the trachea, bronchi or lung substance, spontaneous pneumothorax, tension pneumothorax, or damage by long-standing disease such as emphysema.
4. SKELETAL, resulting from maxillofacial injury with obstruction of the upper airway or secondary to blunt or penetrating trauma to the chest wall causing alterations in the respiratory mechanics, as in flail chest or sucking wounds.

More often than not, the causes of an airway inadequacy are multiple; for example, a patient comatose from an overdose of drugs may have depression of the respiratory center (neurogenic) plus retained secretions or vomitus occluding the pharynx (obstructive). Similarly, a patient with gunshot wounds of the neck and chest may have a penetrating wound of the trachea and the lung with pneumothorax (parenchymal) combines with a sucking wound of the chest wall (skeletal).

The above classification is not absolute, for clinically, one category may overlap another; however, it provides the physician or nurse the means for a rational approach to the care of a patient with an airway problem.

RECOGNITION OF AIRWAY DIFFICULTIES

Prompt identification of compromised or inadequate respiration is the keystone of appropriate airway management, for it will determine the therapeutic measures which must be undertaken to correct the problem. This requires a rapid, but thorough, assessment of the patient.

Complete absence of respiratory activity is readily recognized and usually neurogenic in origin. The skin and nail beds may be cyanotic. Cardiac activity may continue with a normal or increased rate and blood pressure is detectable for a period of time after respiratory arrest.

Interference with air flow, due to partial obstruction of the airway or abnormal conditions in the parenchyma or skeletal structures, will produce respiratory distress. The patient will have an apprehensive facies and appear restless as breathing becomes more labored. The accessory muscles of respiration are seen to become active, the ala nasi flare, and supraclavicular and suprasternal tugging is noted. Respirations may become noisy, and gurgling sounds are often heard. These signs are best seen in a small child or infant in respiratory distress, but are applicable to adults. Once observed, they are not easily forgotten and require prompt action.

Cyanosis is not always present. It is an ominous sign which may develop late and is more readily noted in the ear lobes and nail beds. Although there are many conditions in which cyanosis occurs, the underlying factor is the presence of unsaturated hemoglobin in the amount of 6 to 7 volumes percent in the capillary bed. In a patient with a normal hemoglobin level of 14 to 15 Gm per 100 cc of blood, this would be equivalent to one-third of the hemoglobin being unsaturated. In an anemic patient, it is possible that the total amount of circulating hemoglobin is insufficient to allow this degree of unsaturation and, thus, despite respiratory insufficiency, cyanosis may not be detected.

Noisy respiration is a frequent sign of partial airway obstruction. Perhaps the best example of this is snoring, which is produced by the tongue partially obstructing the hypopharynx.

In patients with chest wall injury, observe the motion of the chest on the injured side. With simple rib fractures the chest will be splinted by the patient and restricted movements noted on the injured side. With extensive rib fractures, when a rib is broken in two places, the normal excursion of the chest wall is lost. The injured segment moves paradoxically. With inspiration, the fractured segment is drawn inward and with expiration it bulges outward (paradoxical respiration). As a result, the lung underlying this flail segment fails to draw in or expel

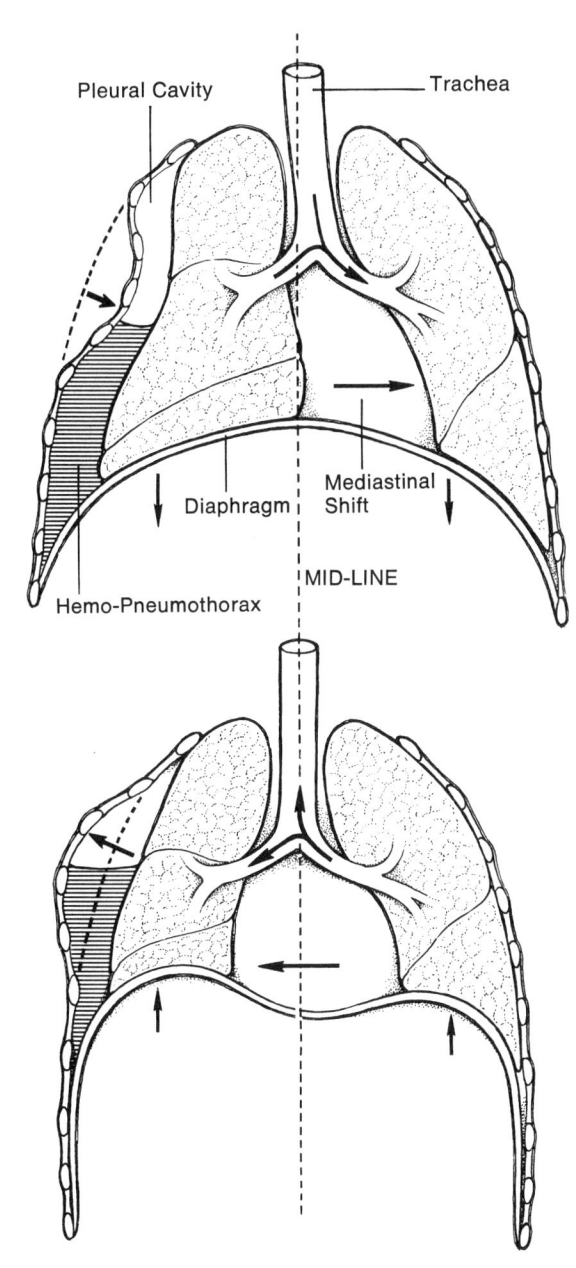

Respiration in a flail chest. Diagram on top shows flail area of right chest wall, which moves in with inspiration. Air moves into the left (normal) lung from the right bronchial tree as well as via normal tracheal inflow. Ventilation of the right lung is compromised. The mediastinum shifts to the uninjured side, further compromising exchange on the normal side. On expiration (bottom), air is driven out through the trachea and into the right (injured) side. This movement of air from one lung to the other is known as "pendulum movement," which leads to further deoxygenation. Hemopneumothorax further compromises oxygen exchange.

air effectively. The severity of respiratory compromise is directly proportional to the size of the injured (flail) segment and the degree of paradoxical respiration that results.

In penetrating wounds of the chest wall, a sucking wound may be present. In this situation, a direct communication exists between the pleural cavity and the atmosphere, with the result that a pneumothorax is invariably present with partial collapse of the lung, causing poor respiratory exchange. A noisy, sucking sound will be heard with inspiration and expiration as air is drawn in and pushed out through the open wound.

TREATMENT

Once the cause(s) of the airway problem are recognized, appropriate corrective measures should be undertaken. In addition to opening the airway, these measures include attempting to reverse the pathophysiology of the problem and even providing artificial ventilation.

The first step in relieving airway obstruction is to position the patient properly; usually the supine position is preferable. This is especially true for comatose patients. This position allows for removal of secretions or foreign bodies from the mouth and pharynx and is suitable for mouth-to-mouth ventilation if required.

After ascertaining that there is no fracture or dislocation of the cervical spine, extend the head and neck by placing one hand behind the patient's neck and raising it, while pushing backwards on the forehead. This head-tilt maneuver may, of itself, correct the situation.

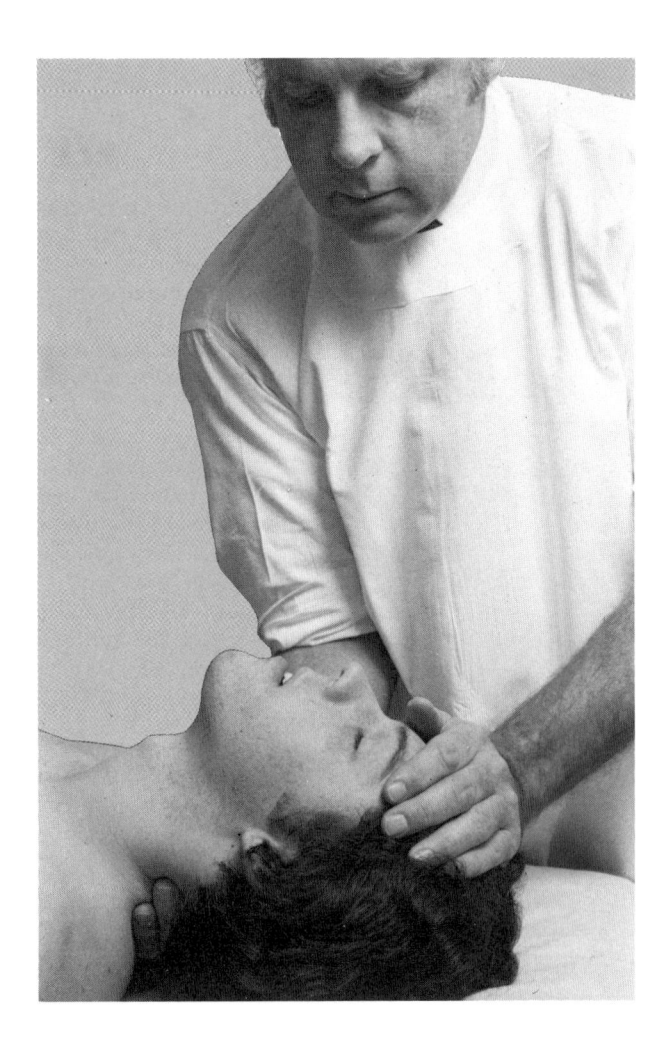

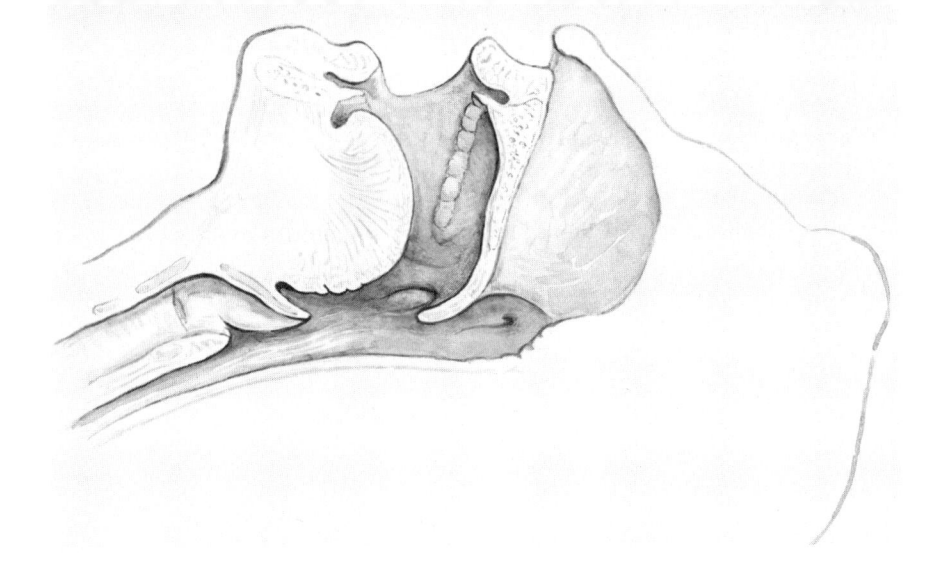

If not, elevate the mandible by upward pressure with the fingers at the angles of the jaw. This will raise the tongue from the hypopharynx. If needed,

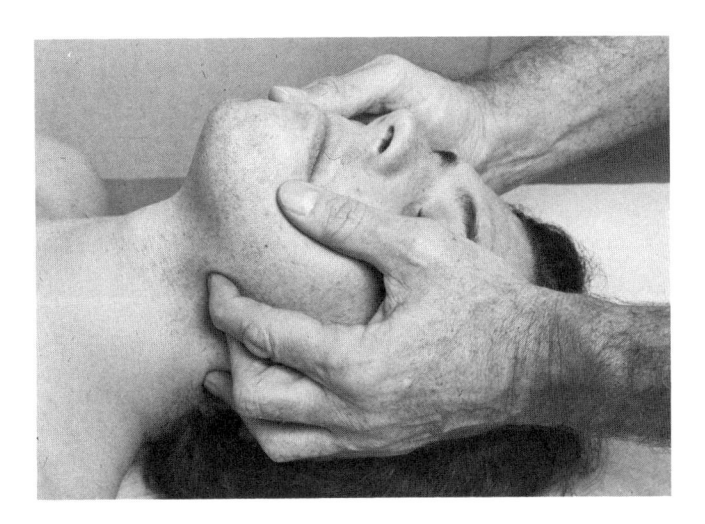

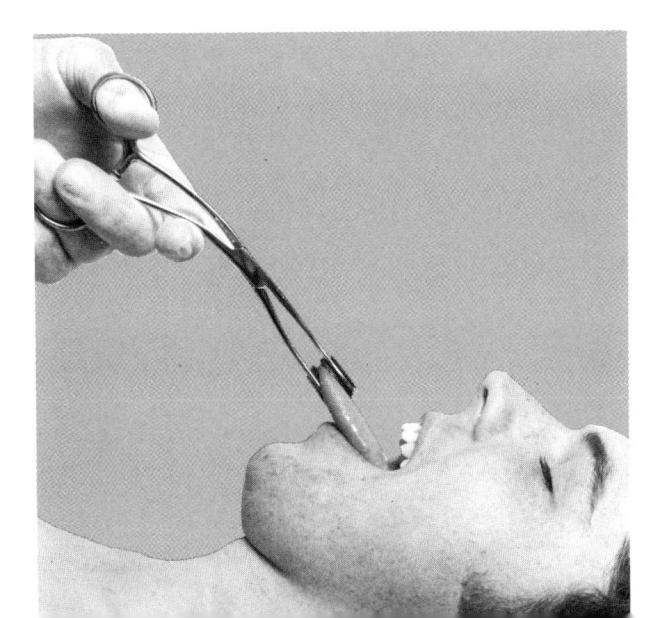

grasp the tongue with a padded forceps and draw it outward. Check the mouth and pharynx, aspirate secretions and remove visible foreign bodies. If the patient is apneic, commence artificial ventilation.

If the patient is breathing spontaneously introduce an oropharyngeal airway. This device is inserted through the mouth over the tongue to the pharynx

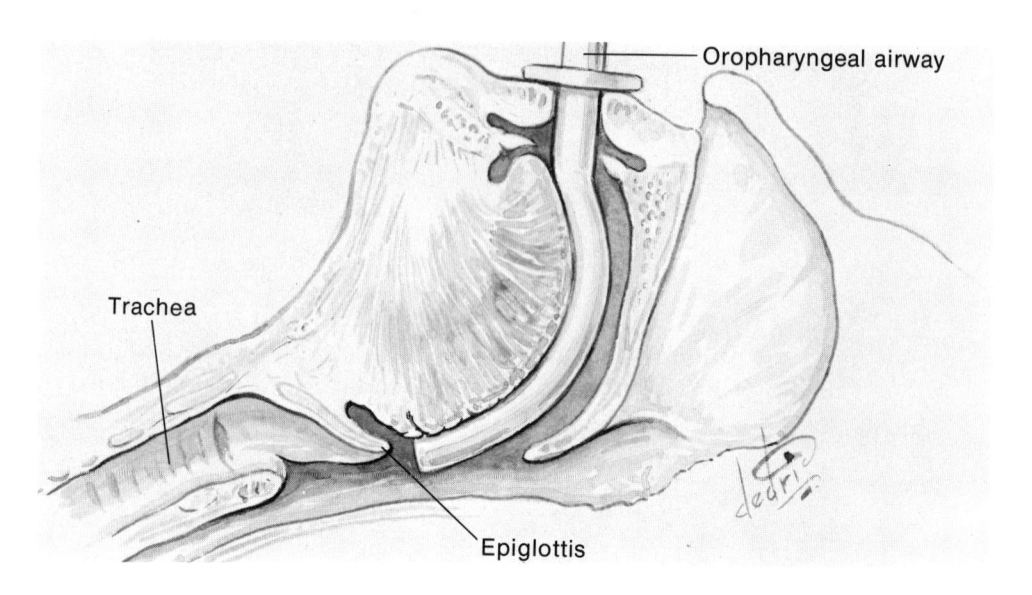

and keeps the tongue in a forward position. These airways are available in varying size and may be inserted via the nose (nasopharyngeal airway).

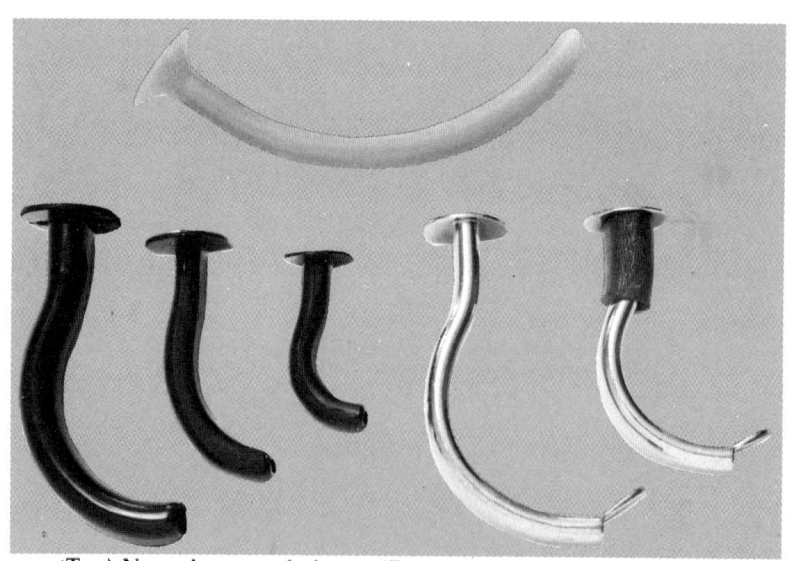

(Top) Nasopharyngeal airway (Bottom) Oropharyngeal airways

Ventilatory assist may be given using a bag-valve-mask unit, such as an Ambu® bag. However, if this is needed for an extended period of time, some other method of airway maintenance is preferable. Prolonged ventilatory assist with the bag-valve-mask may cause gastric dilatation, with subsequent regurgitation and possible aspiration of gastric contents into the airway. In this instance, endotracheal intubation is much better and may be combined with an Ambu bag.

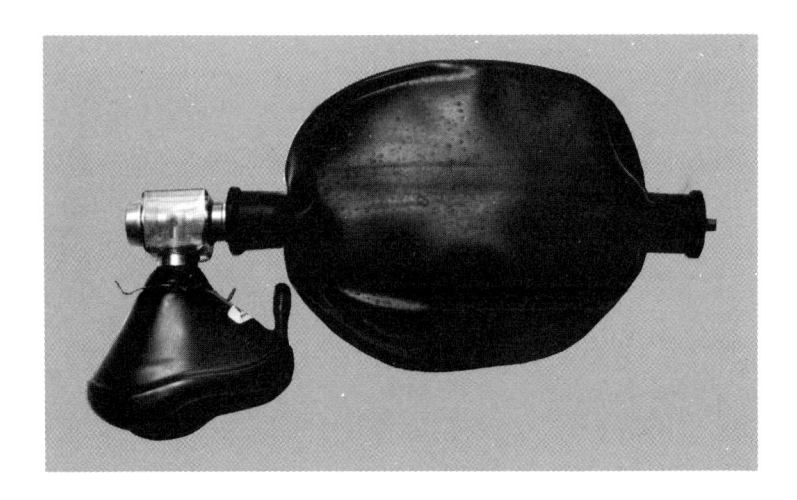

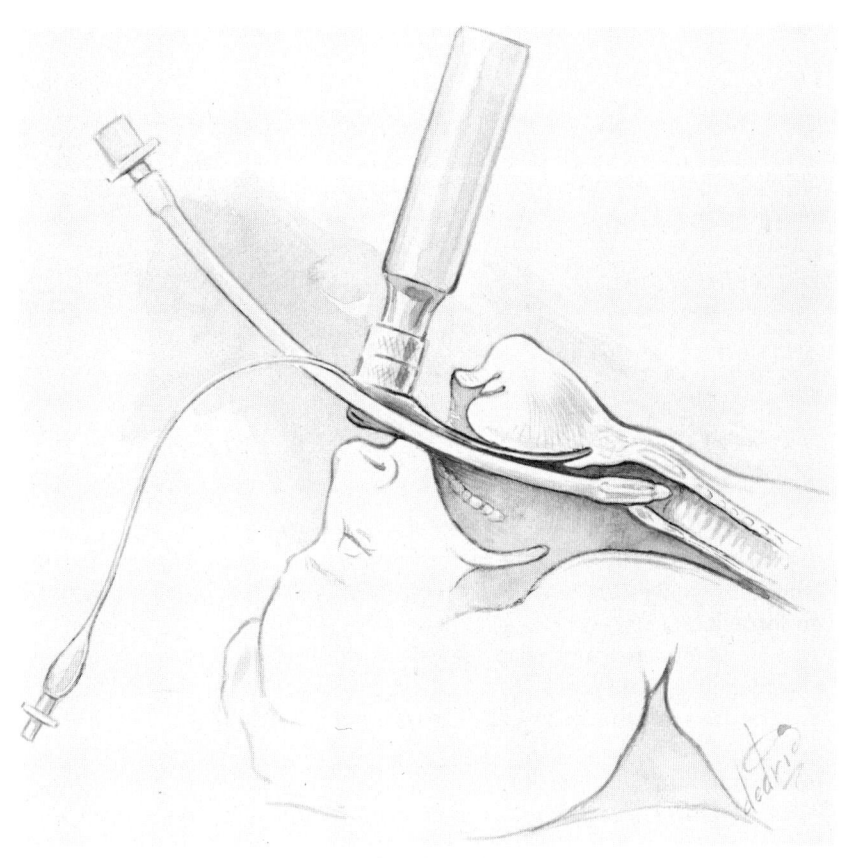

Insertion of endotracheal tube

Other means of establishing and maintaining an airway include cricothyrotomy, esophageal obturator airway, and tracheostomy. As a minimum, any emergency physician or nurse should be skilled in the insertion of a cuffed endotracheal tube.

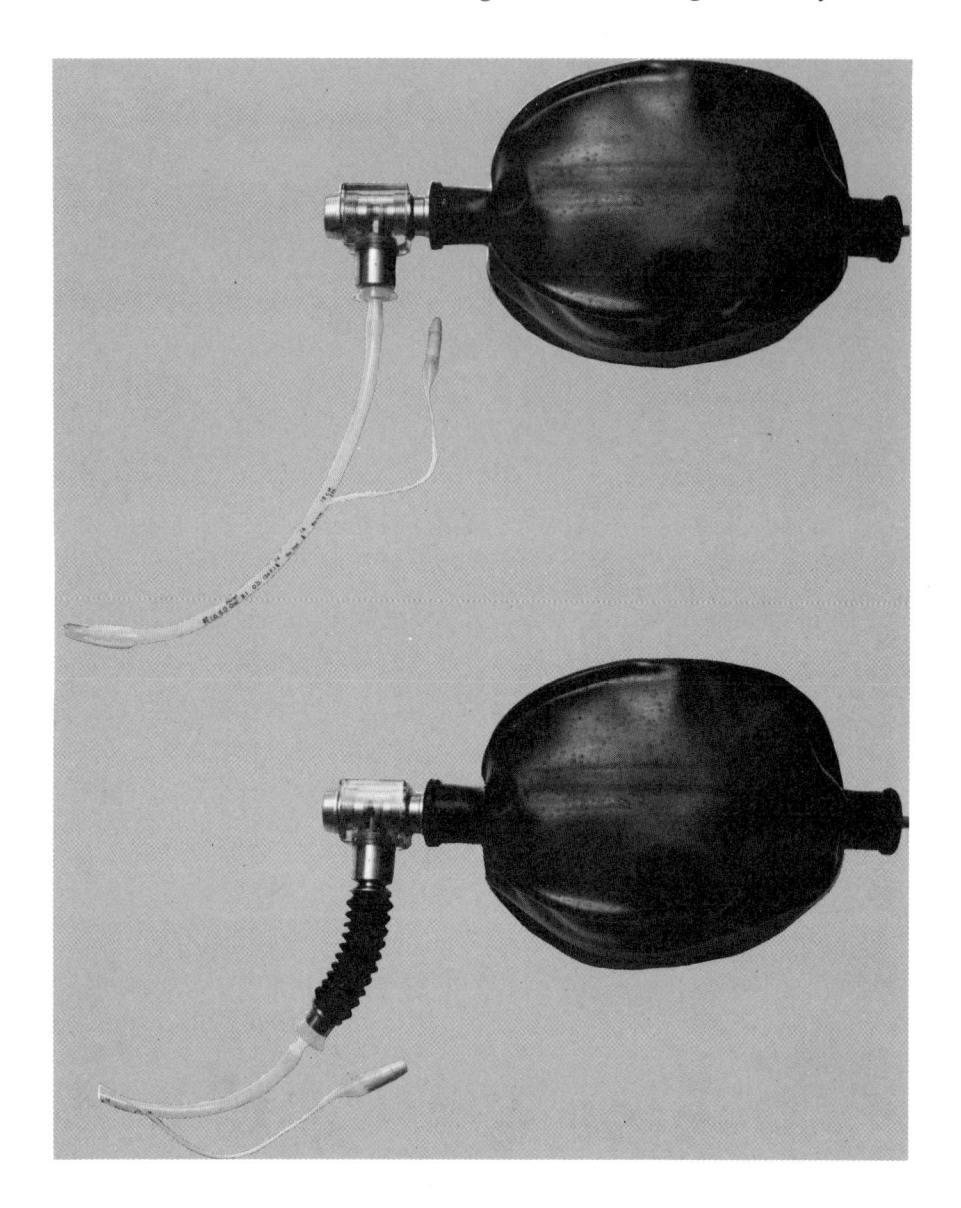

Tracheostomy is a hazardous procedure which should be done in the emergency setting only as a last resort and should not be performed by those unfamiliar with the technical problems which may arise.

These four methods of airway maintenance will be described in detail in later sections.

Other procedures which must accompany correction of airway problems are directed toward restoration of normal pulmonary physiology. For example, a pneumothorax should be evacuated by underwater drainage, a large hemothorax should be drained by closed thoracostomy or simple thoracentesis.

Flail segments of the chest wall must be stabilized and sucking wounds of the chest must be closed. Furthermore, hemorrhage must be controlled and cardiovascular hemodynamics stabilized by restoring circulating blood volume.

Management of the patient with cardiac or cardiorespiratory arrest will be discussed in a later section.

Adjunct laboratory studies which are vital to the treatment of a patient with airway difficult are arterial blood gases (Table 1). These should be done at the onset of treatment and periodically during the time resuscitative measures are being undertaken as one parameter of the patient's progress and response to therapy.

table 1   normal values of arterial blood gases

pH	7.4 ± 0.3
pCO_2	40 ± 4 mm Hg
pO_2	80-100 mm Hg
Standard Bicarbonate	24 ± 2 mEq/L
Base Excess	0 ± 2.5 mEq/L
Oxygen Saturation	95-97%

− base excess >2.5 mEq/L suggests metabolic acidosis
+ base excess >2.5 mEq/L suggests metabolic alkalosis

SUMMARY

Proper airway management constitutes the highest priority of care of the acutely ill or injured patient. The causes of airway problems are many and, in a given patient, multiple etiological factors may be involved.

Appropriate treatment is based on the indentification of the proximate cause(s) of the airway difficulty and the initiation of therapeutic measures to correct the altered physiology. Treatment is directed toward both the establishment and maintenance of a patent airway. In apneic patients, assisted ventilation is required. Baseline arterial blood gas determinations are made at the time of initial assessment of the patient and at intervals during the course of treatment.

2 USE OF ESOPHAGEAL OBTURATOR AIRWAY

INDICATIONS
1. Respiratory arrest.
2. Depressed respiration with need for assist.
3. Unavailability of equipment or personnel for tracheostomy or endotracheal intubation.

EQUIPMENT
1. Esophageal obturator airway
2. 50 cc syringe
3. Lubricating jelly (K-Y or lidocaine jelly)

PROCEDURE
1. Lubricate the airway with K-Y or lidocaine jelly.
2. Grasp the patient's lower jaw and raise it along with the tongue.
3. Insert the tip of the esophageal obturator airway into the mouth with the concave curve toward the patient's feet.

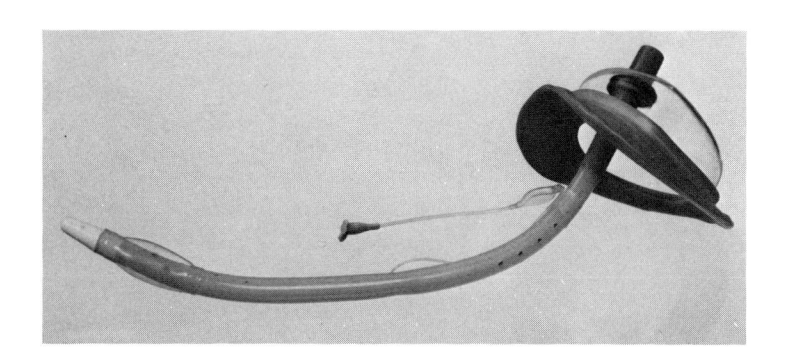

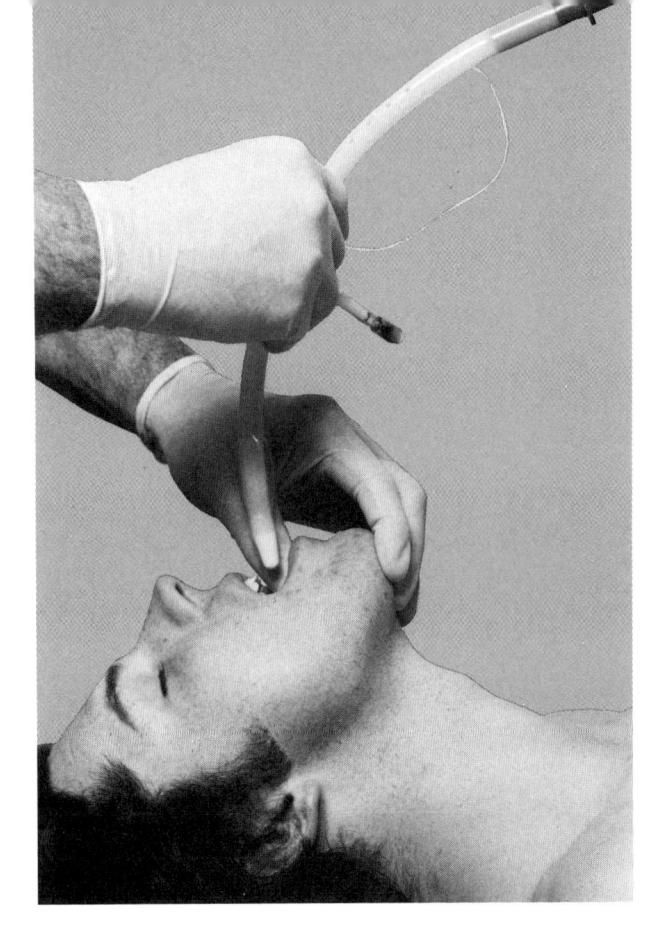

4. Continue to advance the airway into the pharynx and esophagus carefully. Be sure the airway balloon extends below the bifurcation of the trachea.
5. Apply the mask to the airway and seat it firmly on the patient's mouth and nose.
6. Draw 30 to 35 cc of air into the syringe and inflate the cuff.

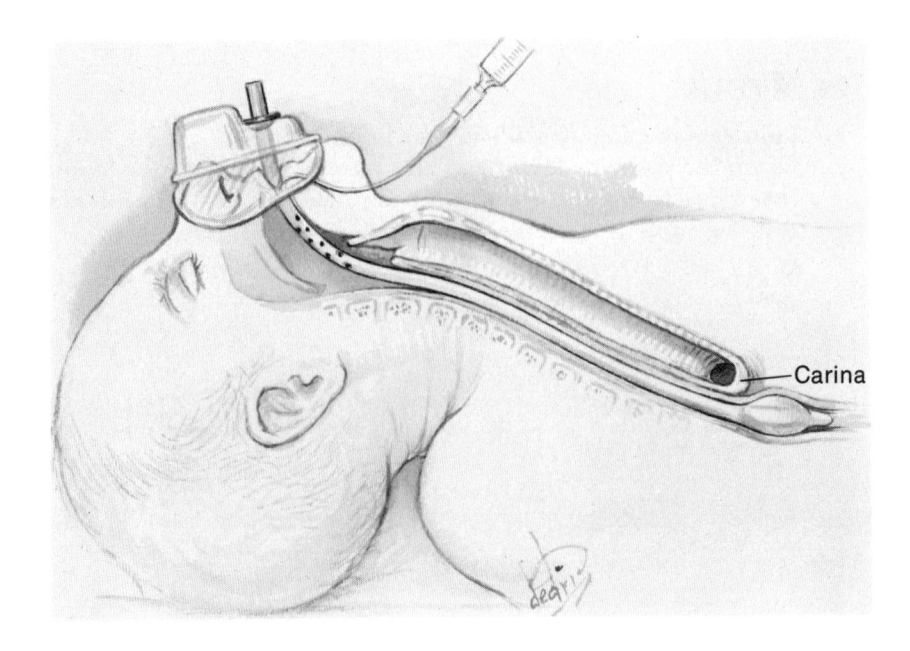

7. Initiate bag-to-mask resuscitation.
8. Once the personnel and equipment for endotracheal intubation are present, an endotracheal tube should be inserted prior to removal of the esophageal airway.
9. When the esophageal airway is to be removed, be sure to deflate the balloon first in order to avoid damage to the esophagus.

NOTE: If gastric aspiration is indicated, the esophageal cuff may be deflated for a brief time and a nasogastric tube inserted.

After the nasogastric tube is in place, the esophageal balloon can be reinflated. The esophageal balloon should not be inflated until it lies below the tracheal bifurcation to avoid airway obstruction by the balloon impinging against the posterior membranous wall of the trachea.

BIBLIOGRAPHY

Don Michael, T. A., Lambert, E. H., and Mettran, A. Mouth to lung airway for cardiac resuscitation. Lancet 2:1329, 1968.

Farley, M. The Esophageal Obturator Airway. Respiratory Therapy. 3:95, Nov. 1973.

Huszar, R. J. Emergency Cardiac Care. Maryland: Robert J. Brady Co., 1974, pp. 73-75.

Johnson, K. R., Genovesi, M. G., and Lassar, K. H. Esophageal obturator airway: Use and complications. JACCP 5:36, Jan. 1976.

Standards for CPR and emergency cardiac care. Supplement to JAMA 227:853, Feb. 18, 1974.

3 ENDOTRACHEAL INTUBATION

INDICATIONS
1. Need to establish and maintain an airway in patients with respiratory insufficiency or hypoxia.
2. Need to provide ventilatory assist.
3. A method of airway control in patient's with flail chest.
4. For control of respirations in patients with damage to the major bronchi.

EQUIPMENT
1. Laryngoscope with handle and lighted blade. The handle contains batteries which serve as a power source. The blades are changeable and of varying sizes and shapes suitable for infants and adults.

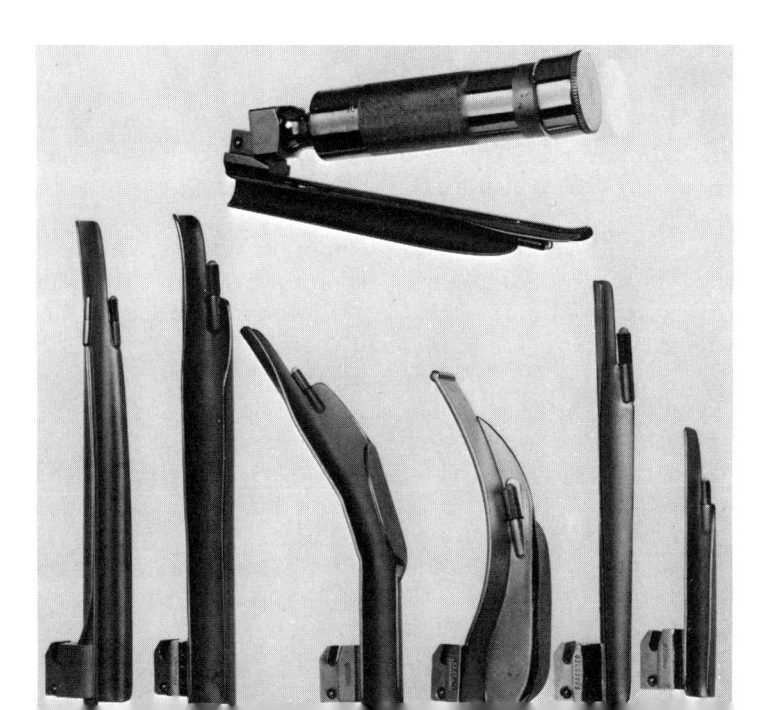

2. Endotracheal tubes. These are available in graduated sizes with an internal diameter of 3.5 to 9 mm which fits all patients. These devices are disposable. Each is fitted with a connector which is adaptable to standard resuscitation equipment. (Some tubes may cause tracheal irritation, particularly in infants and children. A tube should not be used unless it is implant-tested and free of toxicity—these are marked IT and Z79.)

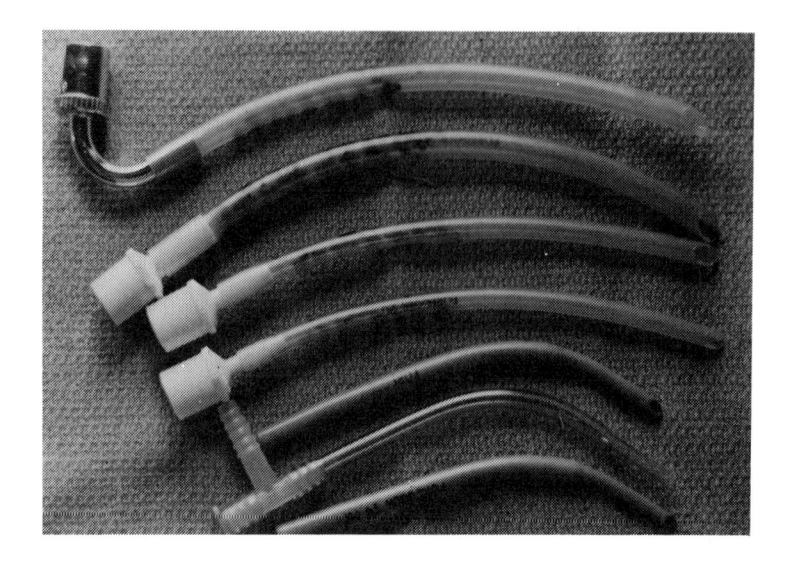

To obtain an airtight fit in the airway, the distal end of the tube is fitted with an inflatable rubber cuff. Cuffs are usually not used on tubes with an internal diameter of less than 7 mm.
3. Water-soluble lubricating jelly
4. 4% topical licocaine spray
5. Stylet (optional)
6. Suction machine—tonsil (rigid) suction tip
7. 10 cc syringe

ANATOMICAL CONSIDERATIONS

The tube may be passed into the trachea via the mouth (orotracheal) or nasal route (nasotracheal). The orotracheal method is most commonly used and performed under direct vision, while the nasotracheal route is essentially a "blind" technique.
1. The trachea is in the midline of the neck, its superior entry being the glottis which contains the vocal cords. In orotracheal intubation, the vocal cords must be visualized before the tube is passed into the trachea.
2. The uvula is identified suspended from the midline of the soft palate to guide the operator to proper placement of the laryngoscope.
3. The epiglottis is attached to the base of the tongue and should be visualized and elevated to expose the glottis and vocal cords. In thick-necked patients, the glottis may be more easily visualized by applying external pressure on the thyroid cartilage while the base of the tongue and the epiglottis are being elevated with the laryngoscope blade.
4. The trachea extends to the level of the second intercostal space anteriorly

and bifurcates into left and right bronchi. The right main bronchus comes off at a very slight angle to the trachea, while the left takes off at a 45-degree angle. This anatomical configuration allows the endotracheal tube to be passed easily into the right bronchus. This point is important, because, if the tube is passed unsuspectedly into the right bronchus, atelectasis of the left lung occurs with aggravation of pulmonary insufficiency.

PROCEDURE

1. Lubricate the endotracheal tube with water-soluble jelly.
2. Stand at the patient's head. The patient is preferably in the supine position. Extend the patient's neck by elevating the neck or jaw and applying pressure on the forehead. Use caution in patients suspected of having an injury to the cervical spine.
3. Retract the lips onto the teeth or gums to avoid pinching them in the blade. 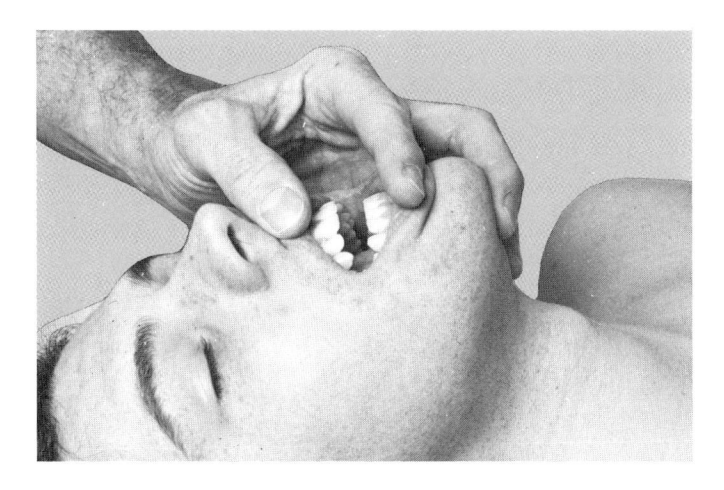
4. Grasp the lower jaw with the right hand and draw it forward and upward.

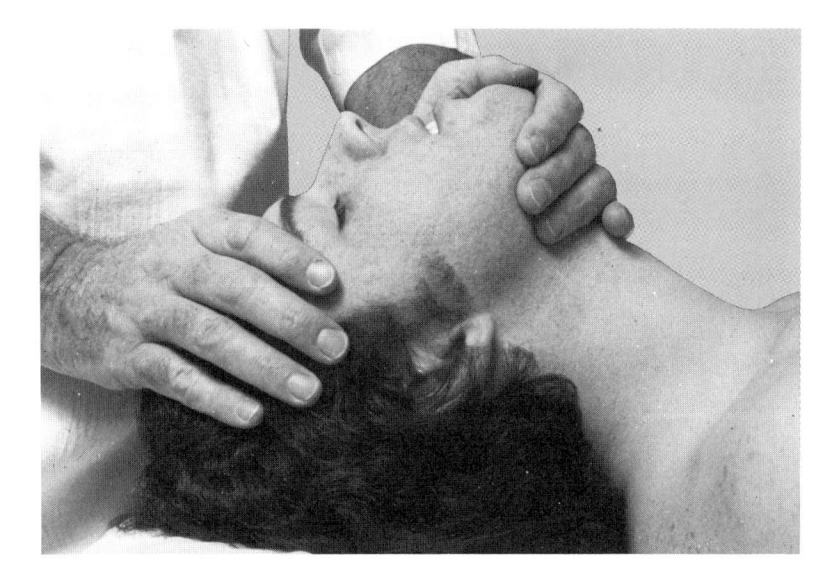

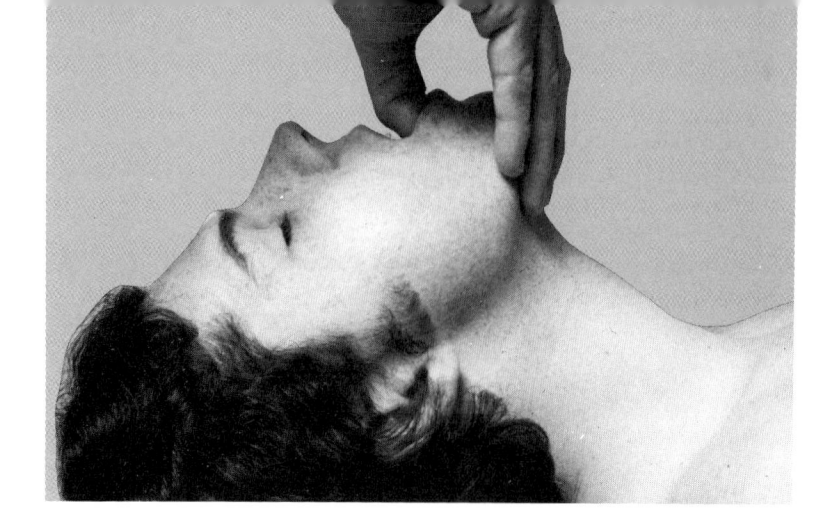

Remove any dentures.
5. With the laryngoscope in the left hand, insert the blade into the mouth over the tongue toward the right side, pushing the tongue to the left. Continue to

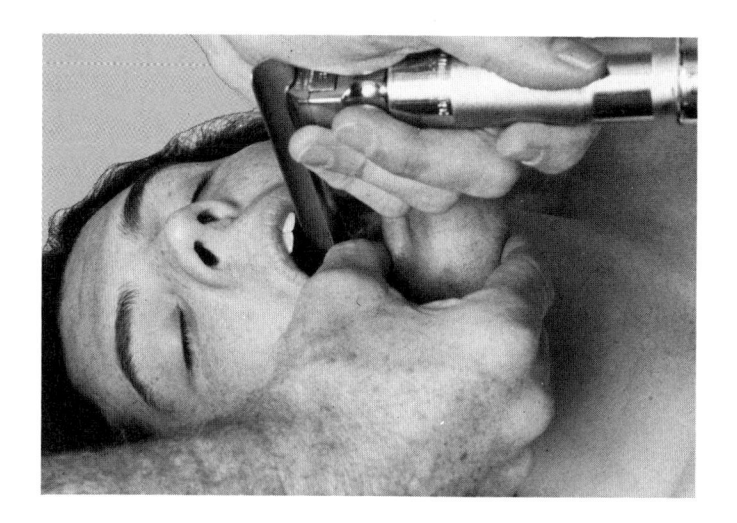

advance the blade into the mouth and identify the uvula.

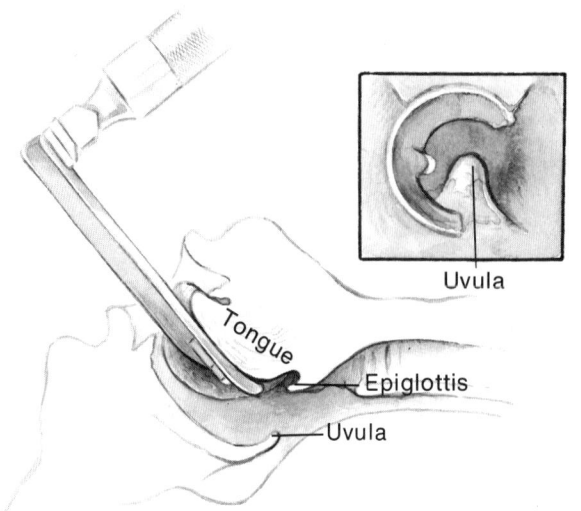

Tongue
Epiglottis
Uvula

Uvula

6. Keep the blade closer to the floor of the mouth. Then elevate the tongue until the epiglottis is visualized. Observe the mouth and oropharynx for any for-

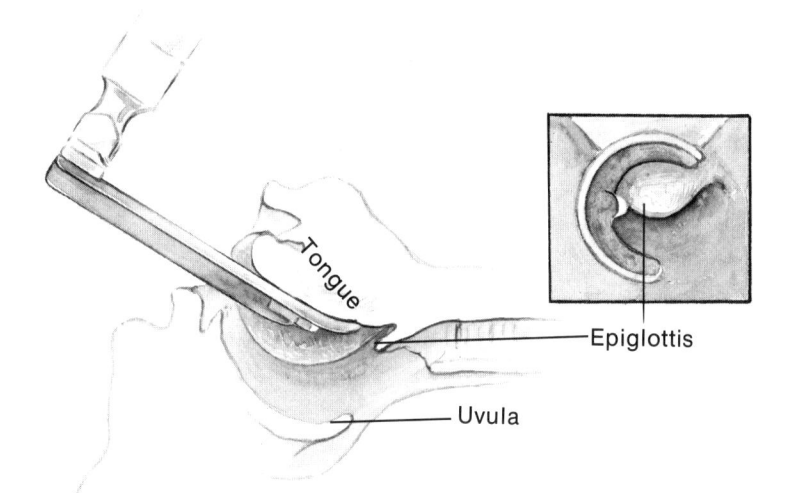

eign bodies or secretions, and, if present, remove them for better visualization of anatomical landmarks and to prevent aspiration into the trachea.
7. Advance the laryngoscope blade over the epiglottis and elevate the tongue and epiglottis by firmly raising the handle of the laryngoscope. Do not lever the laryngoscope blade against the upper teeth to avoid injury or loss of a damaged or carious tooth. With the tongue and epiglottis raised, the glottis should be visualized.
8. If the patient gags or if the vocal cords are closed (in an adducted position), spray the cords with 4% lidocaine solution. If the patient is breathing spontaneously, the cords may open during inspiration.

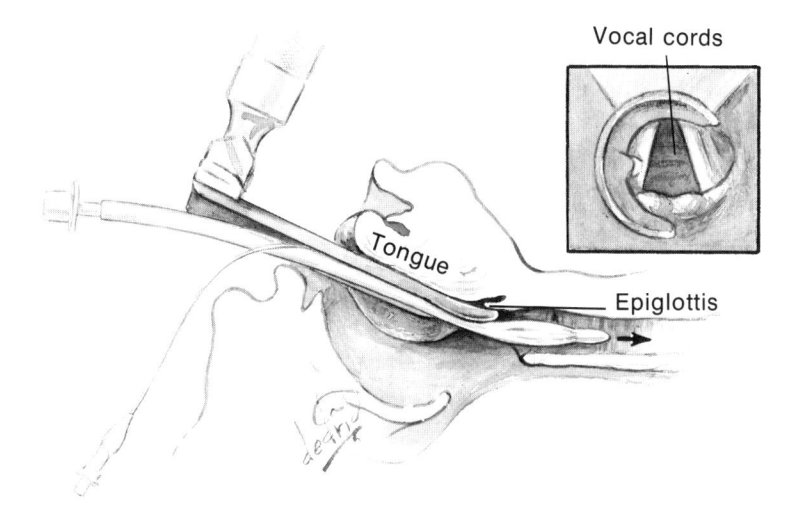

9. With the cords in full view, pass the appropriate size tube into the trachea. In an adult, a 7 mm tube may be used. In infants a size 4 to 5 mm tube is preferable, while in a newborn, a 3.5 mm should be used.

10. Check the position of the tube in the airway by placing the ear next to the end of the tube and compressing the chest. If the tube is properly placed, air will be expelled through it with this maneuver.
11. Inflate the cuff with 5 to 8 cc of air.
12. Attach tube to a mechanical ventilator or resuscitation bag device (Ambu bag) as indicated.
13. Once the patient is being ventilated, ascultate the chest to be certain both lungs are being aerated. If the breath sounds are decreased or absent in the left lung, the tube may have been passed into the right main stem bronchus and may have occluded the origin of the left main bronchus. If this is the case, deflate the cuff, withdraw the tube 1 to 2 cm and repeat the auscultation.
14. Withdraw the tube until both lungs aerate equally; continue as before.
15. Place an oropharyngeal airway in the mouth to prevent the patient from biting the endotracheal tube. Tape the endotracheal and oropharyngeal tubes to the side of the face to prevent expulsion.

BIBLIOGRAPHY

Smith, R. M. Respiratory Arrest and Its Sequelae in the Critically Ill Child. Clement A. Smith, Ed. Philadelphia: W. B. Saunders Co., 1972, pp. 124-138.

4 NEEDLE CRICOTHYROTOMY

INDICATION

Acute upper airway obstruction when suitable equipment or qualified personnel are not available for endotracheal intubation or tracheostomy.

EQUIPMENT

1. Large-bore needle(s) (13- or 14-gauge) with short bevel
2. Prep
3. Large-bore (13- or 14-gauge) cannula-over-needle device (optional)

ANATOMICAL CONSIDERATIONS

1. The cricothyroid membrane provides easy and rapid access to the trachea.
2. The cricothyroid membrane is easily identified on the anterior aspect of the neck. It lies between the inferior margin of the thyroid cartilage and the upper border of the cricoid cartilage (the first tracheal ring).
3. The thyroid notch (Adam's apple) is palpated in the midline of the upper neck.
4. By moving the finger downward on the neck about 4 to 5 cm, the cricoid cartilage is palpated as a prominence in the midportion of the neck.
5. Just above the superior border of the cricoid cartilage is a diamond-shaped depression which is the cricothyroid membrane.

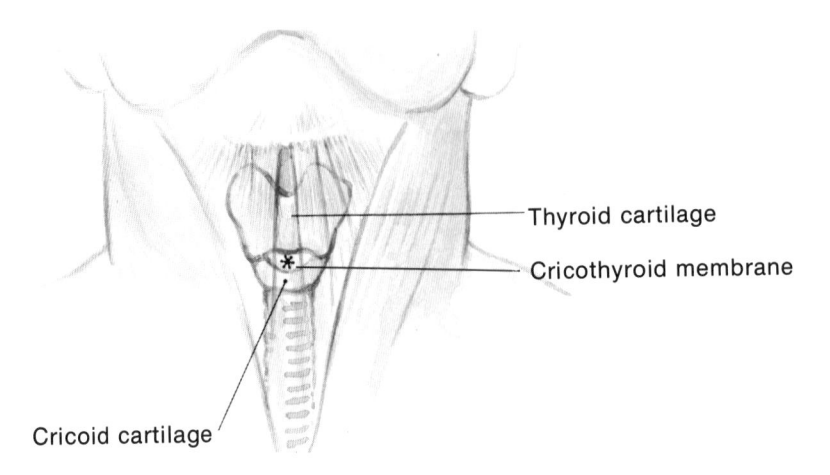

Thyroid cartilage
Cricothyroid membrane
Cricoid cartilage

6. The size of the trachea varies with the individual. The posterior wall of the trachea below the cricoid cartilage is membranous. The esophagus lies immediately behind this area.
7. There are no major vessels in this area, nor is the thyroid isthmus proximate to the cricothyroid membrane.

PROCEDURE

1. Place the patient in a recumbent or semirecumbent position.
2. Extend the neck and prep with povidone-iodine.
3. Palpate the thyroid notch and the cricoid cartilage and identify the cricothyroid membrane.
4. Stabilize the trachea between the thumb and the index and middle fingers of one hand and firmly insert the needle perpendicularly into the membrane.

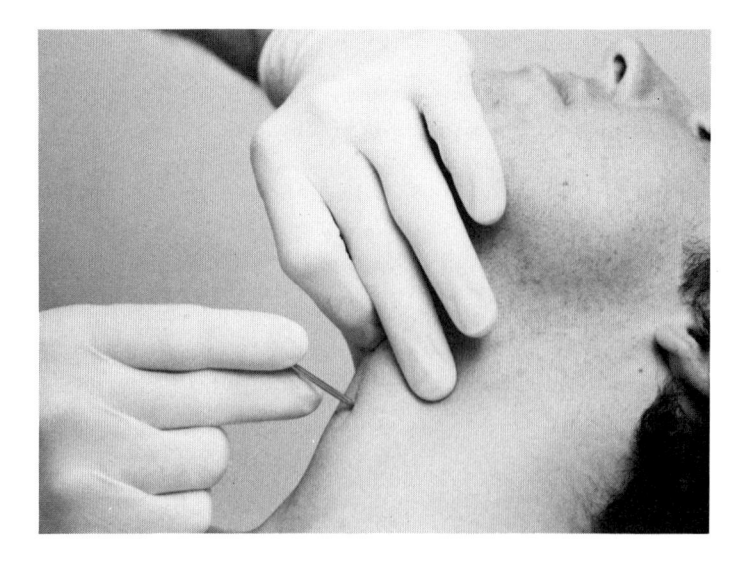

5. As the trachea is entered, air will pass back and forth through the needle with the patient's respiratory activity.
6. Once the needle is inside the trachea, direct it downward and posteriorly, so as not to penetrate the posterior membrane into the esophagus. Place an additional needle if necessary.

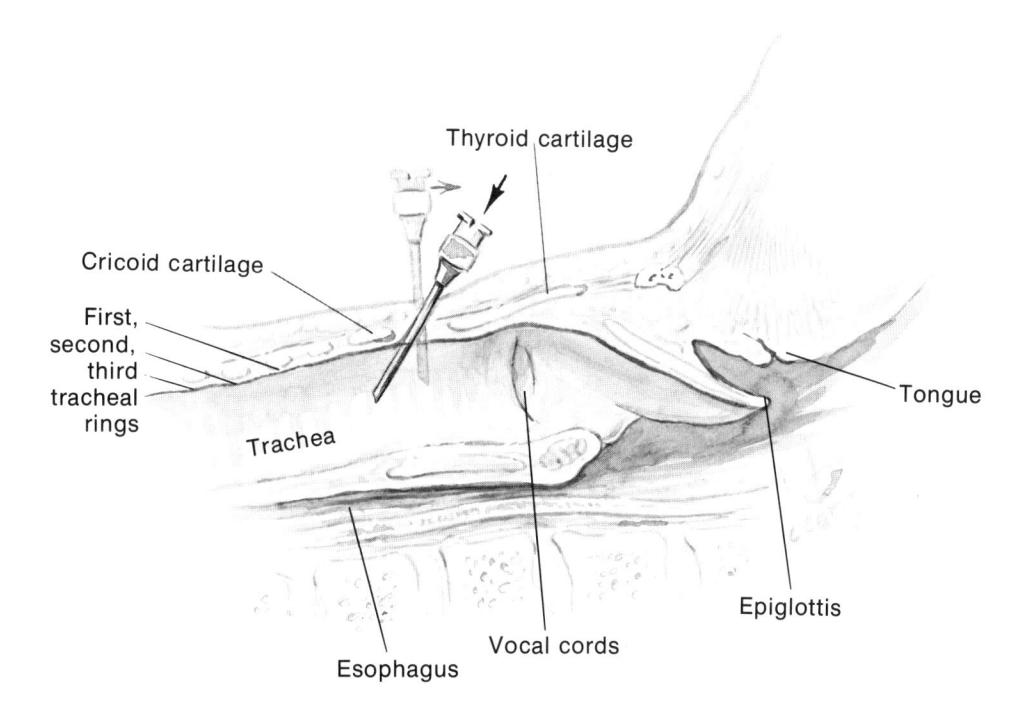

7. Stabilize the needle with adhesive tape.
8. Keep the patient's head relatively immobile.
9. Make preparations for more permanent airway control, using endotracheal intubation or tracheostomy.
10. A variation of this procedure involves the use of a cannula-over-needle combination device. Insert this device into the cricothyroid membrane as indicated in Step 4. Once the needle enters the trachea (air will pass back and forth through the needle), direct it downward and posteriorly as in Step 6. Then remove the needle and leave the plastic catheter in place in the trachea. Place a second such device at an adjacent site if needed for an addition to the airway.

BIBLIOGRAPHY

Craig, D. B. Transtracheal ventilation. JAMA 235:2082, 1976.

Jacobs, H. B. Emergency percutaneous transtracheal catheter and ventilator. J. Trauma 12:50-55, 1972.

Jacoby, J. J., Hamelburg, W., and Ziegler, C. H., et al. Transtracheal resuscitation. JAMA 162:625-628, 1956.

5 TRACHEOSTOMY

A cuffed tracheostomy tube is used almost exclusively for this procedure. The balloon cuff should be tested to be sure no leaks are present prior to use of the tube.

INDICATIONS
1. Upper airway obstruction.
2. Pulmonary insufficiency associated with increased retained secretions.
3. Improvement of pulmonary toilet.
4. Flail chest.
5. Need to provide direct access to the airway in patients who require ventilatory assist or complete mechanical ventilation.

EQUIPMENT
1. Six small curved hemostats
2. Two #3 scalpel handles
3. #15 scalpel blade
4. #11 scalpel blade
5. 10 cc syringe
6. 25-gauge ⅝-inch needle
7. 22-gauge 1½-inch needle
8. Tracheostomy tube (assorted sizes for children to adults), preferably plastic, with inflatable cuff

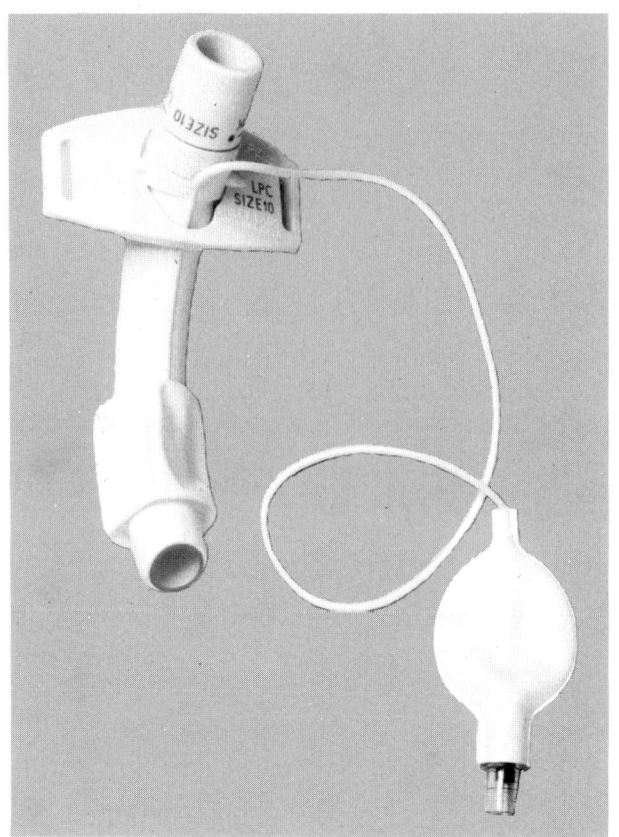

Low pressure cuff   Tracheostomy tube

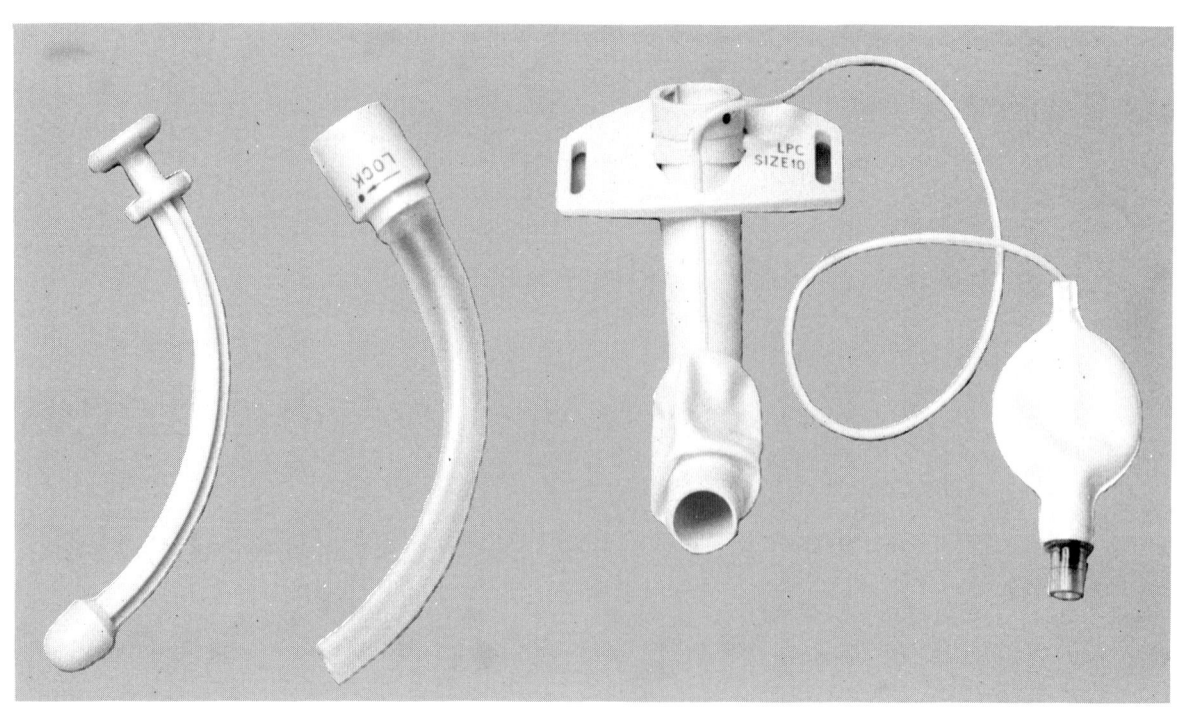

Obturator   liner

9. Four towels
10. Twenty-four 4 × 4-inch gauze sponges
11. Mastoid retractor
12. Two small rake retractors with blunt retractor head on one end
13. Two Allis forceps
14. Two right-angled skin hooks
15. Suture scissors
16. Two Kelly hemostats
17. Two Army-Navy retractors
18. Needle holder
19. Tissue forceps with teeth
20. Tissue forceps without teeth
21. Prep cup
22. 3-0 catgut on needle
23. Catgut tie
24. 4-0 silk on needle

ANATOMICAL CONSIDERATIONS

1. The trachea lies in the midline of the neck and extends from the lower end of the thyroid cartilage to the suprasternal notch.
2. The first tracheal cartilage is the cricoid cartilage and can be easily palpated as a prominence just below the thyroid notch (Adam's apple). This cartilage should not be incised in the course of a tracheostomy since it is a complete ring encircling the trachea. Healing of an incision through this tracheal ring may result in stenosis of the trachea.
3. The lower tracheal cartilages are incomplete, extending approximately two thirds of the circumference of the trachea. The posterior wall of the trachea is membranous. Healing of an incision through such an incomplete ring rarely results in tracheal stenosis in an adult.
4. Tracheostomy should be performed through the second tracheal ring or lower.

PROCEDURE

1. Place the patient in either the recumbent or semirecumbent position.
2. Hyperextend the head and neck with a sandbag, or folded sheet, placed beneath the scapulae.
3. Prep the skin of the neck and supraclavicular areas with povidone-iodine and drape.

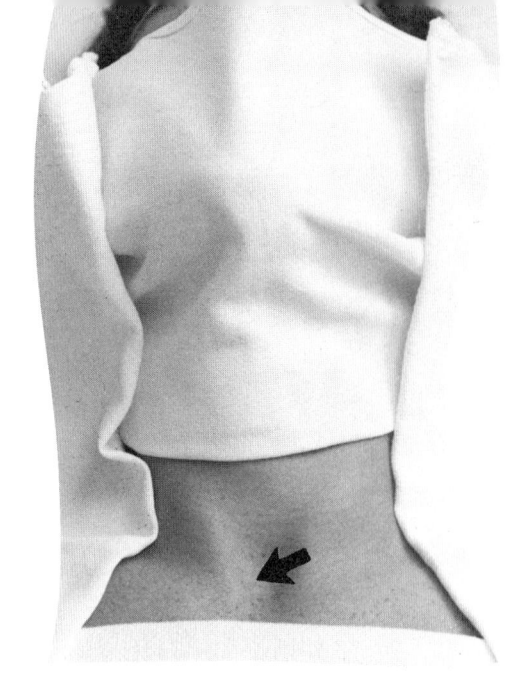

Suprasternal notch

4. The choice of incision (vertical or horizontal) depends on the patient's condition and the urgency of the situation. A vertical incision requires a minimum amount of dissection and avoids most of the superficial venous tributaries. It provides more rapid access to the trachea and allows exposure of a greater length of the trachea without time-consuming dissection of flaps.

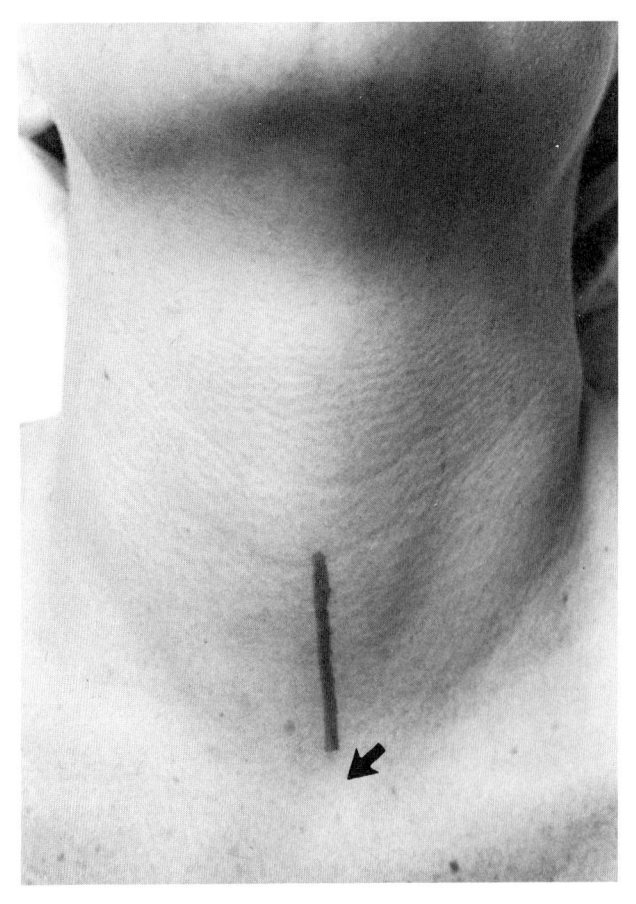

Suprasternal notch

28

A transverse incision, though it heals with a scar which is more cosmetically acceptable, requires more time to develop and therefore is not the incision of choice in an emergency. In a patient with a short, thick neck, this incision may be difficult and prolong the procedure unduly.

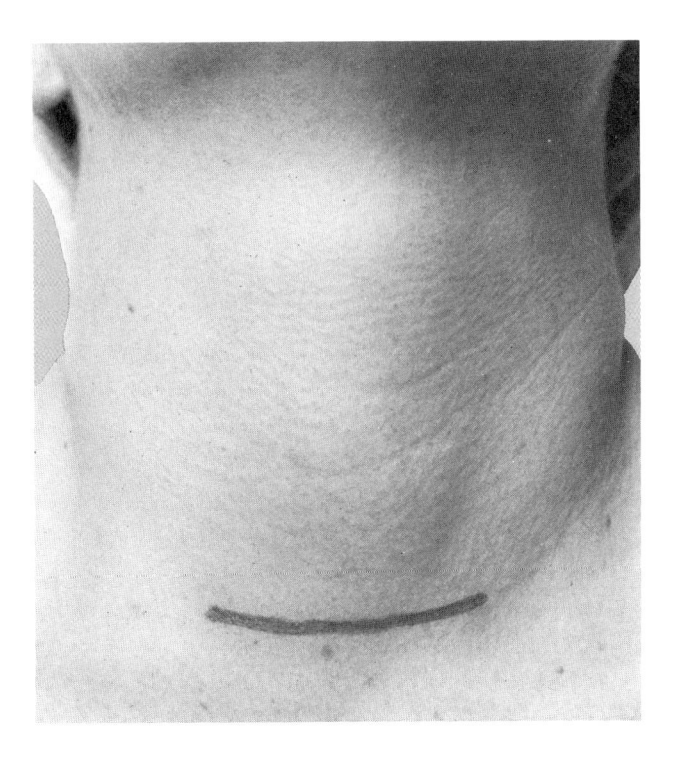

5. The vertical incision should be placed in the midline, starting at the level of the cricoid cartilage and extending to the suprasternal notch.

   The transverse incision is placed approximately 2 cm above the clavicles and should be at least 6 cm long in adults (a shorter incision is required in infants and children.)

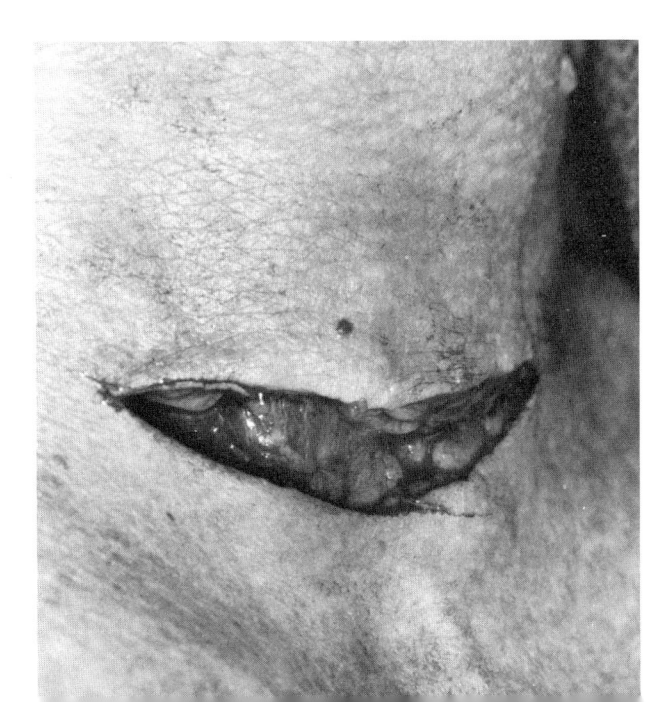

6. Once the choice of incision has been made, infiltrate the skin and subcutaneous tissues with anesthetic agent initially using the 25-gauge needle for the skin wheal and the longer 22-gauge needle for the deeper tissues.
7. Incise the skin, subcutaneous fat, and platysma muscle. If a vertical incision is used, continue to deepen it through the median raphe of the anterior strap muscles of the neck, and the deep cervical fascia.

If a transverse incision is chosen, separate the platysma muscle from the underlying anterior strap muscles until 4 to 5 cm of the median raphe is exposed. Incise the raphe.

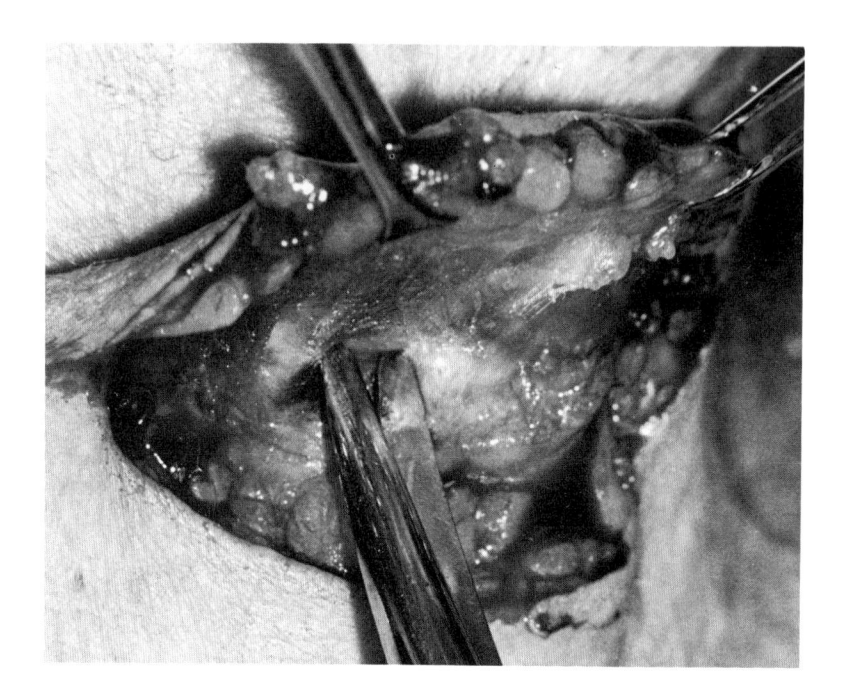

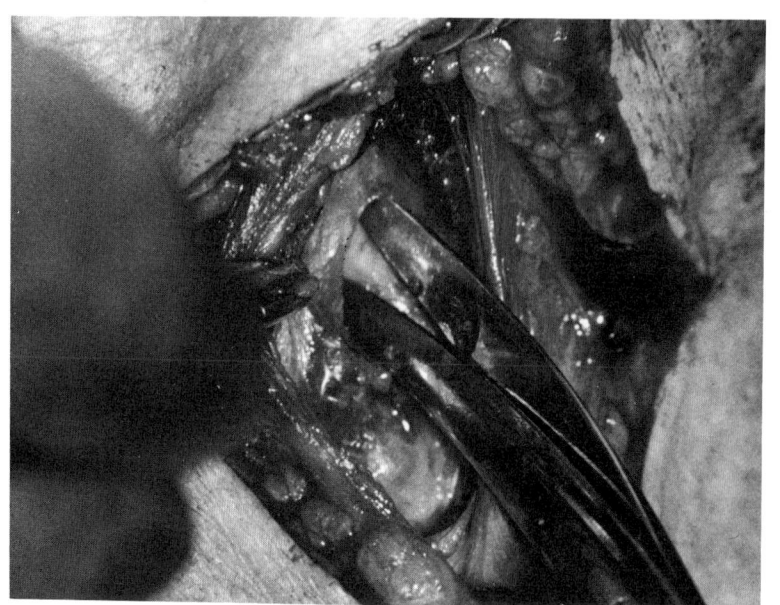

Edge of median raphe

8. Retract the wound edges with a mastoid retractor or the small rake retractors.
9. Palpate the trachea and identify the cricoid cartilage.
10. Identify the thyroid isthmus which crosses the trachea at the level of the second to fourth tracheal rings. In most instances, the isthmus can be retracted upward using a blunt retractor.

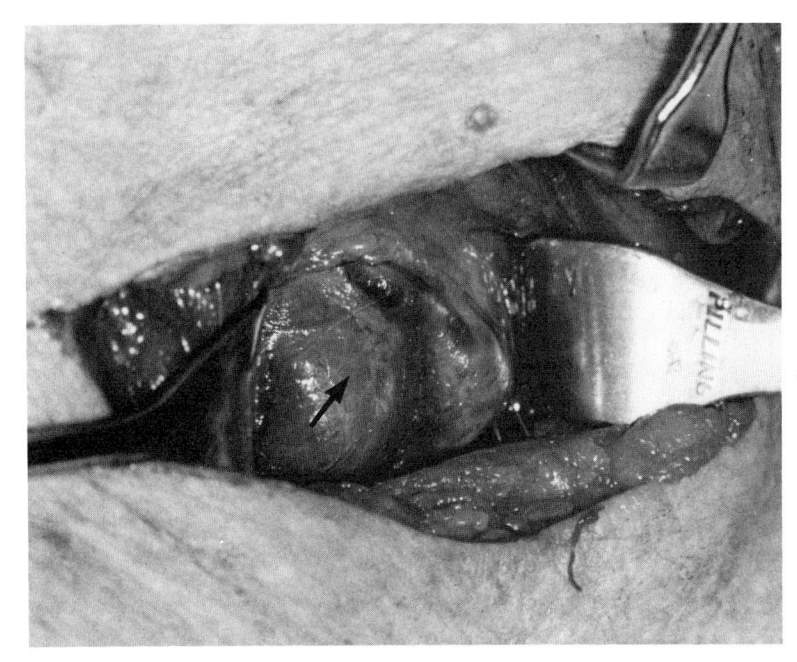

Thyroid gland

If the isthmus cannot be retracted, dissect it from the anterior aspect of the trachea by blunt dissection using a small curved hemostat.

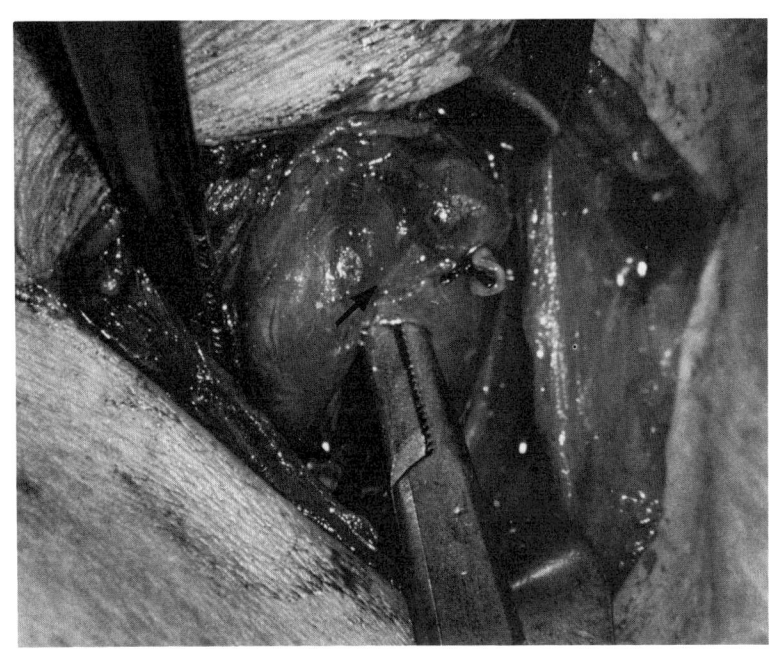

Isthmus of thyroid gland

11. Divide the isthmus between clamps and place suture ligatures of 000 chromic catgut in the cut edges of the gland for hemostasis.

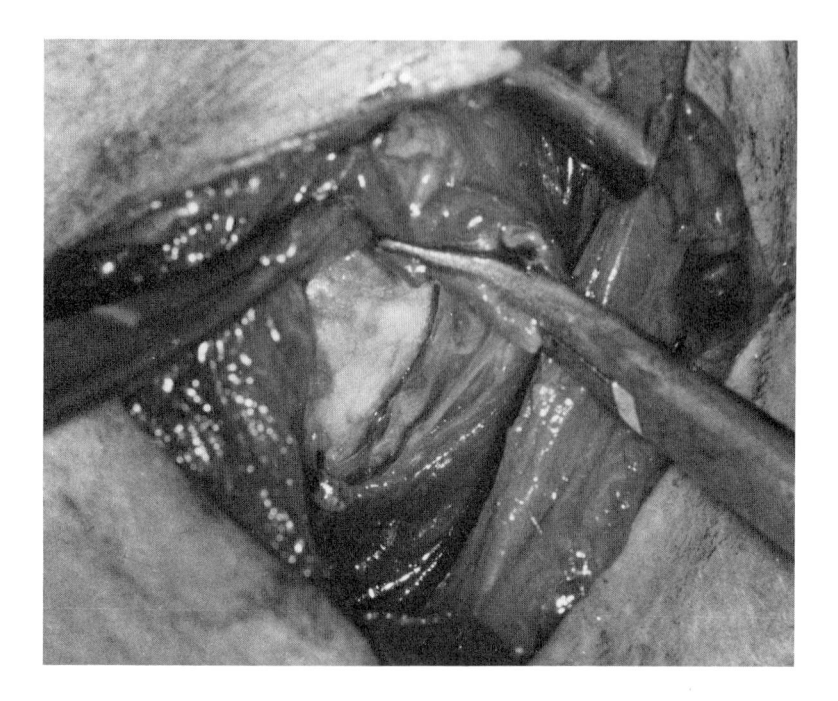

12. Incise the pretracheal fascia and expose the tracheal cartilages.

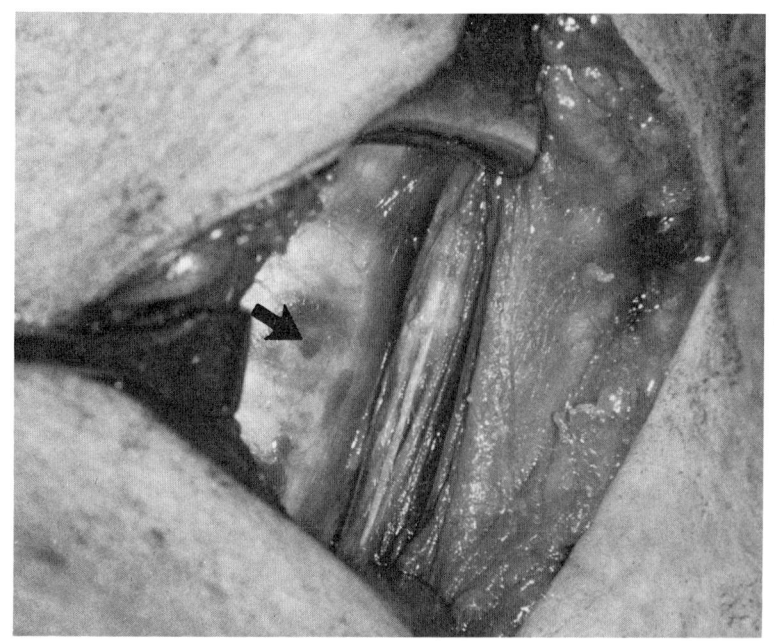

Tracheal cartilage

13. Using a #11 scalpel blade incise the anterior wall of the trachea transversely in the membranous portion above the cartilage(s) to be excised, and extend the incision downward through one or two cartilages and transversely again in the membranous septum. This incised "flap" may be held

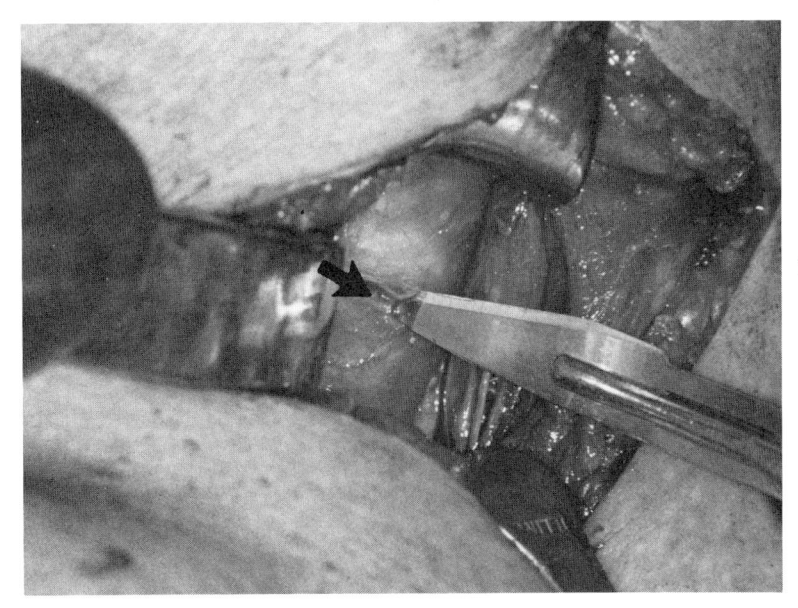

Incision of trachea

by a skin hook or Allis forceps and the incision completed to that a "window" is made in the trachea.

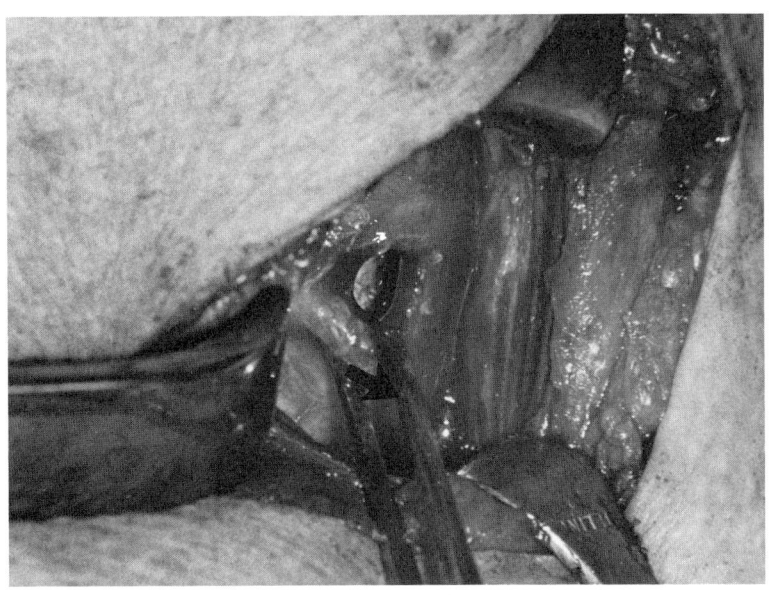

Allis forceps on tracheal flap

14. Remove the "window" in one piece, taking care to see that no portion falls into the trachea and is aspirated into the lower airway.

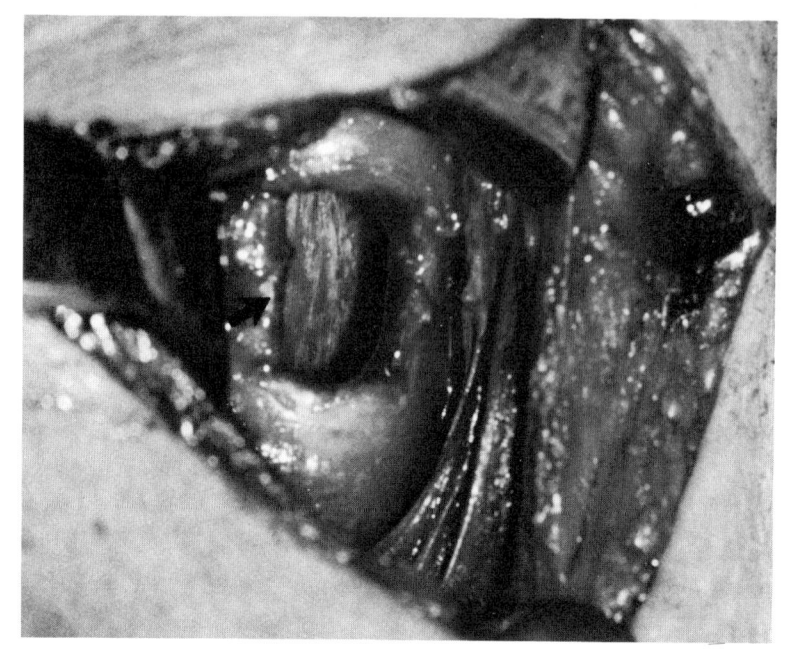

"Window" in trachea

15. Next, remove the secretions from the trachea by suction.

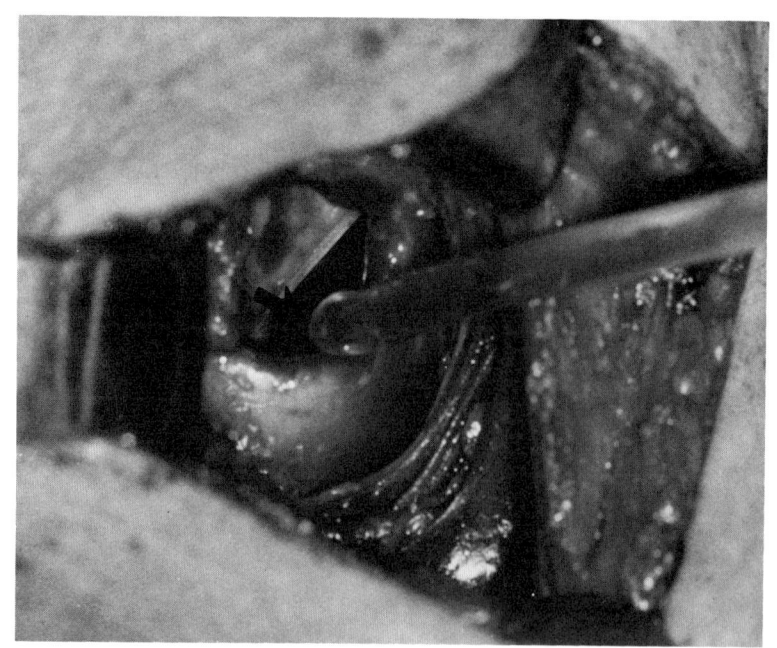

Suction catheter in trachea

16. Insert the sterile tracheostomy tube into the trachea. In adults, a #6, 7 or 8 tube may be used. In children, a smaller-sized tube is used.

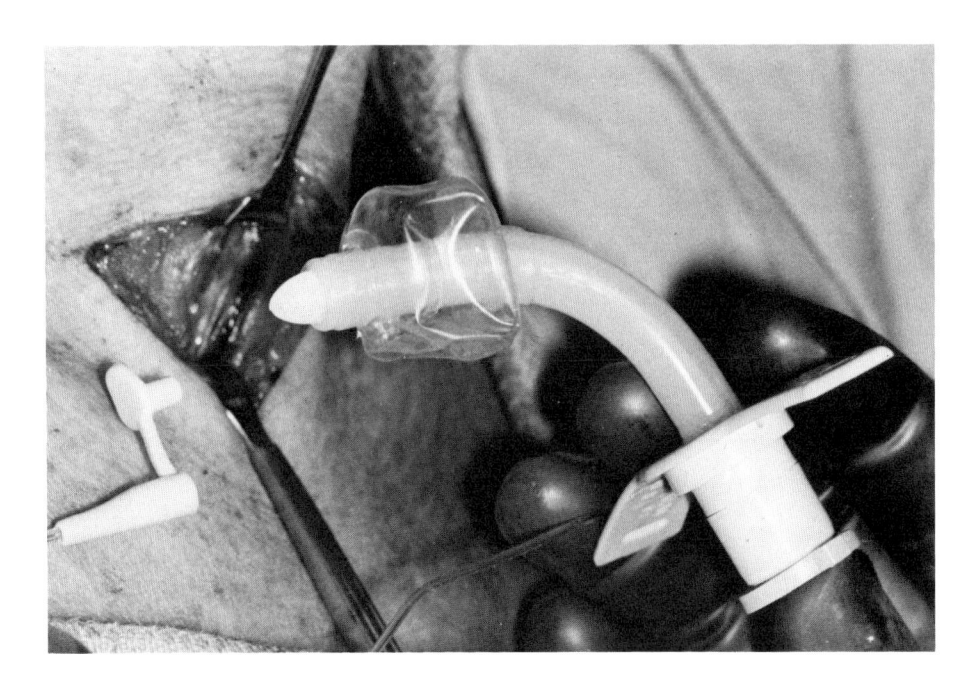

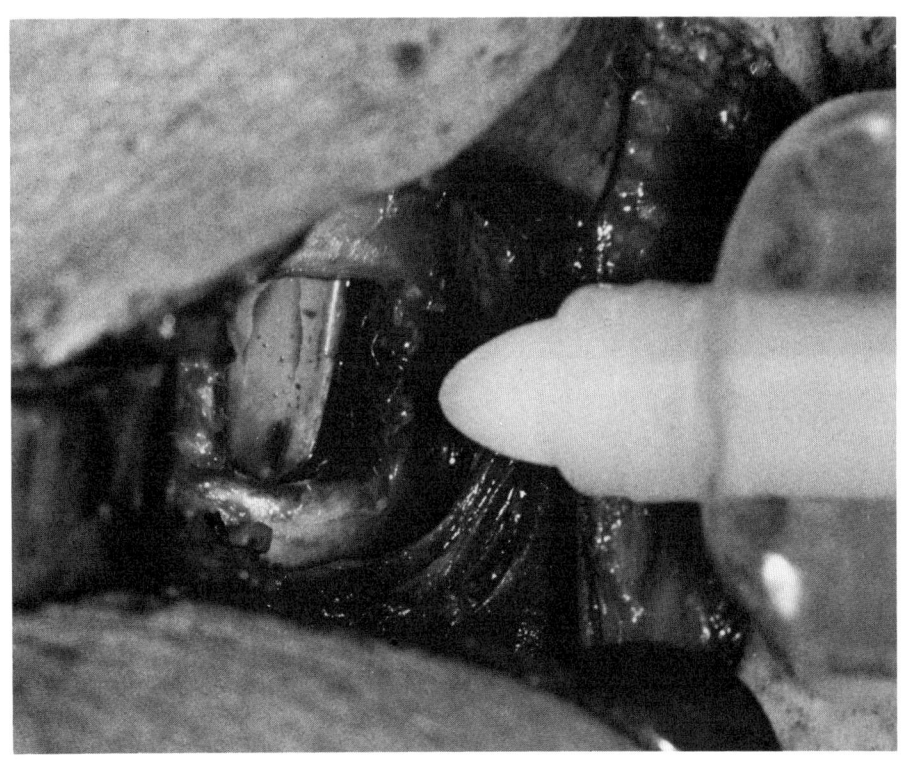

17. Remove the obturator and inflate the cuff. The tube should be long enough to fit comfortably in the trachea, but MUST NOT OBSTRUCT the carina.

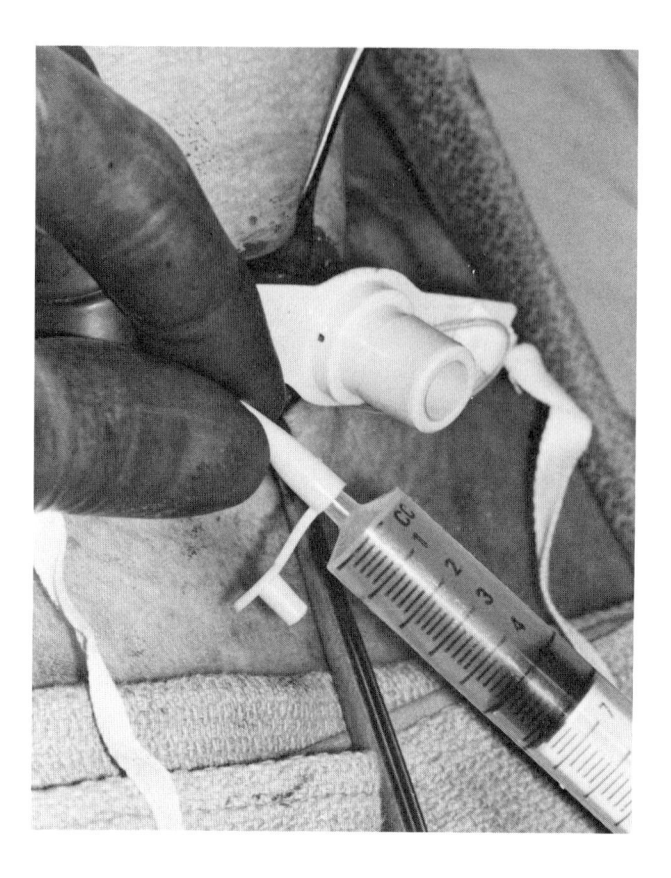

18. Tie the tube in place with umbilical tape, tied behind the neck.
19. Approximate the wound edges loosely using 3-0 catgut in the muscle and subcutaneous tissue and 4-0 silk or mersilene in the skin.

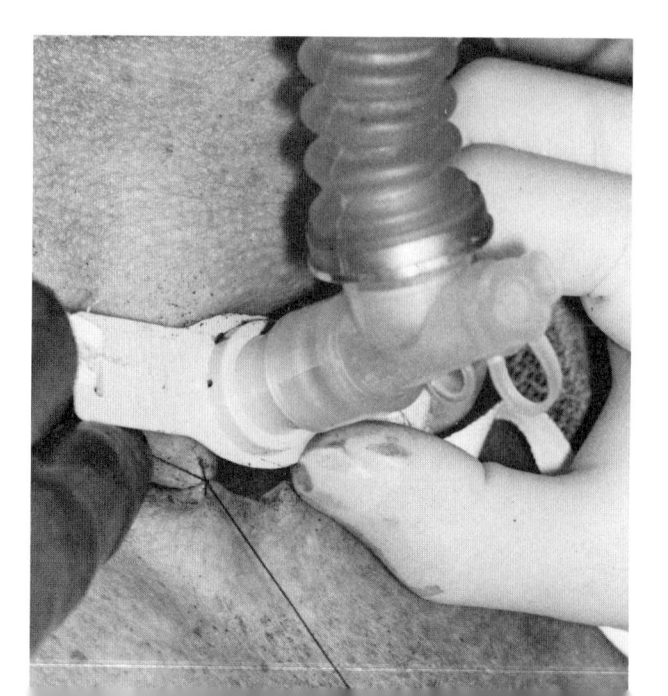

20. Dress the wound with a folden 4 × 4-inch gauze pad. The deeper layer is split to pass around the tube. The outer layer folds over the tube to prevent aspiration or foreign material.

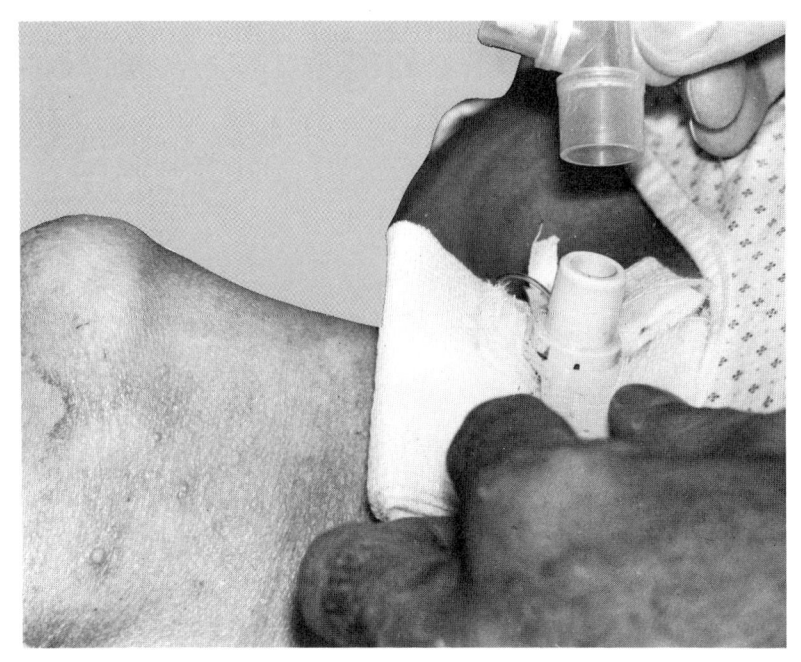

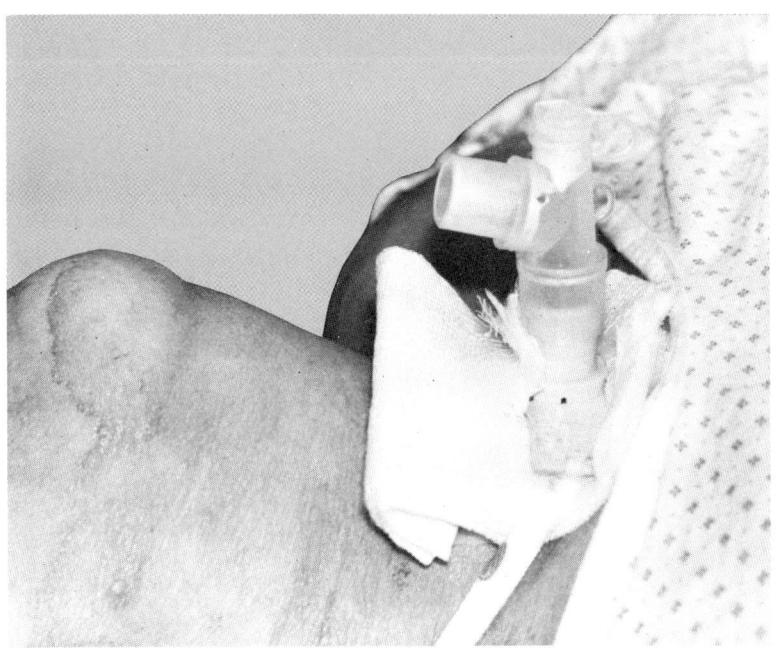

6 HEIMLICH MANEUVER

INDICATIONS
1. Asphyxiation from bolus of food or foreign object occluding the upper airway.
2. Unavailability of personnel and/or equipment for immediate tracheostomy.

EQUIPMENT
None

PHYSIOLOGIC CONSIDERATIONS
When a food bolus is aspirated, the patient invariably has inspired; thus, the lungs are inflated and the diaphragms have descended. In effect, the Heimlich maneuver produces a sudden increase in intra-abdominal pressure which forces the diaphragms upward. This increases the intrathoracic pressure which is then transmitted to the lung, increasing the pressure in the airway and forcing the bolus to pop out of the glottis.

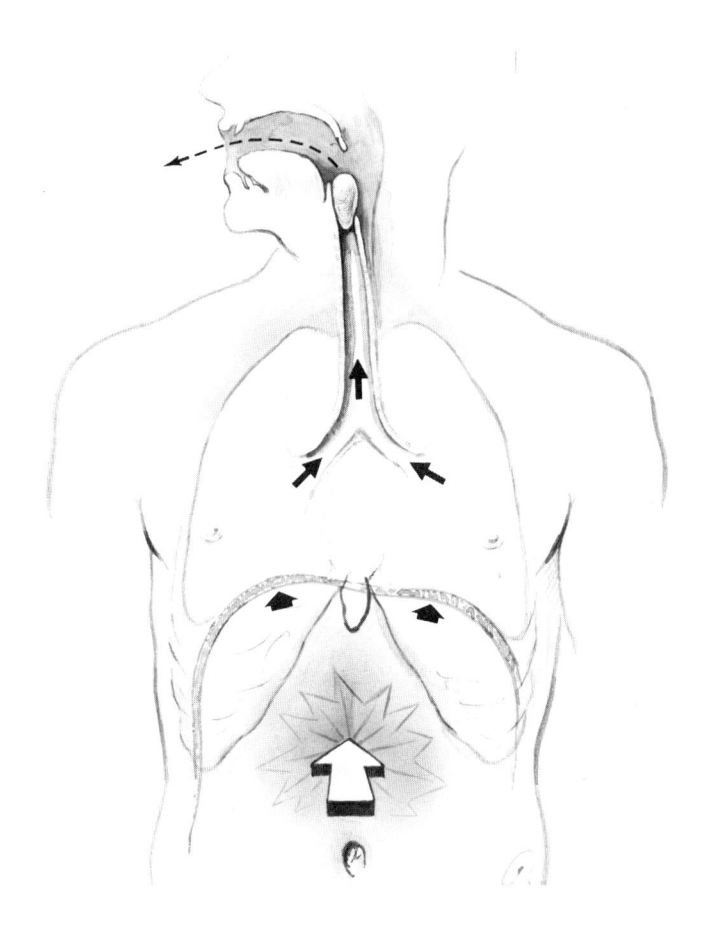

PROCEDURE

IF PATIENT IS SITTING OR STANDING

1. Stand behind the patient and encircle his waist with your arms.
2. Place your fist with the thumb side against the patient's abdomen above the umbilicus, but <u>below</u> the rib cage.

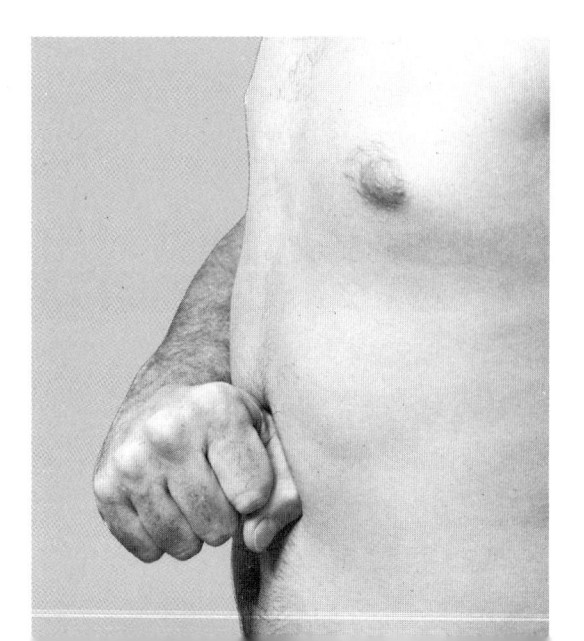

40

3. Grasp your fist with your other hand.

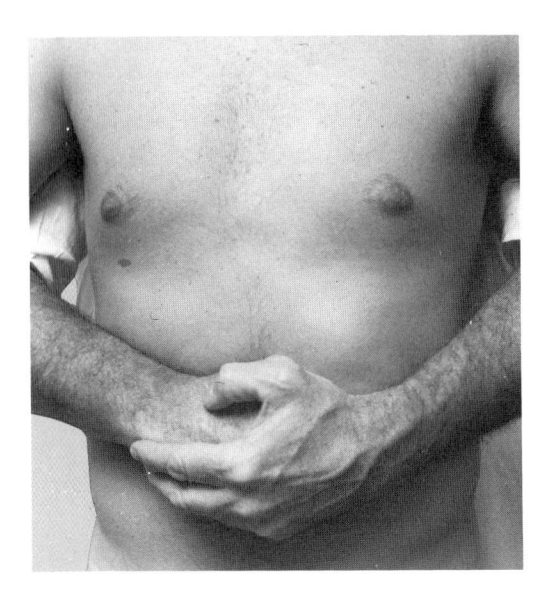

4. Press your fist into the patient's abdomen with a <u>quick upward</u> thrust, toward the diaphragm while the patient is flexed over the forearms.

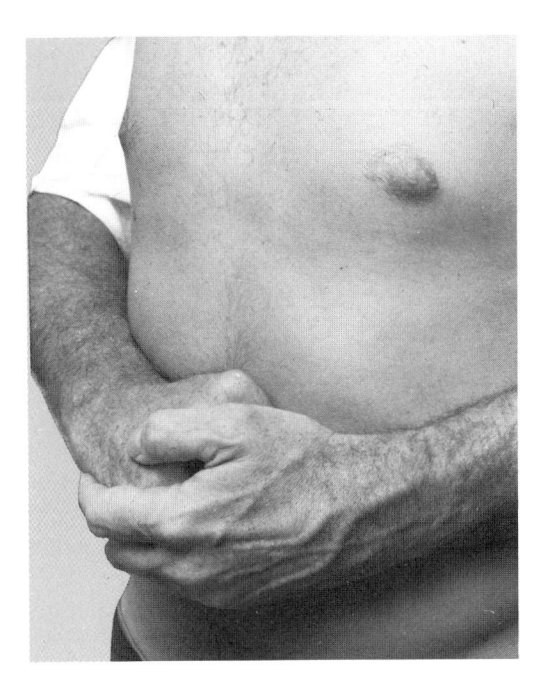

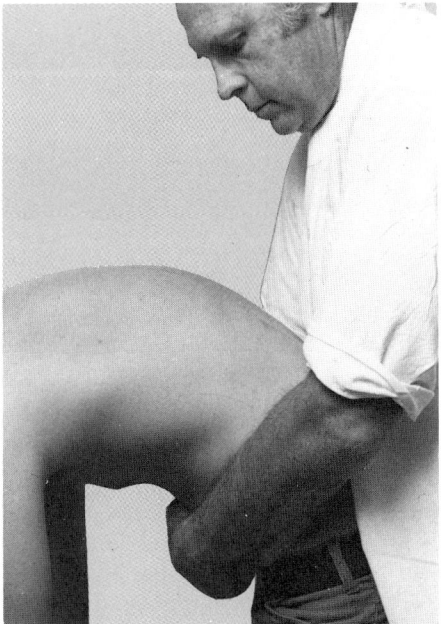

5. The obstructing bolus should "pop" out of the mouth.
6. Repeat the maneuver if necessary.

IF PATIENT HAS COLLAPSED OR IS UNABLE TO BE LIFTED

1. Place the patient in the supine position.
2. Kneel astride or to one side of the patient's hips and face him.
3. Place your fist on the upper abdomen, grasping your wrist with your other hand for stability. The fist must be placed in the midline to avoid injury to the liver or spleen.

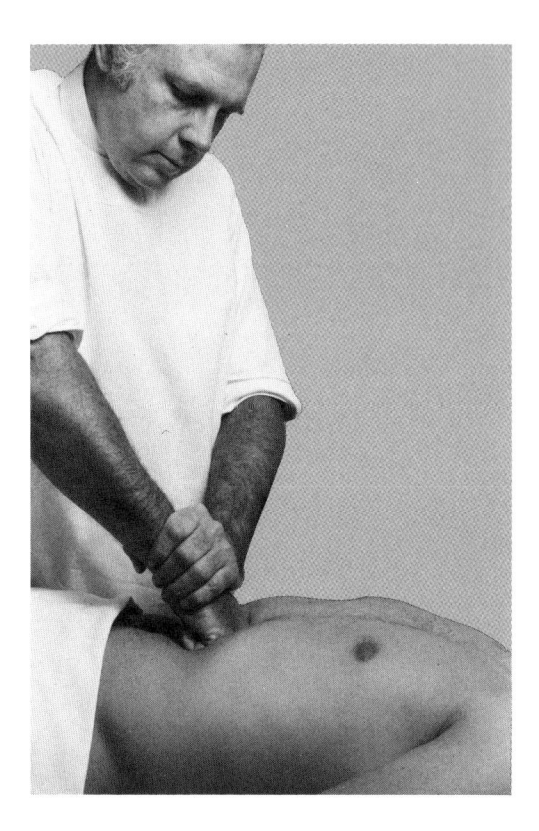

4. Press your fist into the patient's abdomen with a <u>quick</u> <u>upward</u> <u>thrust</u> toward the diaphragm.
5. The obstructing bolus should "pop" out of the mouth.
6. The maneuver may be repeated if necessary.

NOTE: If the patient vomits while in the supine position, turn the patient on his side quickly and wipe out the mouth to prevent aspiration.

Because of the possibility of immediate or delayed complications, a patient successfully resuscitated should be admitted to the hospital for a minimum 24-hour observation.

The above maneuver for the patient in the supine position, is a modification suggested by the author because of the difficulty of performing this astride the patient on a narrow hospital cart. In a personal communication, Henry Heimlich, M.D., stated that he had no personal experience with this modification but questioned its use because of the possibility of injury to solid upper abdominal viscera; hence, the precaution to keep the fist in the midline.

PEDIATRIC PATIENTS
1. For larger children and adolescents, use the technique described for adults.
2. For smaller children, place the child face down and flexed over the rescuer's forearm and deliver a sharp blow to the back. The pressure of the forearm against the child's abdomen combined with the blow to the back should dislodge the obstructing bolus.
3. For infants, grasp the child by the ankles with one hand and hang him in the head down position. Deliver a blow to the interscapular area. The bolus should be expelled.

BIBLIOGRAPHY

Heimlich, H. J. Pop goes the cafe coronary. Emerg. Med. 154, 1974.

———. A life-saving maneuver to prevent food choking. JAMA 234:398, 1975.

———. Personal communication.

Visinting, R. E. and Black, C. H. Ruptured stomach after Heimlich manuever. JAMA 234:417, 1975.

7 SINGLE INJECTION PERCUTANEOUS FEMORAL ARTERIOGRAM

INDICATIONS

1. Suspected recent occlusion (thrombus or embolus) of the common or superficial femoral artery.
2. Suspected injury to an artery of the leg associated with a dislocation and/or a fracture of the extremity.
3. Evidence of acute arterial insufficiency in the leg.

EQUIPMENT

1. 10 cc syringe
2. Two 20 cc syringes
3. 25-guage 5/8-inch needle
4. 22-gauge 1 1/2-inch needle
5. Connecting tubing with Luer-Lok fittings (B-D #8286)
6. 3-way stopcock
7. 19-gauge 3 1/2-inch spinal needle with obturator
8. Curved hemostat
9. 1% Lidocaine
10. 60% Renografin
11. Four towels
12. One dozen 4 × 4-inch sponges
13. Medicine glass
14. Two sterile 250 cc basins
15. Normal saline

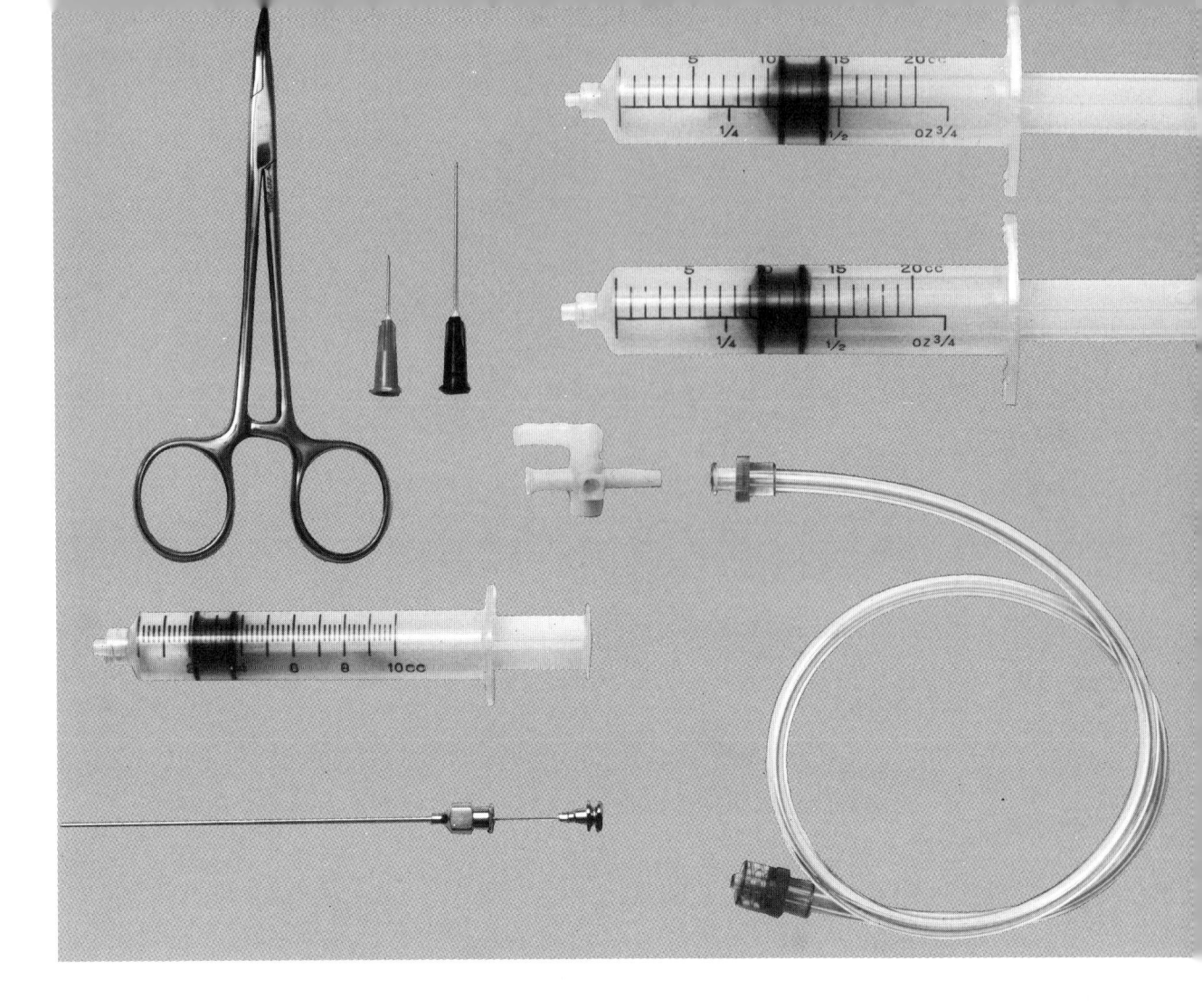

ANATOMICAL CONSIDERATIONS
1. The common femoral artery is identified at the inguinal crease as the vessel passes from beneath the inguinal ligament.
2. The arterial pulse can be palpated approximately in the middle of the crease.

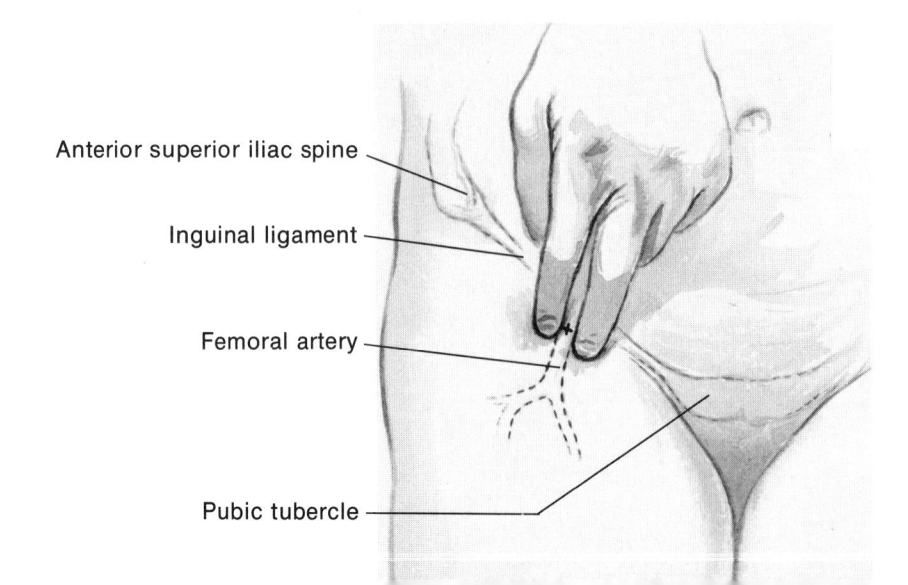

8 SINGLE INJECTION PERCUTANEOUS AXILLARY ARTERIOGRAM

INDICATIONS

1. Suspected recent occlusion (thrombus or embolus) of the axillary or brachial artery.
2. Suspected injury to the axillary or brachial artery in association with a fracture and/or dislocation of the extremity.

EQUIPMENT

1. 10 cc syringe
2. Two 20 cc syringes
3. 25-gauge 5/8-inch needle
4. 22-gauge 1½-inch needle
5. Connector tube with Luer-Lok fittings (B-D #8286)
6. 3-way stopcock
7. 19-gauge 3½-inch spinal needle with obturator
8. Curved hemostat
9. Sponge forceps
10. Local anesthetic agent
11. 60% Renografin
12. Four towels
13. One dozen 4 × 4-inch sponges
14. Medicine glass
15. Two metal basins
16. Saline
17. 3-0 silk suture with cutting needle
18. Suture scissors

47

ANATOMICAL CONSIDERATIONS

1. The axillary artery lies in the anterior aspect of the axilla beneath the pectoralis major.
2. With the patient supine, the arm is abducted and the palm placed on top of the head. The axillary pulse should be palpable at the posterior edge of the anterior axillary fold.

PROCEDURE

1. The axilla does not have to be clean shaven, but should be clean.
2. Place the patient supine on the x-ray table with the arm abducted to 90° and the palm placed on top of the head. Rotate the patient's head away from the side to be studied.
3. Prep the axilla and adjacent areas with povidone-iodine and drape.
4. Locate the axillary artery pulse at the posterior edge of the anterior axillary fold and fix the vessel in position with the index and middle fingers of the left hand (for right-handed operator.

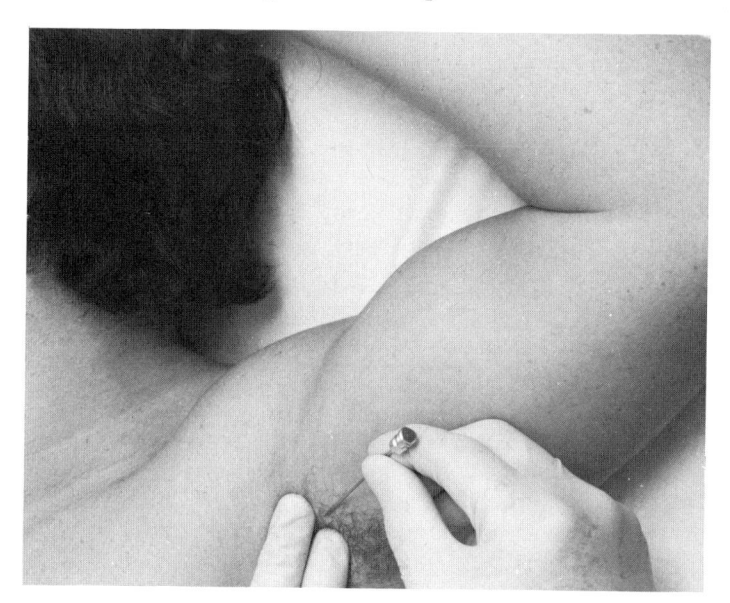

5. Raise a skin wheal with lidocaine using the 10 cc syringe and 25-gauge needle.
6. Insert the 19-gauge needle with obturator through the skin wheal in a plane near 45° to the skin until the tip of the needle may be felt on the artery.
7. While holding the artery in position, quickly thrust the needle through both walls of the vessel.
8. Remove the obturator and slowly withdraw the needle until a free flow of arterial blood spurts out.
8. Fix the needle in position with a suture placed through the skin behind the needle and tied over the needle.
10. Follow the injection procedure outlined for femoral arteriogram from step 10 onward.
NOTE: For this study only 12 to 15 cc of dye are required to adequately visualize the arterial system of the upper extremity.

3. The artery lies between the nerve laterally and the vein medially.

PROCEDURE

1. Place the patient in a supine position on the x-ray table.
2. Prep the inguinal area and upper thigh with povidone-iodine and drape with four towels.
3. Locate the femoral pulsation by palpation just below the inguinal ligament.
4. Raise a skin wheal with lidocaine using the 10 cc syringe and 25-gauge needle.
5. Deposit a small amount of anesthetic agent in the subcutaneous tissue over the artery. Do not place too much, as this will interfere with palpation of the pulse.
6. Using the index and middle fingers of the left hand (for a right-handed person), fix the position of the femoral artery by gentle pressure on either side of the vessel.
7. Introduce the 3½-inch needle and obturator unit at an angle of 60 degrees in the skin wheal and advance it deeper until the femoral pulsation is felt at the tip of the needle.
8. Make sure the artery is fixed by the fingers of the left hand and quickly thrust the needle through the anterior and posterior walls of the artery. If the needle is in proper position through the artery, it will pulsate in a longi-

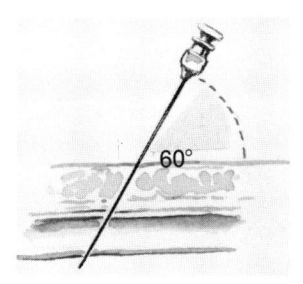

tudinal excursion. If the artery has not been penetrated, lateral movements of the needle will be noted.

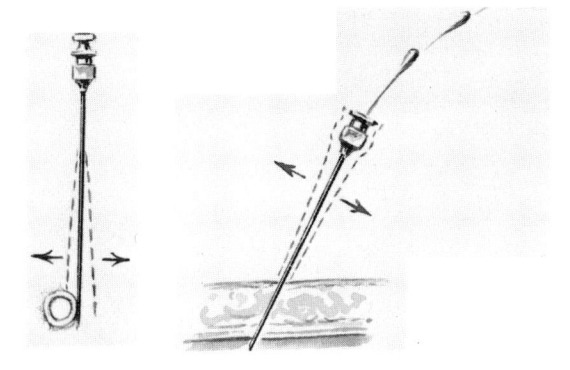

9. Remove the obturator and gradually withdraw the needle until a free flow of arterial blood spurts forth. If blood is not recovered, repeat the puncture.

10. Once arterial blood is obtained, replace the obturator and prepare the dye for injection. Place a hemostat on the needle at the point where it exits from the skin.
11. Fill one 20 cc syringe with normal saline and attach the 3-way stopcock and the Luer-Lok tubing. Remove all air from the system.
12. Remove the obturator and attach the saline syringe–stopcock-tubing assembly to the needle, taking care not to dislodge or rotate the needle.
13. Open the stopcock and flush the artery with a syringe full of saline. Then close the stopcock, remove the syringe and refill it with saline and place aside.
14. Place 20 cc of dye in the other 20 cc syringe and attach to the stopcock-tubing assembly.
15. Open the stopcock and allow a flow of blood into the tubing to be sure the needle is still in proper position. Do not allow the blood to enter the syringe.
16. Alert the x-ray technician that you are now prepared to inject the dye.
17. Alert the patient that the dye injection will cause a severe burning pain in the limb, which will be of short duration (20 to 30 seconds). Admonish the patient to hold the leg in position at all times.
18. Inject the entire 20 cc of dye as rapidly as possible.
19. Call for the x-ray study to be taken as the last of the dye is injected.
20. When the injection is completed, remove the syringe and flush the system with saline.
21. Review the x-ray film and determine if another injection is required.
22. The timing of the x-ray study will vary with the speed of blood flow in the limb. Occasionally the film is delayed for a second or two after the last dye is injected in order to better visualize the vessels of the calf.
23. Two 14 × 17-inch or one 14 × 36-inch x-ray plates are used to visualize the arterial system of the entire leg.

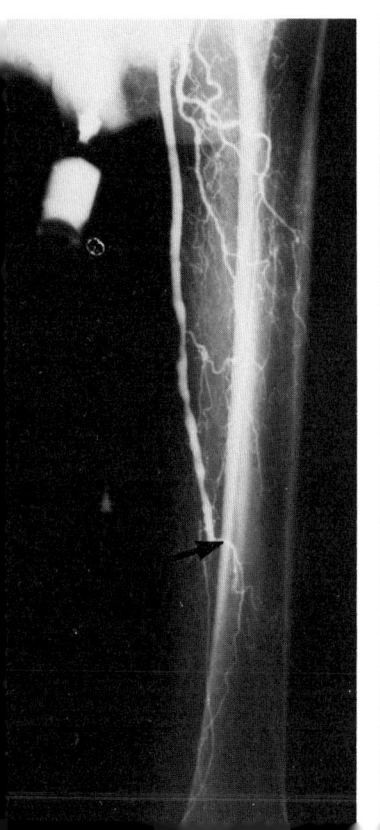

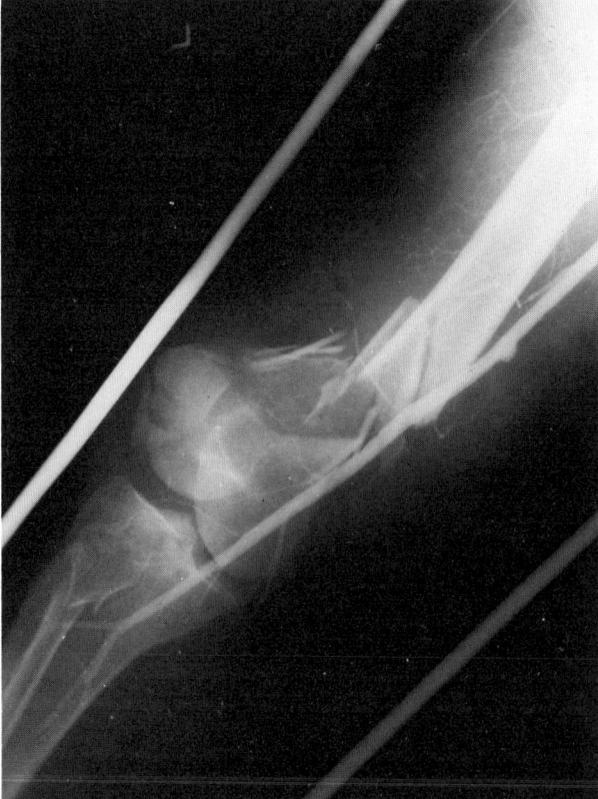

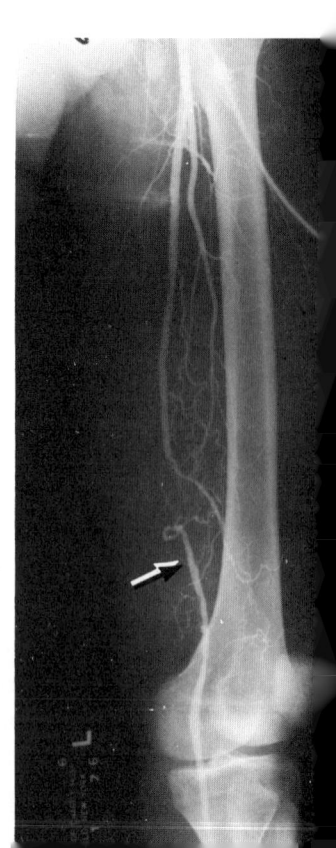

24. Once satisfied with the procedure, withdraw the needle and maintain firm pressure over the injection site for five minutes.
25. Apply a dry sterile dressing.

NOTE: In infants and children a 19- or 20-gauge needle is used. The amount of dye used is 5 to 10 cc, depending on the size of the child.

(Left) Emergency department femoral angiogram of elderly patient with acute occlusion of the superficial femoral artery. Note level of occlusion and sudden cessation of dye column. (Center) Emergency department femoral angiogram of patient with severely comminuted distal femur. The limb was cool below the knee. The femoral artery is intact and there is no evidence of vascular injury. (Right) Emergency department femoral angiogram of patient with sudden occlusion of the superficial femoral artery. Note distal occlusion at adductor hiatus. In this instance, a 36-inch x-ray plate was used.

9 VASCULAR PUNCTURE TECHNIQUES

Percutaneous puncture of a vein or artery is perhaps the most common procedure performed in the hospital setting. This technique may be needed to obtain blood samples for laboratory examination, to monitor venous or arterial pressure, or as a pathway for administering fluids, electrolytes, blood, or medication.

COMPLICATIONS

Whatever the purpose of the vascular puncture, it is considered an invasive technique and thus must be performed using aseptic methods. While the risk of a single vascular puncture, as might be done to obtain blood samples, carries an extremely low morbidity, the risk associated with indwelling intravascular catheters or cannulae is much higher.

The most common complication of an indwelling device is local sepsis; other complications include local damage to the vessel wall with extravasation of blood, thrombus formation, or more rarely embolic phenomena. Less commonly, air embolism or major bloodstream sepsis (septicemia) results. Each of these complications may lead to a more serious and, at times, fatal result. Thus, a seemingly innocuous procedure can precipitate a life-threatening condition if established principles are not followed. Extreme caution must be taken to maintain all precautions, especially in the stress of the emergency setting.

EQUIPMENT

NEEDLES AND CANNULAE

A wide range of devices are available commercially for insertion into the vascular tree. For the most part, these are packaged sterile and disposable, thus reducing to some extent the risk of septic complications.

Available equipment includes hollow needles, plastic cannulae, and cannula-needle combinations. These vary in size from very large diameter (13-gauge) to very small (27-gauge) and from ⅜ inch to 8 inches in length, with and without special devices to simplify insertion. A single- or double-winged needle device (also called a butterfly) is especially suitable for both infants and adults. Generally the smaller bore needles and cannulae are used in infants and children and the larger in adults.

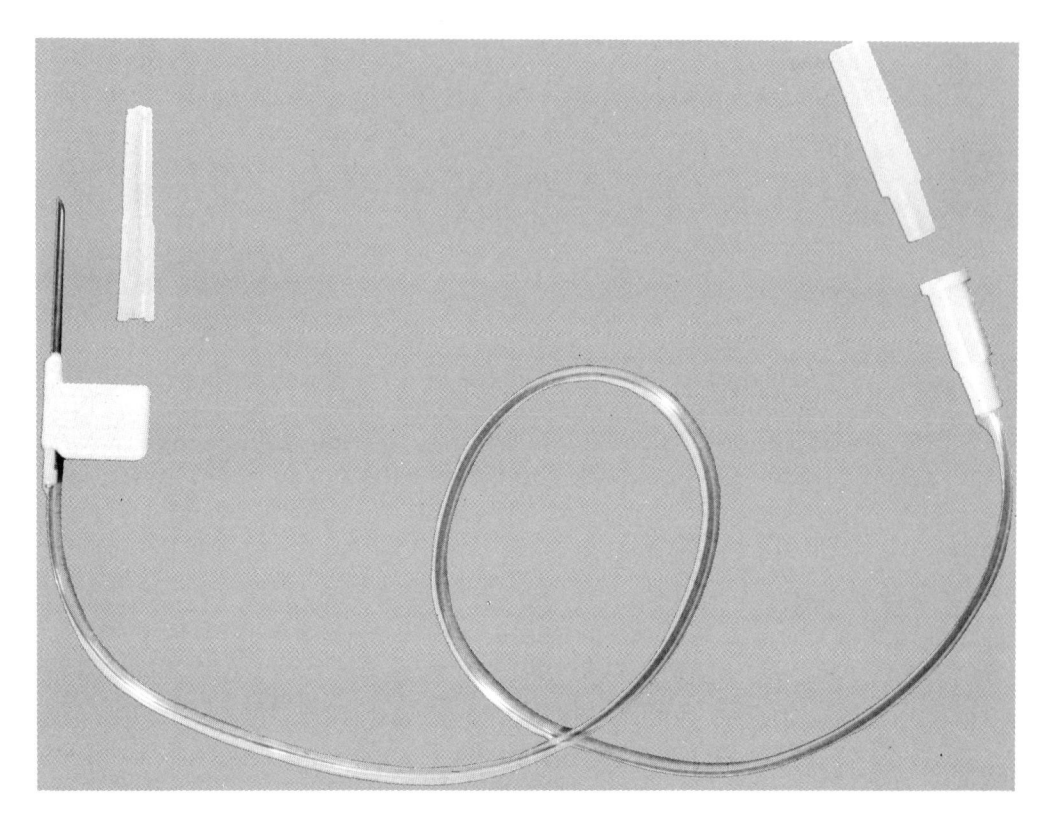

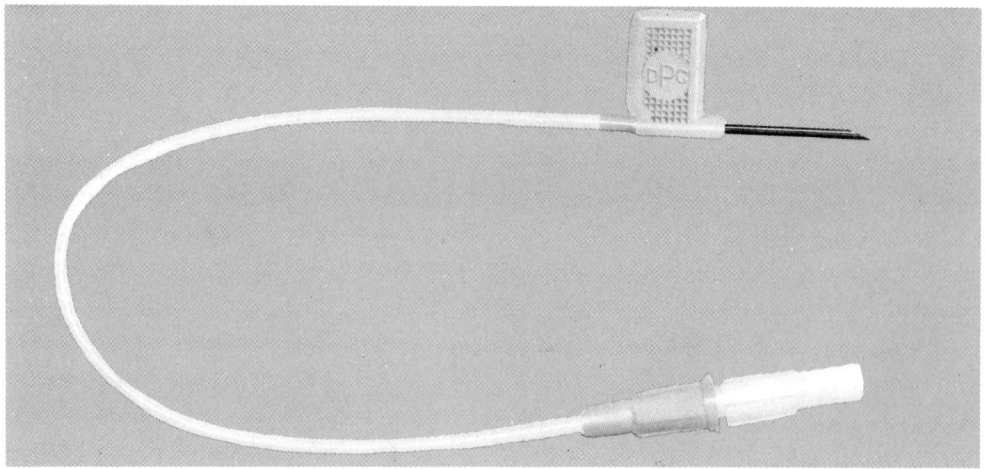

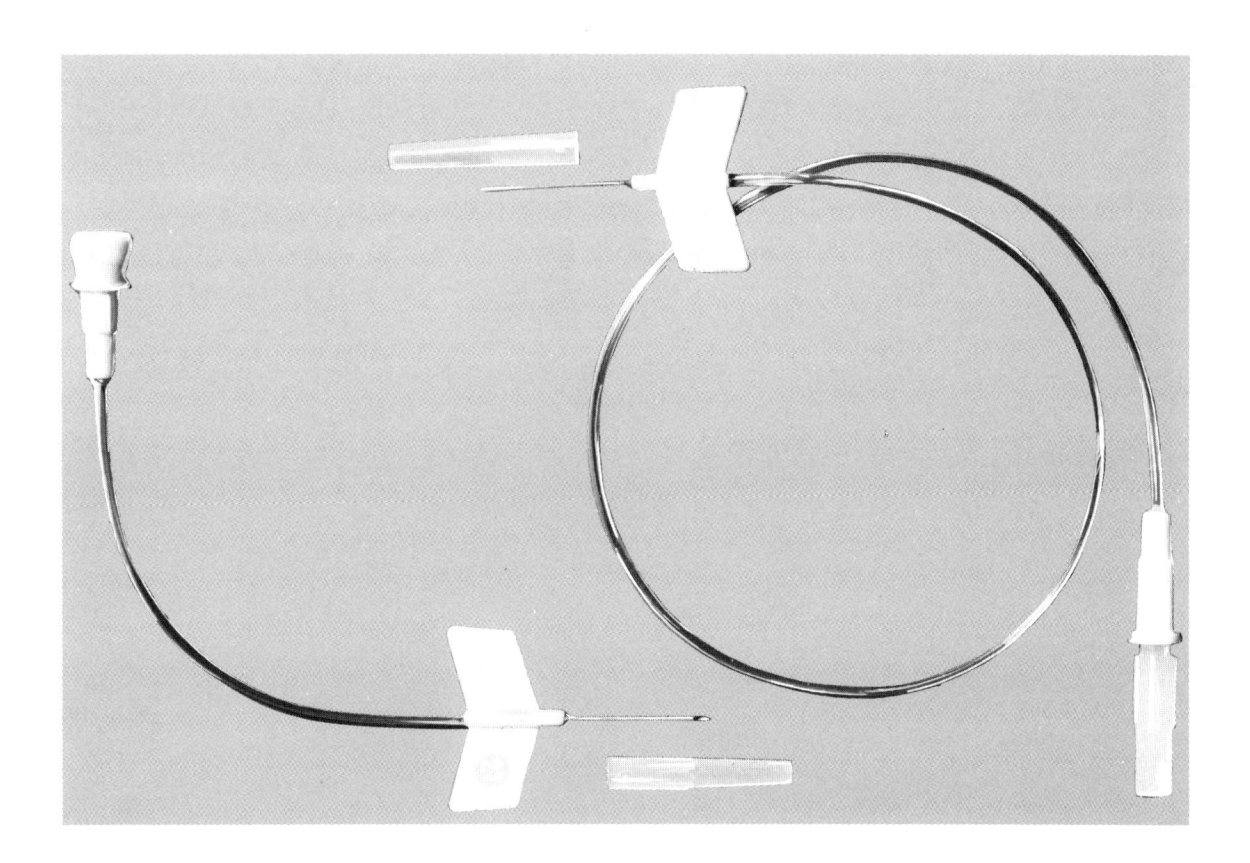

INFUSION SETS

To prevent waste and to function more efficiently, an appropriate infusion set should be utilized from the outset of the procedure when an indwelling device is used. The important parts of an infusion set include a spike tip to penetrate the solution container, a drip chamber, plastic connecting tubing, a male needle adapter and rubber flash chamber, and a roller crimping device which regulates the rate of flow. The standard fluid infusion device is a straight-line set which is used for most electrolyte solutions. A blood infusion set (often called a Y-type) has two spiked tips and a filtered drip chamber, to connect to the blood pack and the isotonic fluid used to administer the blood.

The drip chambers are calibrated to various standards so that the speed of infusion can be regulated accurately and the amount of fluid to be given in a specific period of time determined precisely. For adults, the infusion sets are calibrated to deliver 10 drops per ml; for pediatric patients, the calibration is 50 to 60 drops per ml. One should become familiar with the calibration of the sets available in the hospital. The calibration of the infusion set is marked on the package.

The lower end of the infusion set contains a male fitting needle adapter and immediately proximal to this, a rubber flash chamber. This rubber chamber may be used for the injection of additional medication. The plastic tubing should never be punctured for it will not seal.

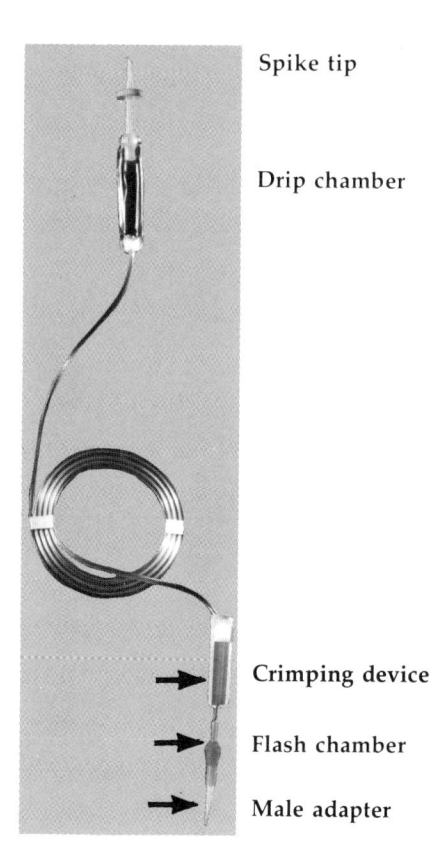

Spike tip

Drip chamber

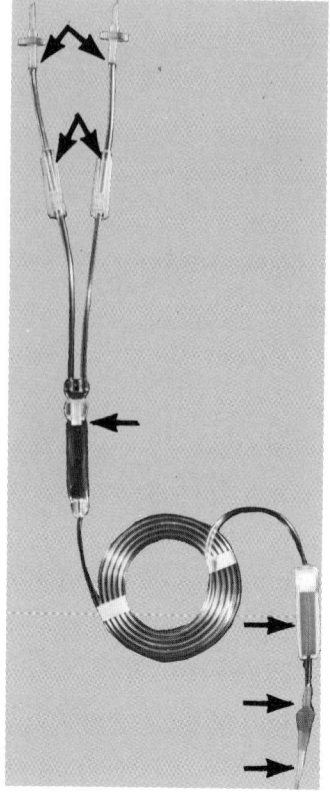

Crimping device

Flash chamber

Male adapter

Spike tip

Crimping device

Drip chamber with filter

Crimping device

Flash chamber

Male adapter

INDICATIONS

The indications for use of specific equipment will depend on the purpose of the procedure and the needs of the patient. For example, if venous blood is to be drawn for hematology studies, at least a 20- or 21-gauge needle should be used to minimize damage to the blood cells passing through. If the purpose is to replenish circulating blood volume, the size of the needle or cannula must obviously be larger and will depend in part on the size and condition of the patient and the type of fluid to be administered.

Infants and small children do not require or tolerate large bore needles. An adult in hypovolemic shock and in need of rapid restoration of blood volume will require a needle or cannula large enough to infuse the fluid rapidly, under pressure if necessary. As a corollary, if the fluid to be administered is of low viscosity, such as 5% dextrose and electrolyte solutions, a relatively small gauge needle (22 or 23 gauge) may be used. If a more viscous solution (blood, serum albumin, or concentrated glucose) is being given, a larger needle or cannula (18 or 19 gauge) is much better suited to the task.

SELECTION OF A SITE

When choosing a location for venipuncture, consideration should be given to the size of the patient and the duration of parenteral fluid replacement.

In an infant, a scalp vein is the ideal site for an infusion. Veins in the wrist or foot are less likely to be suitable.

In an adult, one is tempted to penetrate the large, readily accessible veins of the antecubital space (anterior aspect of the elbow) or the greater saphenous vein at the medial malleolus of the ankle. But, one must remember the purpose of the infusion and the length of time the parenteral fluids may be required. Every effort should be made to cannulate a vein which does not overlay, or one which is located in proximity to, a large joint such as the elbow, wrist, or ankle. Prolonged immobilization of any of these joints can be most uncomfortable to the patient and actually deter recovery.

With experience and care, a vein of suitable size can usually be found on the forearm or the dorsum of the hand which will allow for maximal safety of infusion with minimal discomfort to the patient.

If a patient, child or adult, is in need of special nutrient fluid, such as hyperalimentation fluid, a large central vein must be used, to prevent local vascular complications. Such a vein is the superior vena cava which may be cannulated from a remote vein. A plastic cannula is inserted into the jugular, antebrachial, or subclavian veins and advanced centrally into the cava or right atrium. Central venous catheterization (CVC) requires precise technique to provide maximal benefit to the patient with a minimum of hazard.

This procedure is discussed in more detail in Central Venous Catheterization.

PRECAUTIONS

Site selection for fluid replacement is of particular importance in a patient with multiple injuries. Every effort should be made to avoid placement of an intravenous line in an injured limb.

Generally, in patients with penetrating trauma to the abdomen, fluid replacement should not be via the lower limbs. Similarly, with penetrating wounds of the neck or upper thorax, the upper limbs should be avoided. The reasons for this are several, but the primary one is the possibility of damage to the large venous channels of the abdomen (especially the inferior vena cava) or neck (the subclavian, jugular or brachiocephalic) as a result of the injury. Volume replacement into a peripheral vein draining into a damaged central vein may result in loss of the infused fluid through the rent in the central vessel.

SPEED OF INFUSION

The speed of infusion is established by the physician as the patient's condition requires or allows. While there are several parameters for determining adequacy of fluid replacement, perhaps the most common are the patient's pulse, blood pressure, urine output, and cardiac status. In critically ill or injured patients, other parameters to be monitored are the pulmonary artery and wedge pressures, the central venous pressure, and arterial blood gases.

TECHNIQUES

Details of vascular puncture are discussed with each specific procedure. Once an infusion is begun, the site must be adequately immobilized to prevent dislodgement of the intravascular device and to keep the patient as comfortable as possible.

10 ARTERIAL PUNCTURE

INDICATIONS
1. Need for obtaining samples of arterial blood.
2. Need for monitoring intra-arterial pressure.

EQUIPMENT
1. 20-gauge 1½-inch needle
2. 5 cc (Luer-Lok) syringe rinsed with heparin
3. A small cork or rubber stopper
4. A shallow pan with shaved ice or a plastic bag with ice and a tie
5. Four 2 × 2-inch gauze pads
6. Skin prep (povidone-iodine)

ANATOMICAL CONSIDERATIONS
1. The arteries which are easiest to puncture are those of medium size close to the skin, namely the radial, brachial, and femoral arteries. They are best identified by palpation of the pulse.
2. The femoral artery may be located just below the inguinal crease at a point midway between the anterior superior iliac spine and the pubic tubercle.

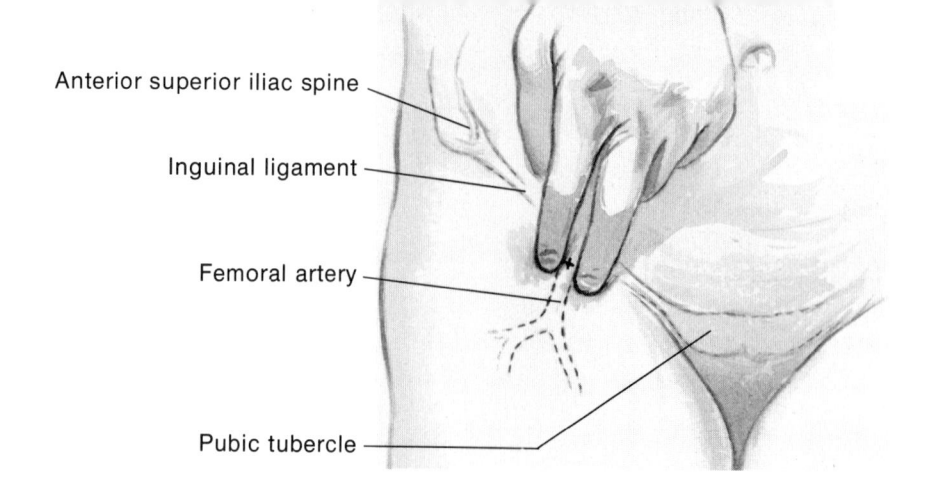

Anterior superior iliac spine

Inguinal ligament

Femoral artery

Pubic tubercle

3. The brachial artery is palpable on the volar (flexor) surface of the elbow in the medial half of the antecubital space. It is brought into a more superficial position by having the patient extend his elbow on a flat surface and rotating the forearm to midposition between pronation and supination with the thumb abducted and pointing toward the ceiling.

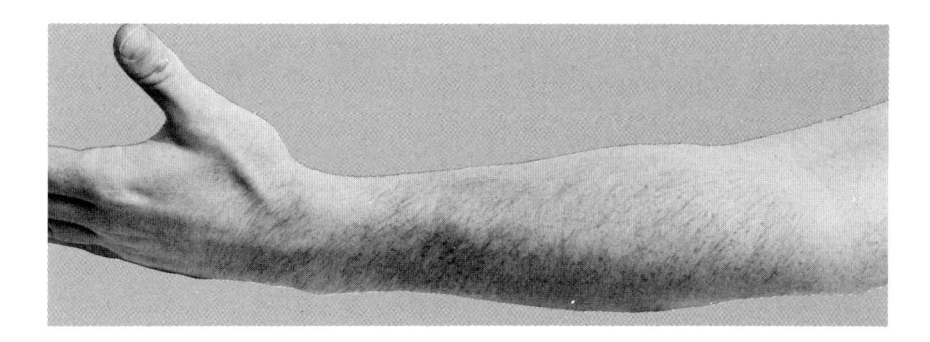

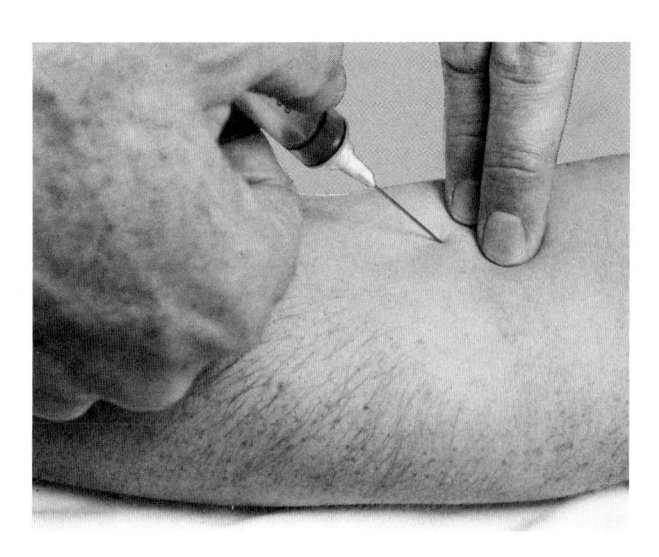

4. The radial artery is palpated on the volar aspect of the wrist just medial to the radial styloid.

PROCEDURE

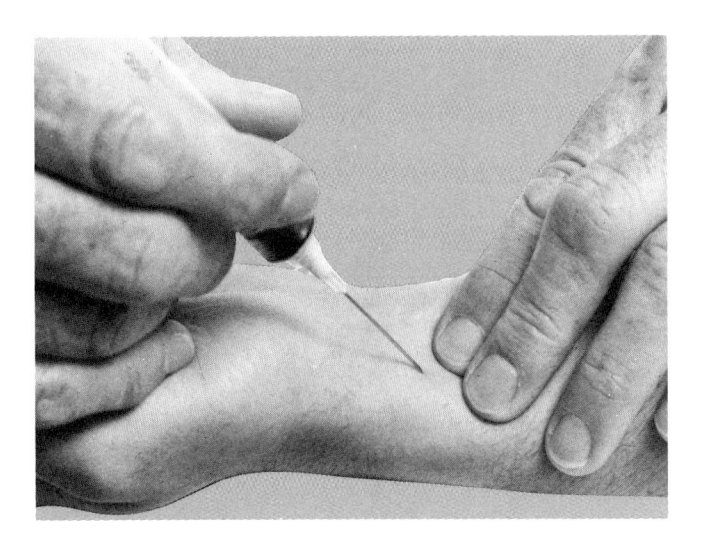

1. Prep the skin of the site with povidone-iodine.
2. Palpate the arterial pulsation.
3. Trap the artery between the index and middle fingers of the free hand to prevent the vessel from slipping away from the needle.
4. Draw 1 cc of heparin into the syringe, then discard it. The small amount of heparin left in the syringe and needle is sufficient for anticoagulation.
5. Introduce the needle, bevel up, through the skin at a 60-degree angle directly over the trapped artery.
6. Advance the needle until the arterial pulsation is felt.
7. While the artery is trapped between the index and middle fingers, advance the needle firmly through the wall of the artery. Both anterior and posterior walls of the vessel are punctured.
8. While aspirating gently, slowly withdraw the needle until a pulsatile flow is seen in the syringe. Usually the syringe will fill readily with a minimum of aspirating pressure.

9. When an adequate amount of blood is obtained, apply finger pressure at the puncture site and withdraw the syringe and needle. The sample must be drawn air-free (without any air in the syringe and needle). Immediately cork the tip of the needle assembly to prevent any air from entering the syringe and mingling with the blood sample.
10. Place the syringe in an ice bath to be taken immediately to the laboratory.
11. Maintain finger pressure on a sterile gauze pad over the puncture site for five minutes to prevent hematoma formation. Pressure may be required for a shorter or longer duration.

FOR ARTERIAL BLOOD PRESSURE MONITORING

1. Use a needle-cannula assembly.
2. Prepare the skin over the arterial pulse selected. (The radial is the artery of choice.)
3. Introduce the needle-cannula assembly as outlined in steps 1 through 8 above. Omit the use of heparin.
4. Once the artery is entered, withdraw the needle from the cannula approximately 1 to 1.5 cm.
5. Advance the cannula in the artery.
6. Once properly seated, remove the needle completely.
7. Attach the cannula to the pressure measuring equipment.
8. Fix the cannula to the skin with a 3-0 silk suture.
9. Apply a sterile dressing with povidone-iodine.

11 VENIPUNCTURE

INDICATIONS
1. Need to obtain blood samples, for study (single puncture).
2. Need to administer fluid, blood, medication (indwelling device).

EQUIPMENT

SINGLE PUNCTURE
1. 20 to 21-gauge needle
2. 5, 10, or 20 cc syringe (as needed)
3. Tourniquet
4. Alcohol swab
5. Sample tubes

INDWELLING CANNULA
1. Cannula-needle assembly with or without attached syringe
2. Tourniquet
3. Povidone-iodine
4. 2 × 2-inch gauze pad
5. Armboard
6. Adhesive tape

ANATOMICAL CONSIDERATIONS
1. When a needle will not be left indwelling in the vein, the site most often used for venipuncture is a vein in the antecubital space of the elbow.
2. When a needle or cannula is to be used for prolonged intravenous administration, it is preferable to select a vein on the forearm or dorsum of the hand.

3. The vessel should not be entered by direct puncture through the overlying skin into the vein wall. The preferred technique is to penetrate the vein on its lateral or medial wall at a point remote from the site of skin penetration.

PROCEDURE

SINGLE PUNCTURE OF THE UPPER EXTREMITY

1. Apply a tourniquet to the extremity, between the site of venipuncture and the heart. The tourniquet should be tight enough to occlude outflow from the superficial veins of the limb without occluding arterial inflow.
2. Ask the patient to make a fist several times to produce venous engorgement. If this is unsuccessful, gently slap the skin of the forearm or elbow.
3. Select a vein suitable for puncture in the antecubital space or on the forearm.
4. Prep the skin with alcohol or povidone-iodine.
5. Introduce the needle, bevel up, at the site selected for venipuncture, through the skin into the subcutaneous tissue to one side of the vein.
6. Pass the needle parallel to the vein for a distance of 1 to 1.5 cm.
7. With the thumb of the free hand, apply pressure to the vein distal to the skin puncture to fix the vein in position and prevent it from rolling away from the needle.
8. Once the vein is fixed, maneuver the needle to enter the side wall of the vessel at an angle of 20 to 35 degrees and firmly pass the point of the needle into the vein.

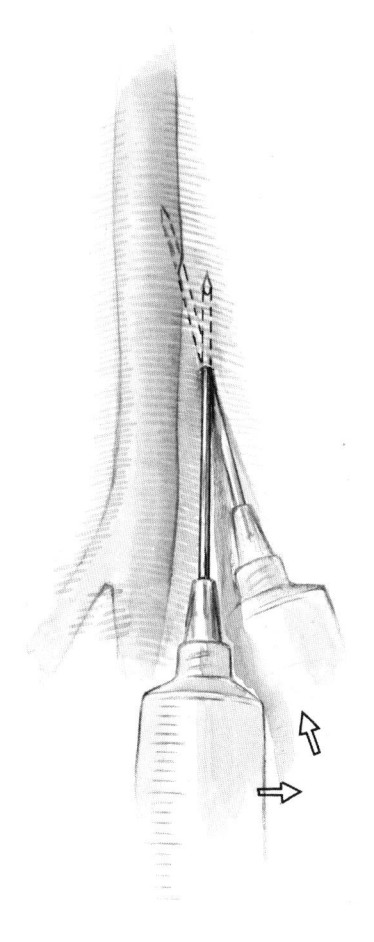

9. After the vein is entered, aspirate the syringe gently. A free flow of blood should be obtained. Withdraw the amount required for study and place it in appropriate tubes.
10. Remove the tourniquet.
11. Place the alcohol swab over the site of skin puncture and apply mild pressure while simultaneously withdrawing the needle.
12. Apply pressure with the swab over the puncture site for 1 to 2 minutes to minimize hematoma formation. If the antecubital space was used, ask the patient to maintain the elbow in acute flexion for the same period.

PUNCTURE OF THE FEMORAL VEIN

ANATOMICAL CONSIDERATIONS

The femoral vein lies medial to the femoral artery as it passes into the thigh beneath the inguinal ligament.

The femoral artery pulse may be palpated on the anterior aspect of the thigh just below the midportion of the inguinal crease.

PROCEDURE

1. Palpate the femoral pulse distal to the middle of the inguinal crease.
2. Prep the skin with alcohol or povidone-iodine.
3. Plunge the needle-syringe assembly through the skin in a perpendicular direction just medial to the femoral pulse. The needle should penetrate at least to a depth of 1 to 1½ inches, to pass through the anterior and posterior walls of the vein.
4. Gently aspirate the syringe. If the needle is in the vein, a free flow of blood will be obtained. Aspirate in two planes.
5. If no blood is recovered, slowly withdraw the needle, aspirating gently during the process. As the needle is withdrawn, it should pass through the vein. If blood is aspirated, maintain the needle in position and collect the necessary amount of blood.
6. When a sufficient amount of blood is collected, quickly withdraw the needle and apply pressure over the puncture site for 3 to 5 minutes.

PLACEMENT OF INDWELLING CANNULA IN A VEIN

PROCEDURE

1. Either a cannula-over-needle or cannula-in-needle device may be used. Choice of one or the other is usually a matter of personal preference.

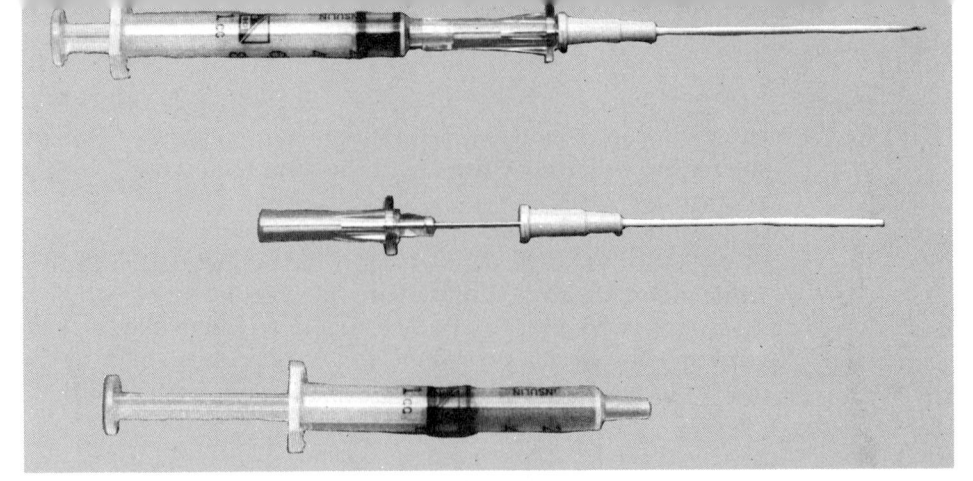

Cannula-over-needle device

2. Follow steps 1 through 4 described under "Single Puncture." Prep the skin with povidone-iodine.
3. Introduce the cannula-needle device through the skin into the subcutaneous tissue, adjacent to the vein.

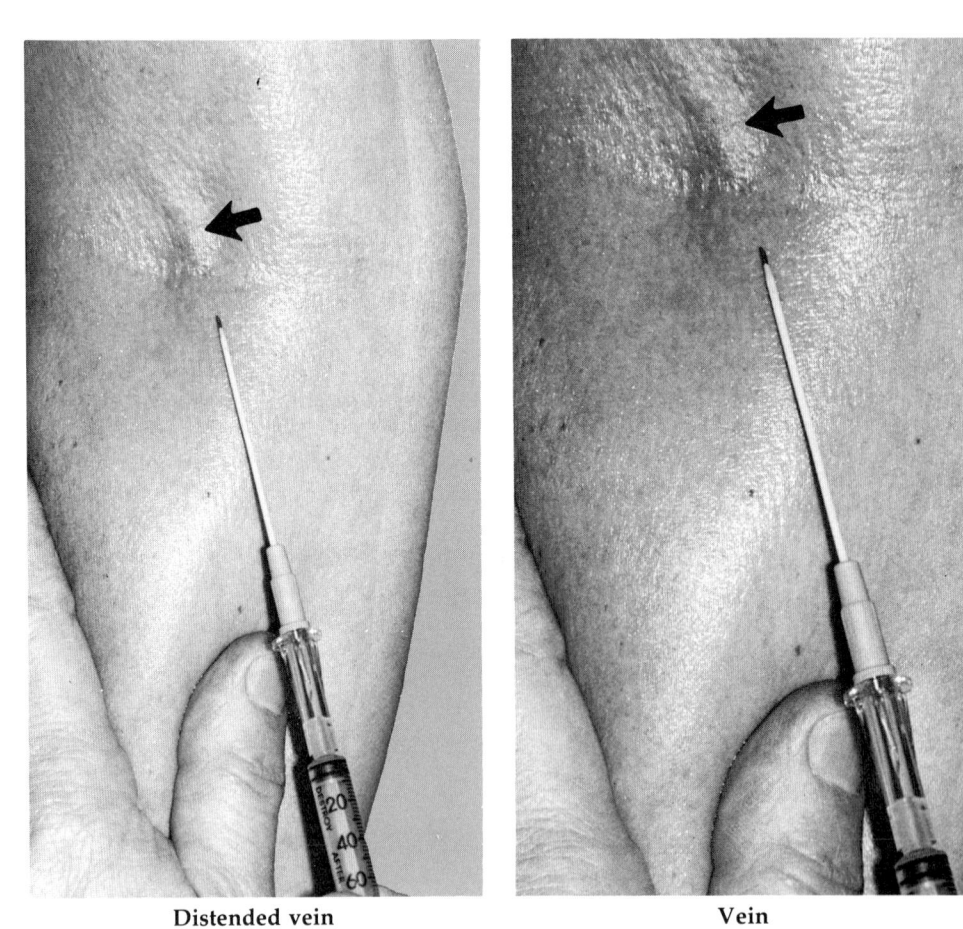

Distended veinVein

4. Pass the cannula-needle assembly parallel to the vein for a distance of 1 to 1.5 cm.

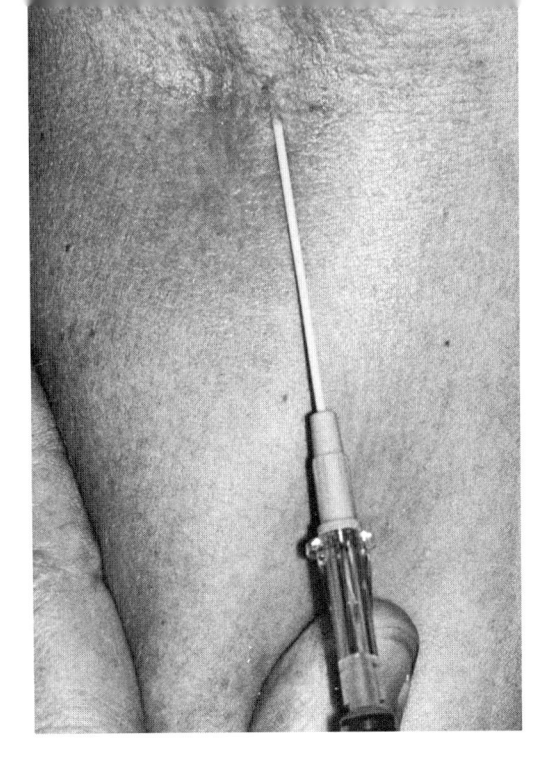

5. Fix the vein in position with the thumb of the free hand to prevent it from rolling away from the needle.
6. With the vein fixed, maneuver the cannula-needle assembly into the side wall of the vein at an angle or 20 to 25 degrees.

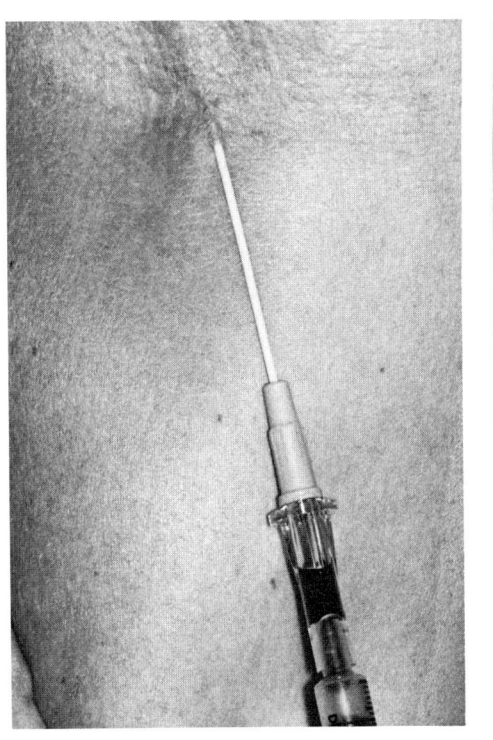

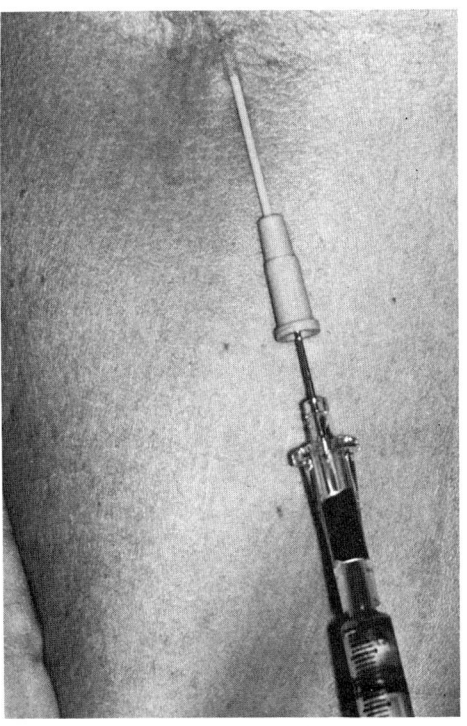

Blood drawn into flash chamber

7. If the vein is entered, blood will appear in the flash chamber. If a syringe is attached, gently aspirate to determine if the needle is properly placed. Remove the touniquet.
8. Once the vein is entered, hold the cannula in position and gently withdraw the needle 1 to 1.5 cm, then advance the cannula a short distance into the vein.
9. Completely remove the needle and pass the cannula to its hub.

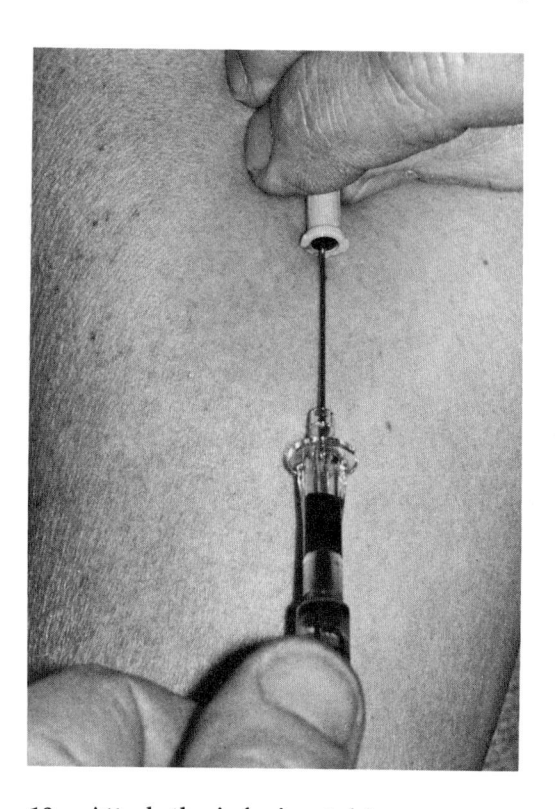

10. Attach the infusion tubing.

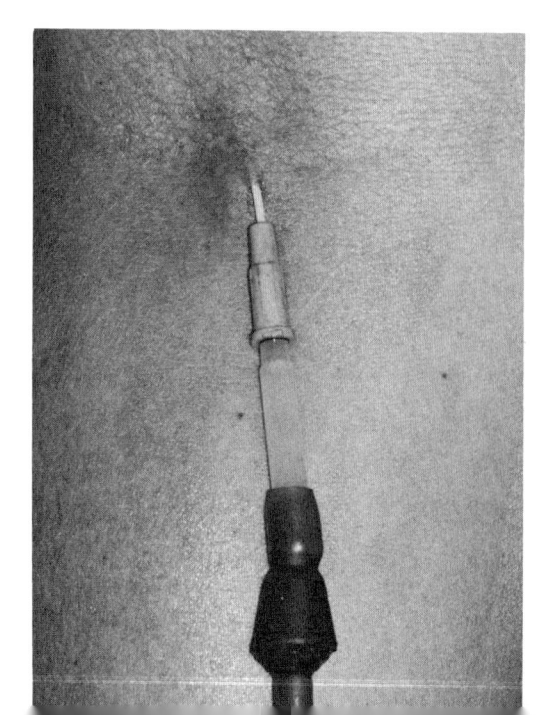

11. Apply a 2 × 2-inch gauze with povidone-iodine ointment to the puncture site.

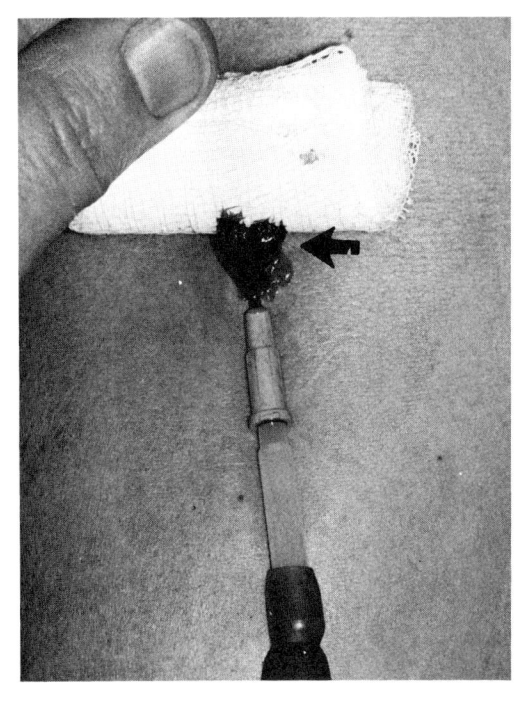

Povidone-iodine ointment

12. Secure the cannula in place with adhesive tape.
13. Tape the extremity to an armboard, to minimize the chance of dislodging the cannula. Avoid immobilizing the elbow joint if possible.
14. Record on the dressing the type and size of the cannula and the date and time of insertion.

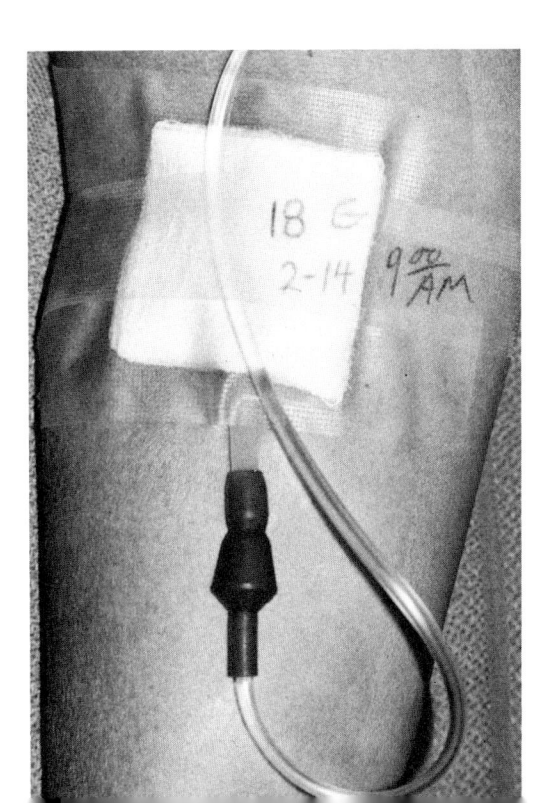

12 VENOUS CUTDOWN

INDICATION
Need to open a veinway, when superficial venous channels are not of sufficient size for percutaneous puncture.

EQUIPMENT
1. Local set (see page 181)
2. #3 scalpel handle and #15 blade
3. Four small hemostats
4. Needle holder (Webster type)
5. Adson forceps with teeth
6. Plastic cannula from 14- to 24-gauge, depending on patient's age (may be taken from a needle-cannula device)
7. 3-0 chromic catgut ties
8. 4-0 silk with swedged needle
9. Four towels
10. Gauze pads

ANATOMICAL CONSIDERATIONS
1. The primary site for cutdown is the greater saphenous vein at the ankle.
2. It is easiest identified at a point approximately 2 cm anterior and 2 cm above the inferior tip of the medial malleolus.
3. A secondary site is the antecubital (median basilic) vein which is located in the medial aspect of the flexion crease of the elbow.

PROCEDURE

1. The technique is basically the same in pediatric and adult patients. Exceptions are noted below.
2. The primary site of cutdown is the saphenous vein at the ankle.
3. To prevent damage to the cannula or vein by ankle movements, infants and children need restraining during the procedure. This can be done by strapping the foot and lower leg to a padded armboard or Papoose Board.
4. Apply a rubber tourniquet to the upper half of the calf.
5. Prep the skin of the ankle with povidone-iodine and drape.

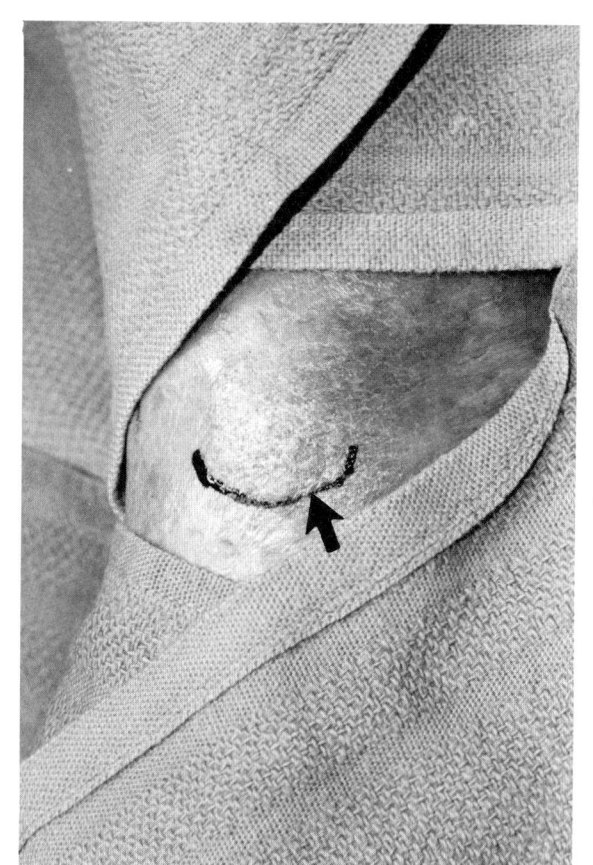

Tip of medial malleolus

6. Infiltrate the skin overlying the saphenous vein with 0.5% lidocaine.
7. Make a transverse incision through the area of anesthesia. A 2 to 2.5 cm incision should suffice.
8. Once the skin is incised full thickness, spread the subcutaneous fat gently with a curved hemostat.
9. Identify the saphenous vein traversing the incision in a slightly oblique direction.
10. Free up the vein from its surrounding tissue by gentle spreading movements with a small curved hemostat. The saphenous nerve is attached to the anterior wall of the vein.

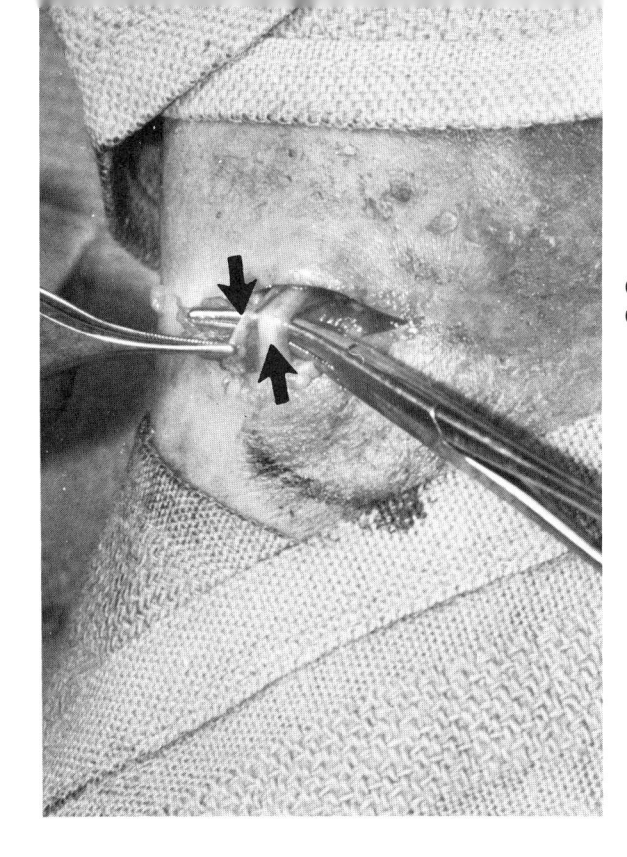

(Top) Saphenous nerve
(Bottom) Saphenous vein

11. Elevate the vein from its bed for a distance of 1.5 to 2 cm and separate the saphenous nerve from the vein.
12. Place a catgut tie at the lower end of the mobilized vein and leave it in place for traction.

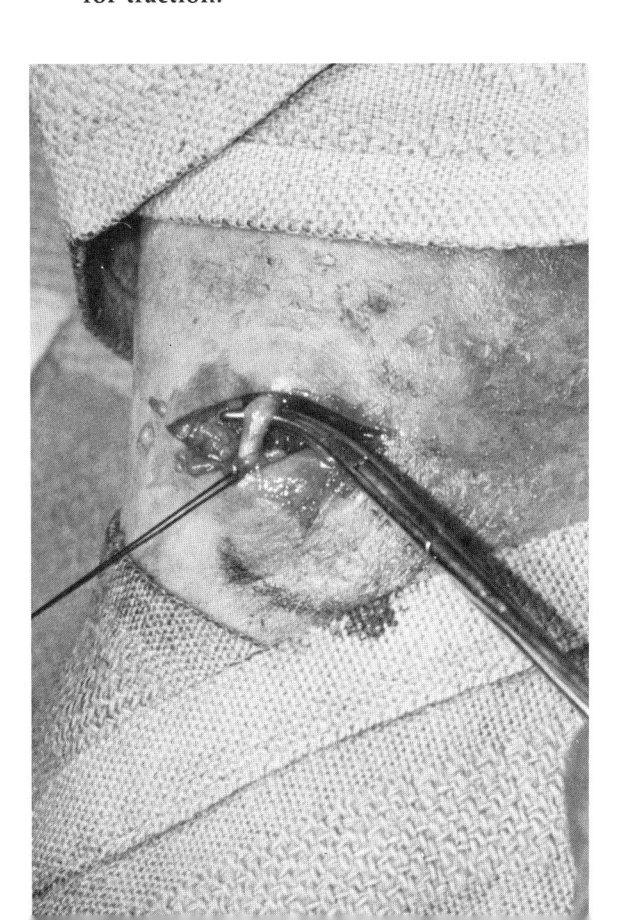

13. Pass a catgut tie behind the vein above the lower tie.
14. Make a small transverse incision in the anterior wall of the vein. A brisk flow of blood will occur because of the tourniquet applied above. Control the bleeding by slight traction on the upper loose tie.

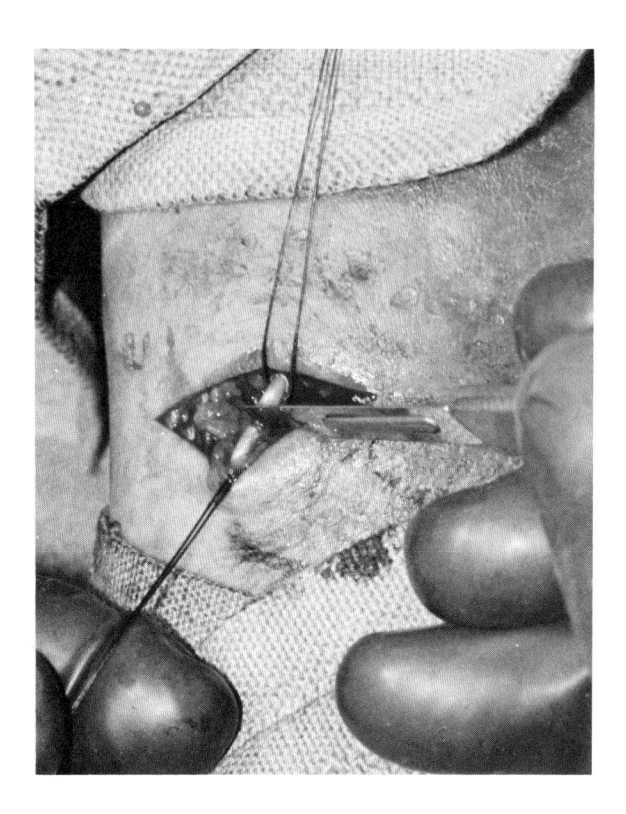

15. The vein when manipulated frequently will go into spasm, making cannulation difficult. Dilate the venotomy gently with the tip of a closed hemostat.

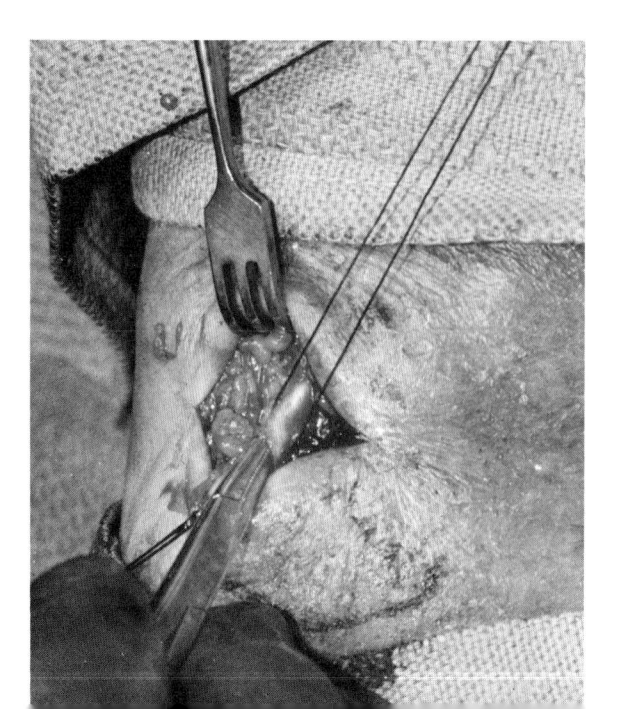

16. Introduce a plastic cannula into the vein through the venotomy and hold it in place by tying the upper tie about the vein. The cannula should be inserted almost to its hub.

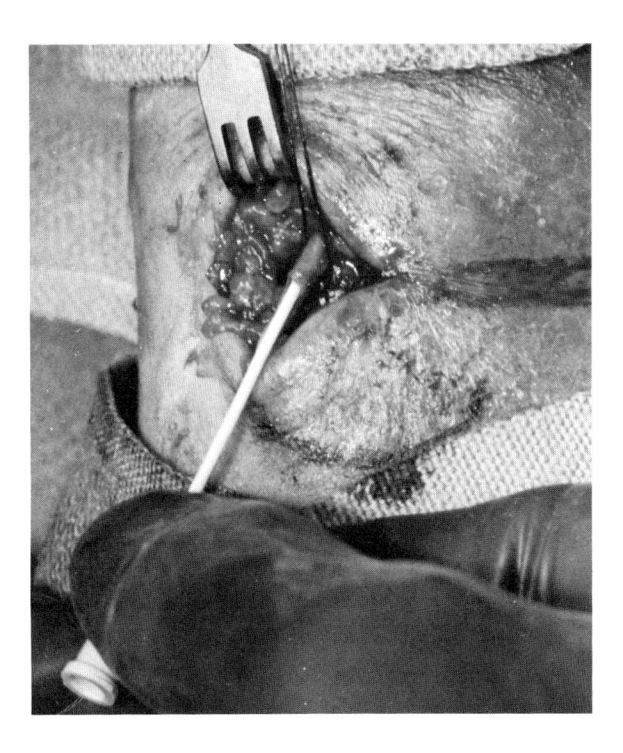

17. Remove the tourniquet.
18. Attach IV tubing to the cannula.
19. Close the skin incision with three or four silk sutures.

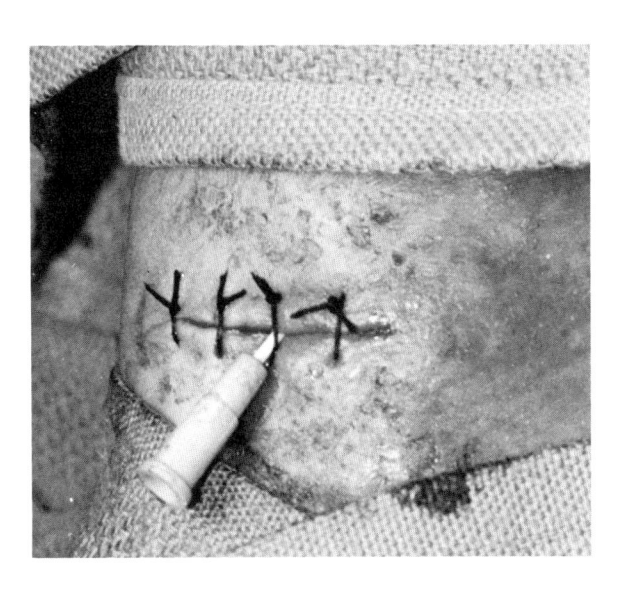

20. Apply a sterile dressing with a topical antibiotic ointment.

75

13 INJECTION OF BICIPITAL TENDON SHEATHS

INDICATIONS

Bicipital tenosynovitis (tendonitis). This condition must be distinguished from subdeltoid bursitis. Familiarity with the anatomy of the shoulder and the location of the short and long heads of the biceps will be helpful in making the correct diagnosis.

EQUIPMENT

1. 10 cc syringe
2. 5 cc syringe
3. 25-gauge ⅝-inch needle
4. 22-gauge 1½-inch needle
5. Local anesthetic agent (0.5% lidocaine or bupivacaine)
6. Hydrocortisone or methylprednisolone

ANATOMICAL CONSIDERATIONS

1. The short tendon of the biceps is enclosed in a fibrous sheath and arises from the inferior aspect of the coracoid process of the scapula. The coracoid process may be found as a bony prominence which lies just below the junction of the middle and outer thirds of the clavicle. It may be somewhat difficult to palpate in muscular males.
2. Palpation along the course of the tendon will reveal marked tenderness in acute inflammatory conditions.
3. The long tendon of the biceps arises from the superior and posterior rim of the glenoid cavity of the scapula. It then courses downward across the front of the head of the humerus, enters the bicipital groove, and is encased in a sheath. Just below the groove, the tendon joins the muscle belly.

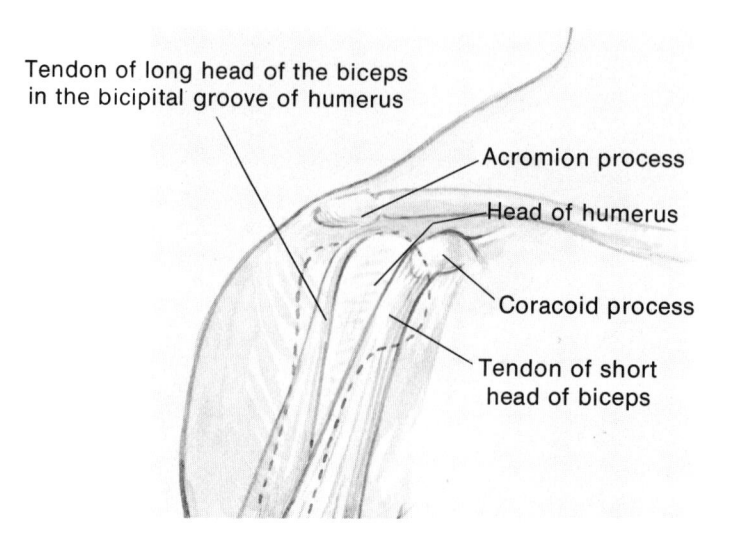

Tendon of long head of the biceps in the bicipital groove of humerus

Acromion process

Head of humerus

Coracoid process

Tendon of short head of biceps

4. To locate the long tendon of the biceps, the anterior aspect of the shoulder is palpated with the patient's arm at his side and the elbow flexed to 90 degrees. The patient's hand is grasped in the handshake position, the shoulder rotated internally and externally, and the long tendon of the biceps will be felt as a linear prominence rolling beneath the palpating finger.
5. Marked tenderness is present when acute inflammation is present.

PROCEDURE

INJECTION OF SHORT TENDON OF THE BICEPS

1. Prepare the skin overlying the coracoid process with povidone-iodine. Palpate the coracoid process with the left thumb.

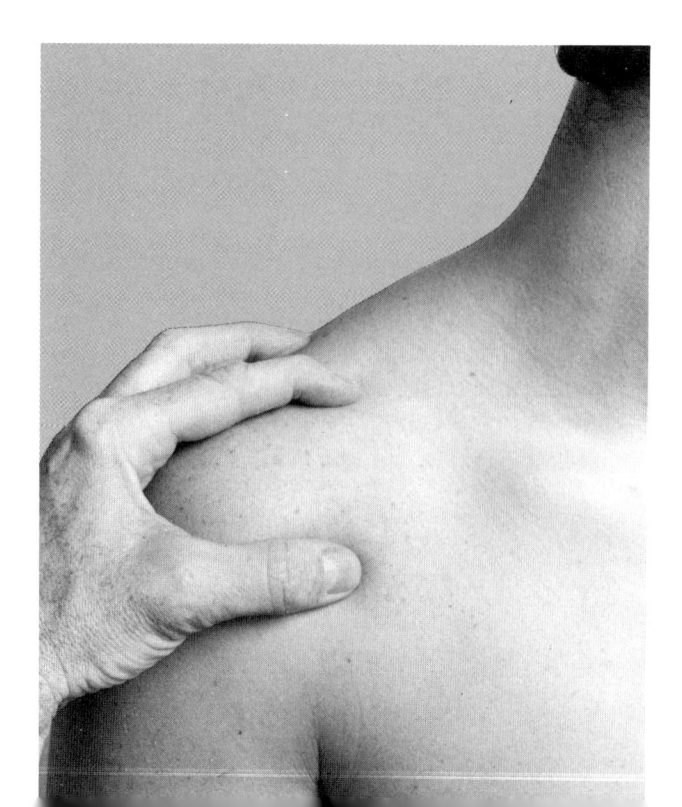

2. Raise a skin wheal just inferior to the tip of the coracoid process with 0.5% lidocaine, using the 5 cc syringe with a 25-gauge needle. Infiltrate the deeper tissue over the point of maximal tenderness. Since the needle must penetrate the pectoralis muscles, care must be taken not to deposit the anesthetic in a blood vessel. This can be prevented by aspirating the syringe in two planes (180 degrees apart) prior to injection of the solution. If blood is recovered, reposition the syringe 1 to 2 mm and reaspirate.
3. Fill the 10 cc syringe with 9 cc of anesthetic solution and 1 cc of steroid and attach the 21-gauge needle.
4. Insert this needle through the skin wheal, directing it toward the biceps tendon. As the biceps tendon is encountered, a slight grating sensation may be felt. The depth to which the needle is inserted varies with the thickness of the pectoralis muscles.

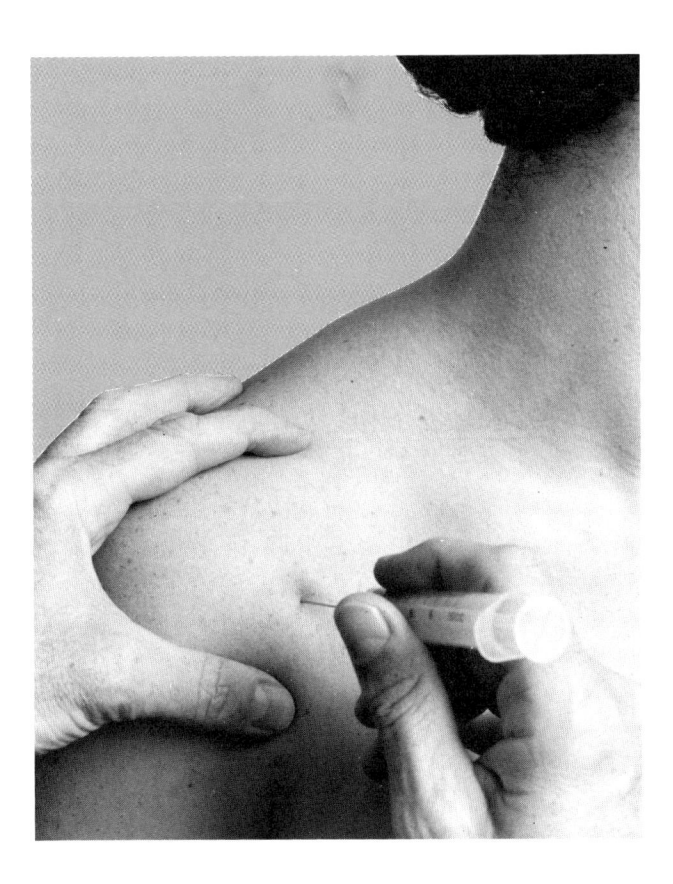

5. Withdraw the needle 1 to 2 mm, aspirate gently in two planes and if no blood is recovered, slowly inject the contents of the syringe into the tendon sheath.
6. Upon completion of the injection, withdraw the needle and apply a dry sterile dressing over the site.

INJECTION OF LONG TENDON OF THE BICEPS

1. Prepare the skin of the anterior aspect of the shoulder with povidone-iodine. With the thumb, palpate the long tendon of the biceps in the bicipital groove and determine the point of maximum tenderness.

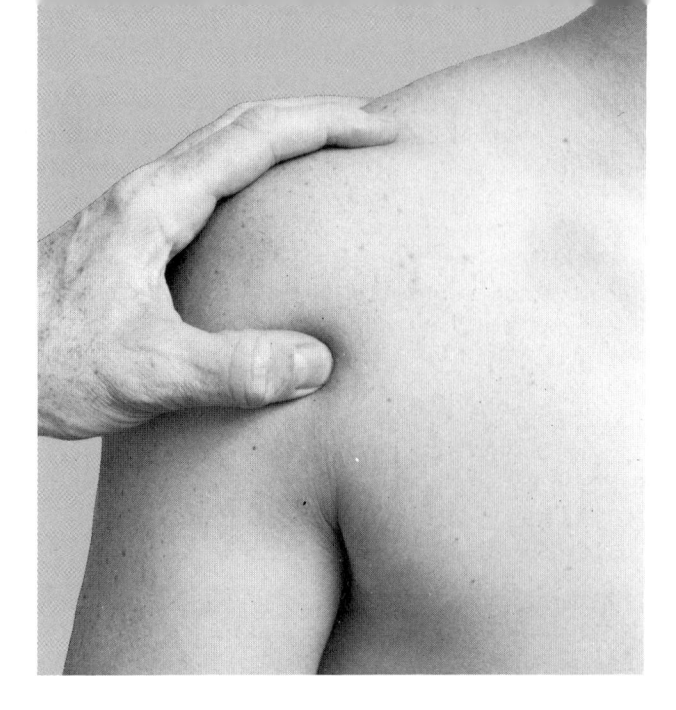

2. Raise a skin wheal and infiltrate the deeper tissues of the anterior aspect of the shoulder with 0.5% lidocaine, following the technique outlined above.
3. Attach the 22-gauge needle to the 10 cc syringe filled with 9 cc of anesthetic solution and 1 cc of steroid. Insert the needle into the skin wheal to the biceps tendon. A slight grating sensation may be noted as the tendon is encountered.

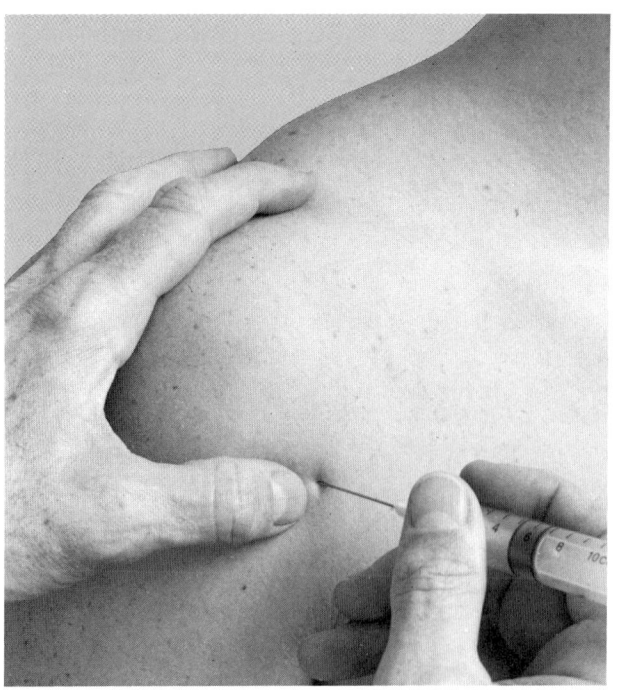

Needle inserted to bicipital tendon

4. Withdraw the needle 1 to 2 mm, aspirate gently in two planes and if no blood is recovered, slowly inject the anesthetic-steroid solution in the area.
5. Withdraw the needle and apply a dry sterile dressing over the site.

14 ASPIRATION OF OLECRANON BURSA

INDICATION
Collection of fluid in the olecranon bursa (olecranon bursitis).

EQUIPMENT
1. 19- or 20-gauge 1½-inch needle
2. 10 cc syringe
3. Prep
4. Hydrocortisone or methylprednisolone (optional)

PROCEDURE
1. Prepare the skin over the extensor aspect of the forearm just distal to the olecranon process with povidone-iodine.
2. Puncture the bursa and aspirate the fluid until the bursa is dry.

Lateral condyle of humerus

Olecranon process

Olecranon bursa

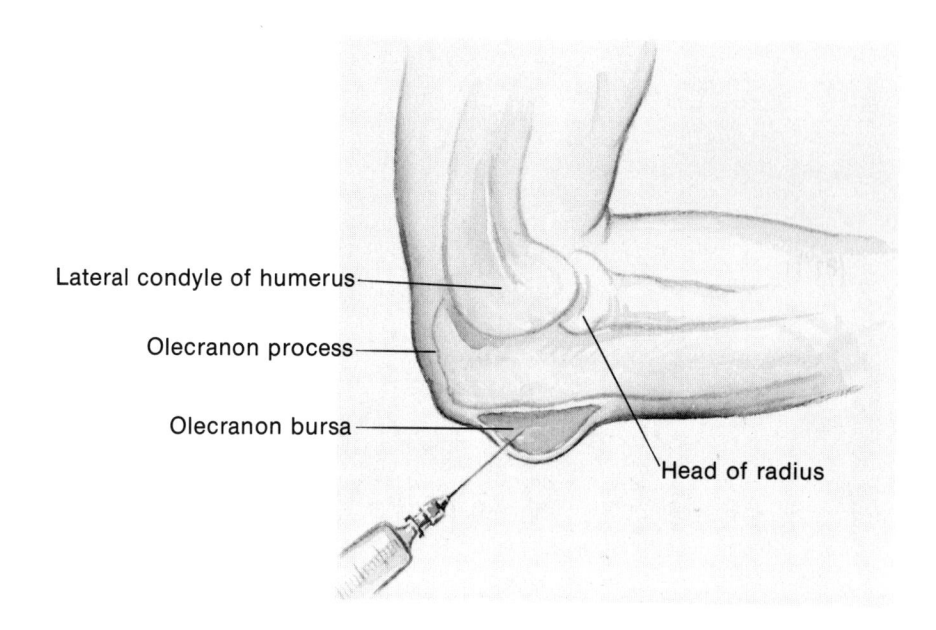

Head of radius

3. Inject hydrocortisone or methylprednisolone into the bursa prior to removal of the needle—this is an optional addition to the procedure.
4. Apply a pressure dressing to the elbow at the termination of the procedure. Place a sterile gauze dressing on the skin and wrap the elbow in a 3-inch elastic bandage. Wrapping should be done with the elbow in approximately 15 to 20 degrees of flexion.

15 ASPIRATION OF PATELLAR BURSA

INDICATION
Acute or chronic bursitis with fluid accumulation in the prepatellar bursa.

EQUIPMENT
1. 25 gauge 5/8-inch needle for the skin wheal
2. 19-gauge 1 1/2-inch needle for aspiration
3. 5 cc syringe for anesthetic medication
4. 10 cc syringe for aspiration of the bursa
5. 0.5% lidocaine
6. Hydrocortisone or methylprednisolone (optional)

ANATOMICAL CONSIDERATION
The patellar bursa is located superficial to the lower half of the patella, superficial to the infrapatellar tendon.

PROCEDURE
1. Prep the skin overlying the swelling with povidone-iodine.
2. Raise a skin wheal over the bursa with the 25-gauge needle and 0.5% of lidocaine.
3. Introduce the 19-gauge needle on a 10 cc syringe through the skin wheal into the bursa and gently aspirate its contents.

Patella

Patellar bursa

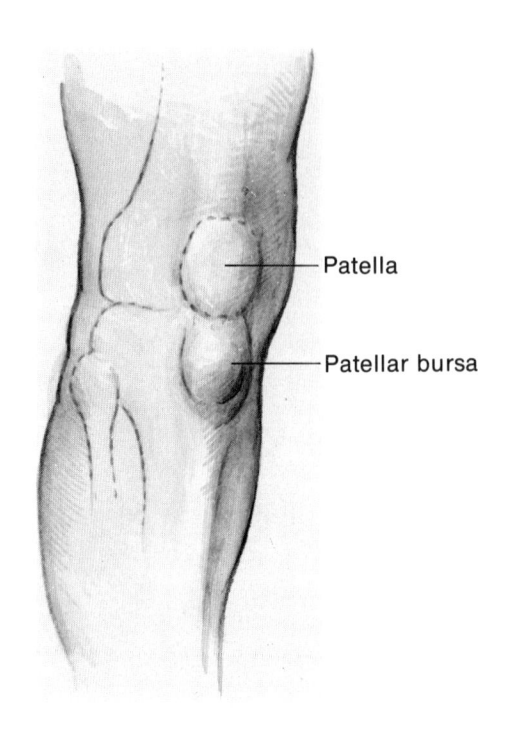

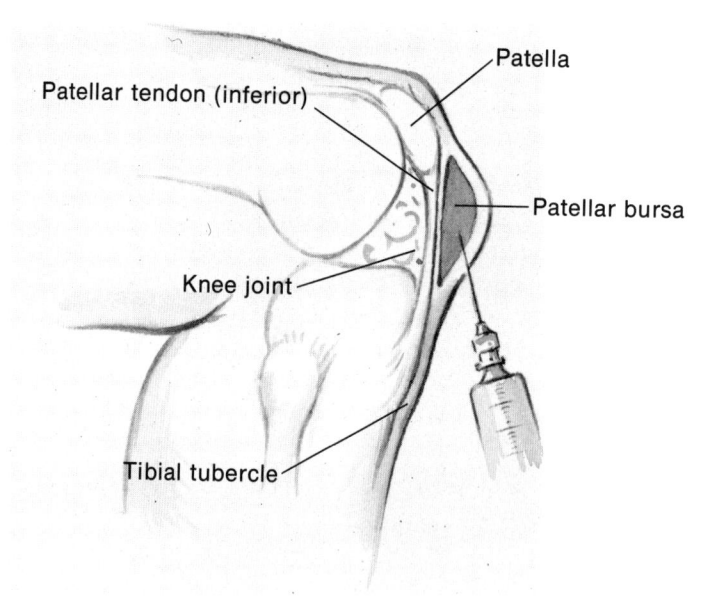

Patella
Patellar tendon (inferior)
Patellar bursa
Knee joint
Tibial tubercle

4. If the fluid is serous or bloody, no additional studies are necessary. If purulent material is recovered, save a portion for bacteriologic study.
5. Hydrocortisone or methylprednisolone may be injected into the bursa prior to removing the needle if pus is not obtained.
5. At the completion of the procedure, apply a pressure dressing using a sterile gauze pad and a 4- or 6-inch elastic bandage.
6. When applying the elastic dressing to the knee, maintain the joint in approximately 30 degrees of flexion.

16 INJECTION OF RADIOHUMERAL BURSA

INDICATION
Acute or chronic bursitis (tennis elbow; epicondylitis).

EQUIPMENT
1. 2 cc syringe
2. 5 cc syringe
3. 25-gauge 5/8-inch needle
4. 22-gauge 1 1/2-inch needle
5. 0.5% lidocaine
6. Hydrocortisone or methylprednisolone

ANATOMICAL CONSIDERATIONS
1. The area to be injected is the point of maximal tenderness which usually is found on the anterior aspect of the lateral epicondyle of the humerus or the extensor tendons overlying the radial head.
2. The two points to be identified are the lateral epicondyle of the humerus and the head of the radius.

Head of radius

Epicondyle of humerus

Olecranon process of ulna

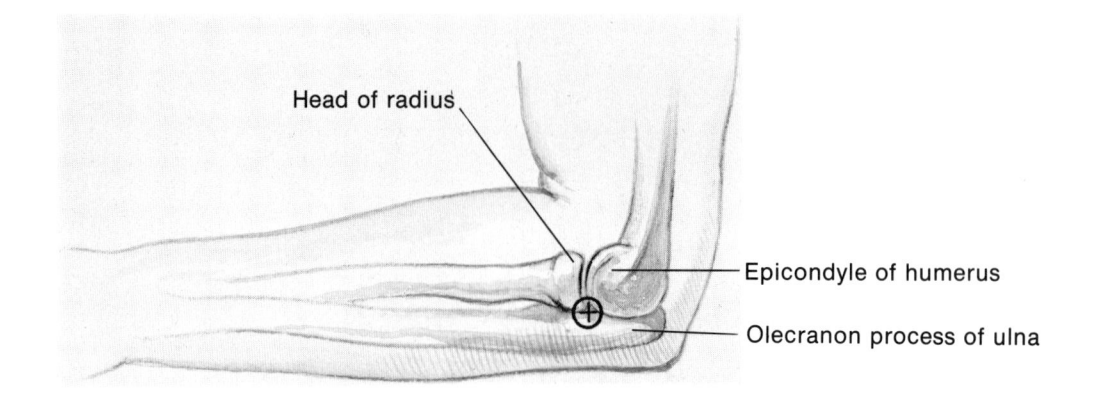

3. Identify the point of maximal tenderness by holding the patient's hand in the handshake position with the elbow flexed at 90 degrees. At the same time, passively pronate and supinate the forearm and palpate the lateral epicondyle and radial head. The radiohumeral joint is identified as a shallow groove distal to the humeral condyle. The radial head is palpable as a small hard protuberance just distal to the joint.
4. The structures to be injected are the extensor aponeurosis and the radial collateral ligament. Occasionally, a periostitis of the epicondyle is present at the origin of the common extensor tendons and is the area to be injected.
5. The symptoms can be reproduced by asking the patient to make a fist and extend the wrist against the resistance of the examiner's hand.

PROCEDURE

1. Identify the point of maximal tenderness in the area of the radiohumeral joint.
2. Keep the patient's elbow flexed at 90 degrees with the palm down on the table for stability.
3. Prepare the skin with povidone-iodine.
4. Raise a skin wheal with lidocaine at the point of maximal tenderness, using the 2 cc syringe and the 25-gauge needle. Insert the needle into the deeper tissues immediately under the wheal, injecting small amounts of the anesthetic agent.
5. Fill the 5 cc syringe with 1 cc of steroid and 4 cc of lidocaine.
6. Using the 22-gauge needle, infiltrate the area, alternately injecting, withdrawing, and redirecting the needle until the entire area is flooded. Avoid striking the bone with the needle to minimize damage, unless maximal tenderness is noted over the lateral epicondyle, indicating the need for infiltration.
7. Apply a sterile elastic bandage dressing over the injection site.

17 INJECTION OF SUBACROMIAL (SUBDELTOID) BURSA

This condition must be distinguished from bicipital tendonitis. Familiarity with the anatomy of the bursa will allow one to make the correct diagnosis.

INDICATIONS
1. Acute or subacute bursitis.
2. Painful calcific bursitis.

EQUIPMENT
1. 10 cc syringe
2. 5 cc syringe
3. 25-gauge ⅝-inch needle
4. 20-gauge 1½-inch needle
5. 0.5% lidocaine
6. Hydrocortisone or methylprednisolone

ANATOMICAL CONSIDERATIONS
1. The subacromial bursa is located on the superior and lateral aspect of the shoulder, deep to the acromion process and the deltoid muscle, overlying the capsule of the shoulder joint.

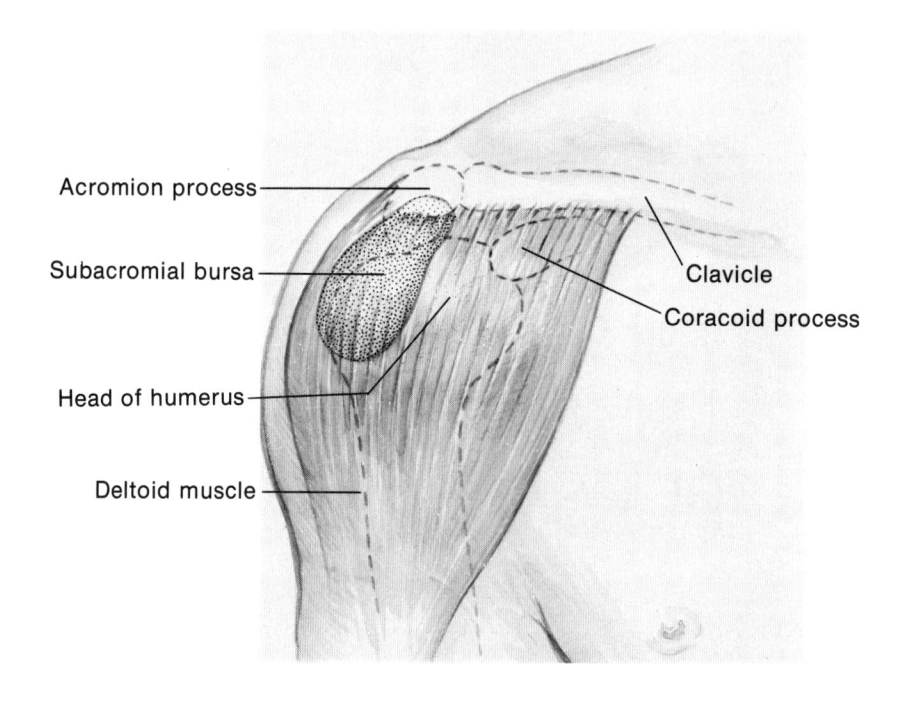

Acromion process
Subacromial bursa
Head of humerus
Deltoid muscle
Clavicle
Coracoid process

2. Careful examination by palpation will reveal a point of maximal tenderness on the shoulder. This is the point of election for injection of the bursa.
3. Identify the anterior tip of the acromion process. The needle should be inserted in a horizontal plane immediately below the tip of the acromion.

PROCEDURE

1. Prepare the skin of the shoulder with povidone-iodine.
2. Palpate the tip of the acromion process with the thumb on the lateral aspect of the shoulder.

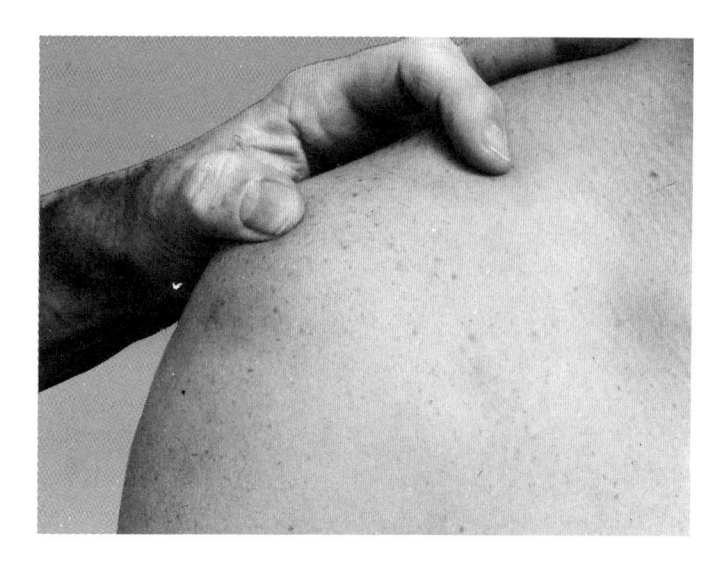

3. Raise a skin wheal over the point of maximal tenderness with 0.5% lidocaine using the 5 cc syringe with the 25-gauge needle and then infiltrate the deeper tissues to the periosteum of the humerus.
4. Fill the 10 cc syringe with 9 cc of anesthetic solution and 1 cc of hydrocortisone or methylprednisolone.
5. Insert the longer 20-gauge needle attached to the 10 cc syringe just beneath the acromion process in the bursa. Occasionally the bursa will be distended with fluid. Therefore, prior to injecting the anesthetic-steroid solution, aspirate the bursa. Some recommend multiple punctures of the bursa to allow for better drainge of the fluid contents.
6. If fluid is recovered, leave the needle in place and change syringes to aspirate the bursa until no more fluid can be recovered.
7. When no more fluid can be aspirated, reattach the filled 10 cc syringe and slowly inject the anesthetic-steroid. The solution may also be injected into the muscles and structures of the shoulder cuff.
8. Upon completion of the injection, withdraw the needle and place a dry sterile dressing over the site.

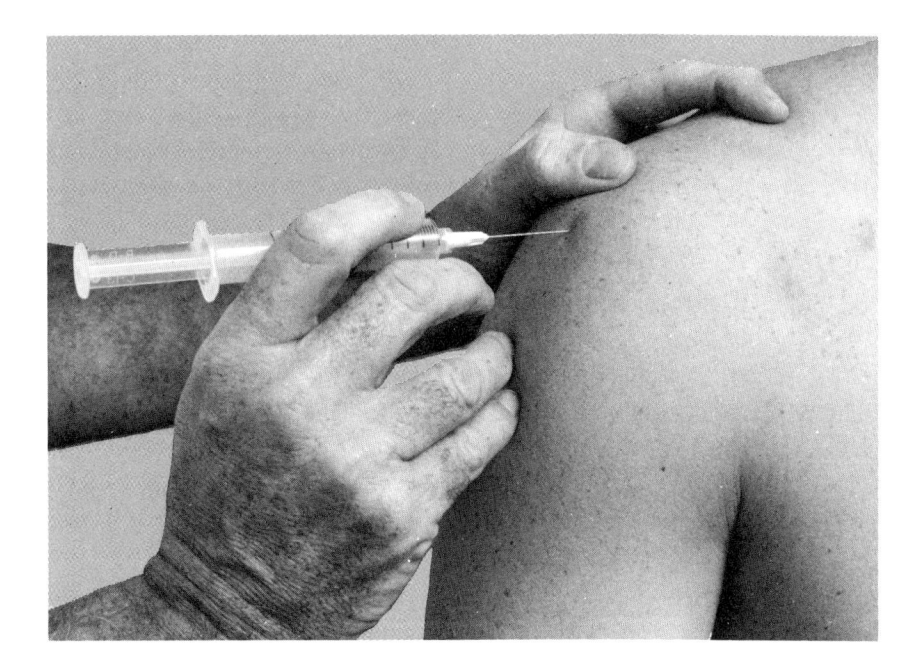

18 ASPIRATION OF GANGLION

INDICATION

Symptomatic ganglion which causes pain or increases in size.

EQUIPMENT

1. 10 cc syringe
2. 19- or 20-gauge 1½-inch needle
3. Prep
4. Hydrocortisone or methylprednisolone (optional)

ANATOMICAL CONSIDERATIONS

1. A ganglion is a cystic structure which is attached to the exterior of a tendon sheath or tendon. More commonly, ganglia arise from a joint as a herniation or outpouching from the joint capsule.
2. A ganglion of the tendon sheath occurs primarily on the flexor surfaces of the fingers or toes. Ganglia are usually small (less than 0.5 cm) and must be distinguished from solid tumors in these areas. The latter are not usually suitable for aspiration.
3. Ganglia arising from a joint usually occur in the wrist or ankle among the carpal or tarsal bones. They vary in size up to several cm in diameter.
4. A ganglion cyst contains thick mucoid fluid similar to that found in a joint space.

PROCEDURE

1. This procedure can usually be performed without local anesthesia. If anesthesia is required, a skin wheal may be raised over the most prominent por-

tion of the mass.
2. Prep the site with povidone-iodine.
3. Flex or extend the part to cause maximal protrusion of the cystic mass.
4. Hold the part firmly and introduce the syringe–needle assembly through the skin at the periphery of the ganglion at an angle roughly parallel to the skin surface.
5. Introduce the needle into the ganglion and simultaneously apply pressure on the apex of the mass while aspirating the fluid. Because of the high viscosity of the content of the cyst, aspiration may be difficult.

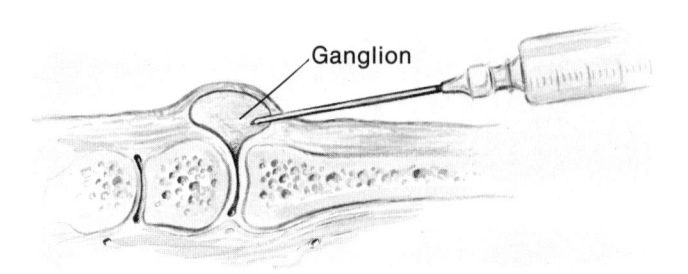

6. The cyst may be punctured in an adjacent site. The combination of external pressure and aspiration will evacuate the cyst. The fluid will be recovered in the syringe, while the continued pressure will cause more fluid to escape through the puncture site into the subcutaneous tissue.
7. After the ganglion is evacuated, leave the needle in place, disconnect the syringe, and inject 1.0 cc of methylprednisolone or hydrocostisone—this is an optional addition to the procedure.
8. At the close of the procedure, withdraw the needle and apply a small, folded gauze dressing for pressure.

19 CARDIOPULMONARY RESUSCITATION (CPR)

Cardiopulmonary resuscitation (CPR) is one aspect of emergency medical care which has broad applicability. It can be performed successfully anywhere, both in and outside of the hospital, by anyone familiar with the technique.

The two types of CPR are
1. Basic life support
2. Advanced life support

BASIC LIFE SUPPORT is essentially a first aid measure which requires one to recognize airway obstruction, respiratory arrest, and cardiac arrest and then initiate proper cardiopulmonary resuscitation. It can be used in the hospital setting before the "resuscitation cart" or similar rescue equipment arrives. No equipment is needed to *initiate* basic life support. Fundamentally, CPR includes establishing and maintaining a patent airway, and providing artificial ventilation by rescue breathing techniques and artificial circulation by closed chest, external cardiac compression. These fundamentals may be expressed as the ABC's of basic life support: A referring to the airway, B referring to breathing, C referring to circulation. Details of this technique will be discussed in the following pages.

ADVANCED LIFE SUPPORT refers to basic life support *plus* adjunctive measures such as endotracheal intubation, placement of veinways for intravenous infusion and drug administration, placement of electrodes for cardiac monitoring, defibrillation, and arrhythmia recognition and control. Generally, advanced life support requires a variety of equipment and supplies which are utilized only by a physician or nurse or a trained paraprofessional acting under their guidance. Advanced life support methods are not reserved or limited to the hospital setting, but are used commonly in sports stadia, industrial health settings, and mobile intensive care units. For the most part, however, advanced life support is used in the hospital setting.

Any physician or nurse whose duties include the care of the acutely ill or injured must be familiar with the techniques of both basic and advanced life support. Furthermore, any hospital must have the personnel, equipment, and supplies available for initiation of life support techniques at any hour of the day or night. It has been demonstrated conclusively that a large number of sudden deaths from acute heart attack may be prevented by prompt and appropriate therapy. It is the purpose of this section to describe both types of life support measures.

BASIC LIFE SUPPORT (BLS)

This procedure should be initiated and maintained until advanced life support is available. It must be started as soon as the following indications are recognized.

INDICATIONS

Respiratory arrest and cardiac arrest.
Cardiac arrest is caused by
1. Cardiovascular collapse (electromechanical dissociation
2. Ventricular asystole
3. Ventricular fibrillation

EQUIPMENT

None.

GENERAL CONSIDERATIONS

The fundamentals (ABC's) of BLS were enumerated earlier but will be repeated here. These include
1. Airway—establish and maintain a patent airway.
2. Breathing—initiate artificial ventilation.
3. Circulation—initiate artificial circulation.

ANATOMICAL CONSIDERATIONS

These will be discussed as they apply to the ABC's.

AIRWAY

Airway obstruction may result from a variety of causes (see "Airway Management"). In patients considered candidates for BLS, the most common findings are retained secretions, vomitus, or dentures in the mouth or pharynx, or relaxation of the temporomandibular joint with collapse of the tongue into the pharynx. Techniques will be described to correct airway obstruction. Foreign bodies may be identified by examining the mouth and oropharynx or sweeping the oral cavity with the index and middle fingers.

BREATHING

Artificial ventilation should be initiated only if the patient is not breathing and after the airway is clear. Observe the chest wall for evidence of respiratory motion or place your ear next to the patient's mouth and nose to check for air movement. The patient may breathe spontaneously upon relief of airway obstruction. If not, artificial ventilation may be started by the mouth-to-mouth or mouth-to-nose technique in large children and adults or the mouth-to-nose in small children and infants. Both techniques will be described. A tight seal must be made between the mouths of the rescuer and patient. If the patient is wearing good fitting dentures, leave them in place to effect a better seal. The number of ventilations per minute will vary with the availability of one or two rescuers. Proper artificial ventilation requires the patient to be in a supine position.

CIRCULATION

Artificial circulation is not begun until after a patent airway is established, artificial ventilation given, and the status of the circulation assessed. A palpable peripheral pulse is a good sign of adequate cardiac action and contraindicates beginning closed chest external cardiac massage. Since the rescuer is usually near the head of the victim working on the airway, the most accessible pulse is the carotid. The carotid pulse may be palpated in the lateral aspect of the neck on either side of the thyroid cartilage in the groove between the cartilage and the anterior aspect of the sternomastoid muscle. Palpate the artery gently at this level to avoid undue pressure on the carotid sinus which may of itself cause alterations in the heart rate and/or rhythm. Remember, initiate cardiac compression only if the carotid pulse is not palpable.

An awareness of the location of the heart in the thorax is essential to proper external cardiac massage. It is the very fact of its anatomical location that makes the heart suitable for external compression. At the same time, the proximity of other structures—the rib cage, lungs and upper abdominal viscera, especially the liver—may result in serious, sometimes fatal, injury in instances when inappropriate resuscitation methods are used.

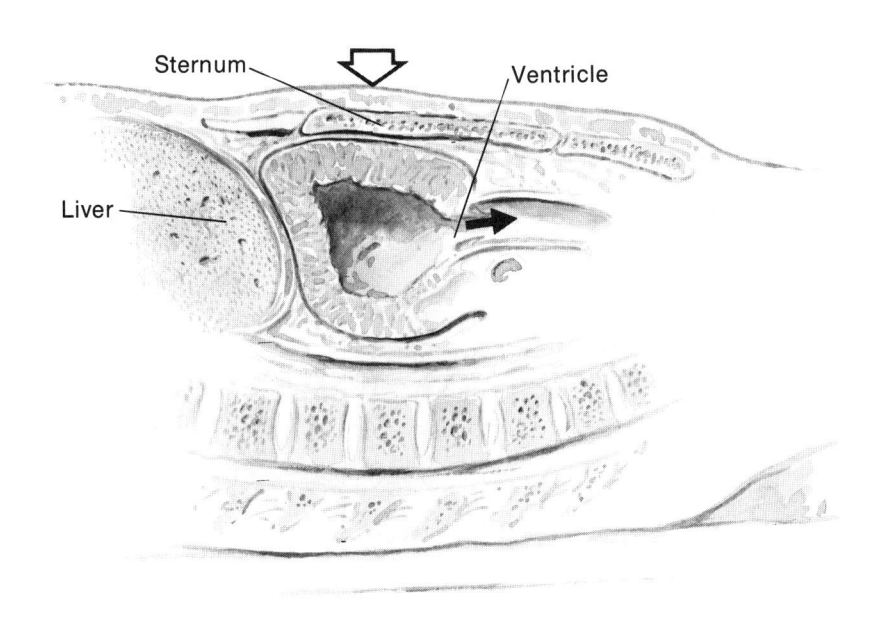

The heart is positioned in the mediastinum, in the center of the chest, between the sternum and vertebral column. In the cephalocaudad direction (head to foot), the heart may vary in its location in relation to the sternum, xiphoid, and costal cartilages, depending on the age of the patient. The portion of the heart of primary concern is the area of the ventricles. In an infant this point lies behind the midportion of the length of the sternum. In an older child this point lies slightly lower, and in an adult at the lower $1/3$ of the sternum.

The amount of force necessary to effect adequate external cardiac compression will vary from an infant to an adult because of the thickness and flexibility of the chest wall. Infants require compression of the sternum to a depth of $1/2$ to $3/4$ of an inch; in a child, 1 to $1\frac{1}{2}$ inches is needed, while in an adult, the sternum must be depressed $1\frac{1}{2}$ to 2 inches.

The frequency of cardiac compression will vary from 60 to 100 per minute depending upon the age of the patient and whether one or two rescuers are present.

For external artificial circulation to be effective, the patient should be in the supine position on a firm support. In the emergency setting, a board should be handy which can be placed beneath the patient's chest to provide the necessary firmness. The padded mattresses on emergency carts and beds are much too soft. For ease of application, the patient may be raised by lifting the sheet under him and sliding the board between the sheet and mattress.

METHOD

For easier learning, the technique of CPR will be discussed in the A, B, C fashion used above. After all, this is the natural sequence of application of the resuscitation maneuvers.

AIRWAY

Perhaps the single most important factor in successful resuscitation is opening an airway. Several methods are used, including the head-tilt, jaw-thrust, and jaw-pull maneuvers.

HEAD-TILT MANEUVER. The patient is supine and the rescuer at one side. The neck is raised by placing one hand beneath the neck and simultaneously pushing posteriorly on the frontal area with the other. This in effect hyperextends the neck and reduces the acute angulation of the pharynx and pulls the tongue forward. This maneuver must be avoided or used with extreme caution in patient's suspected of having a fracture-dislocation of the cervical spine.

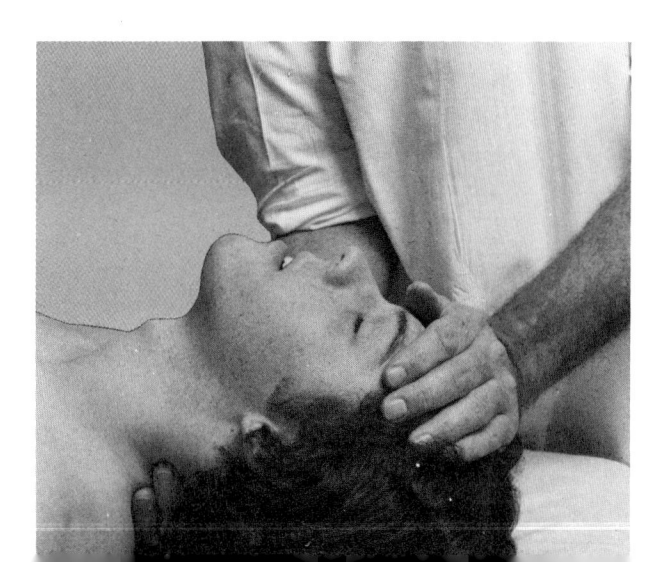

JAW-THRUST MANEUVER. The rescuer is positioned at the head of the patient and elevates the jaw and floor of the mouth by upward pressure with the fingers on the angles of the jaw. With this move, the head is tilted upward, the neck extended, and, thus, the tongue raised from the pharynx.

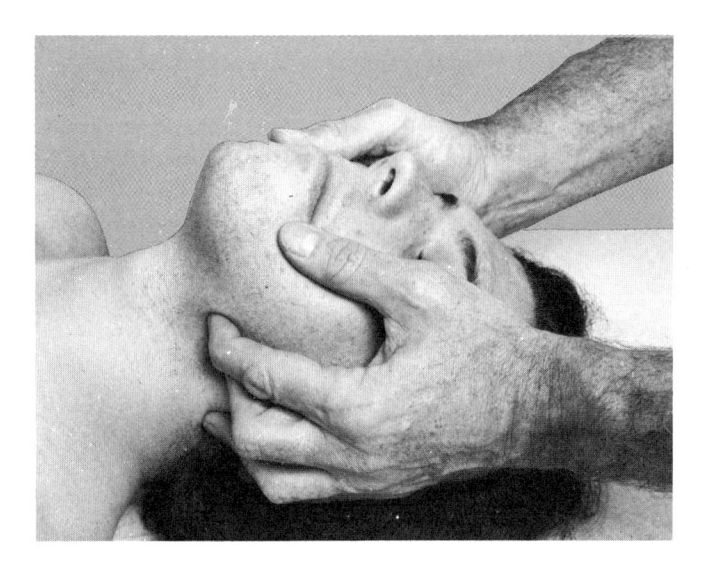

JAW-PULL MANEUVER. The rescuer positioned at the side or head of the patient, grasps the lower jaw with the thumb in the mouth and the fingers under the chin and pulls the jaw forward while at the same time extending the neck by tilting the head posteriorly.

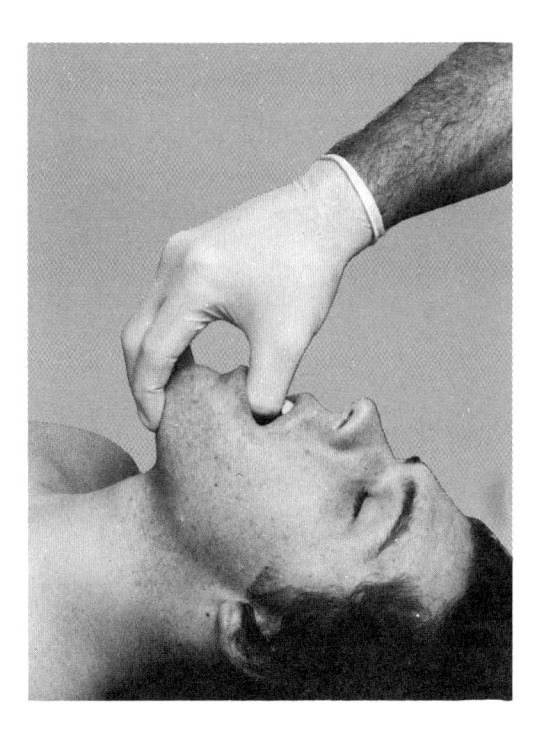

Following one or more of the above maneuvers, a patient's obstructed airway may be relieved and spontaneous respirations may ensue.

BREATHING

The rescuer determines whether the patient has spontaneous respiratory activity by looking for movement of the chest wall or listening at the victim's mouth and nose for any sound of air movement. If spontaneous breathing is lacking or appears ineffective, the rescuer begins artificial breathing.

This is best done with the rescuer to one side of the patient, supporting the head and neck using the head-tilt technique. The hand on the patient's forehead should be used to pinch the patient's nostrils closed; the rescuer should then take a deep breath and place his mouth over the patient's mouth so that a tight seal is made and forcibly exhale into the patient's mouth, taking note of the passive movement of the patient's chest wall. If the chest wall rises, the airway

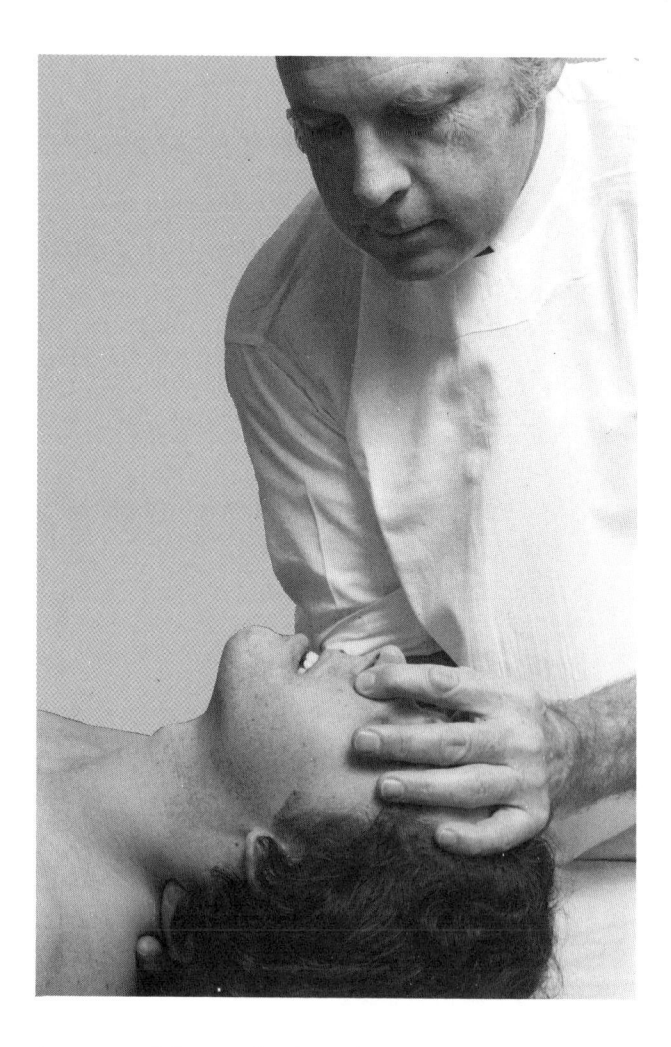

is patent. After expiration, the rescuer should remove his mouth from the patient's and allow passive expiration before repeating the cycle.

If the rescuer is unable to establish adequate ventilation, he must assume the airway is obstructed. The patient's mouth should be opened and any obstructing foreign body identified and removed. Secretions or vomitus in the mouth and pharynx may be removed by the fingers or with a cloth. If this is not successful, the rescuer should turn the patient on his side and strike a sharp blow between the scapulae to dislodge the foreign body.

Once artificial breathing is begun, the rescuer should deliver four quick breaths, allowing the patient to exhale passively between each, and then commence closed chest massage. Ventilation and cardiac massage should alternate continuously in a ratio of 1:5.

In a patient with full dentures, it is easier to perform artificial breathing if these are left in position. When removed, the lips are more flaccid making it difficult to get a tight mouth-to-mouth seal.

The amount of air blown into an adult patient's mouth will be equivalent to the normal tidal volume, about 500 cc. In children, and especially infants, the breaths are necessarily smaller and given faster, usually one every 3 seconds. Care must be taken not to overexpand the pediatric patient's lungs by too aggressive ventilatory efforts.

In the emergency setting, most hospitals will have a resuscitation cart which contains all needed equipment, supplies, and drugs to initiate and maintain life support. Basic life support should be started as soon as it is indicated. Once the resuscitation equipment is at hand, an endotracheal tube should be inserted and respiration maintained with a bag-valve-tube system.

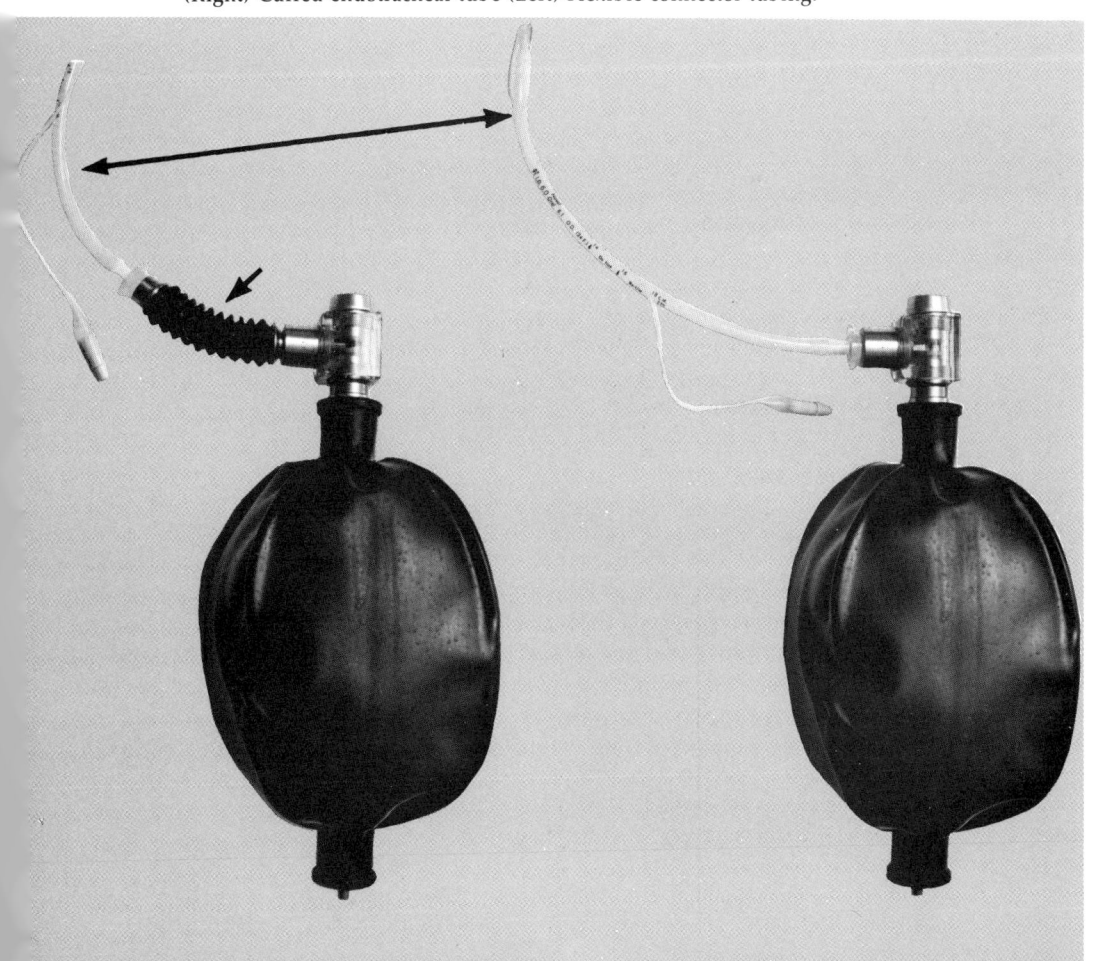

(Right) Cuffed endotracheal tube (Left) Flexible connector tubing.

CIRCULATION

External closed chest cardiac massage should be initiated once it has been determined the carotid pulse is not palpable. If the arrest has occurred in the presence of the physician or nurse or a patient already on a cardiac monitor (a witnessed arrest), the first maneuver is the "precordial thump." A sharp blow is delivered to the patient's midsternal area using the ulnar side of the closed fist. This blow should be initiated from 8 to 12 inches above the sternum. If spontaneous cardiac activity does not begin immediately, BLS should be started.

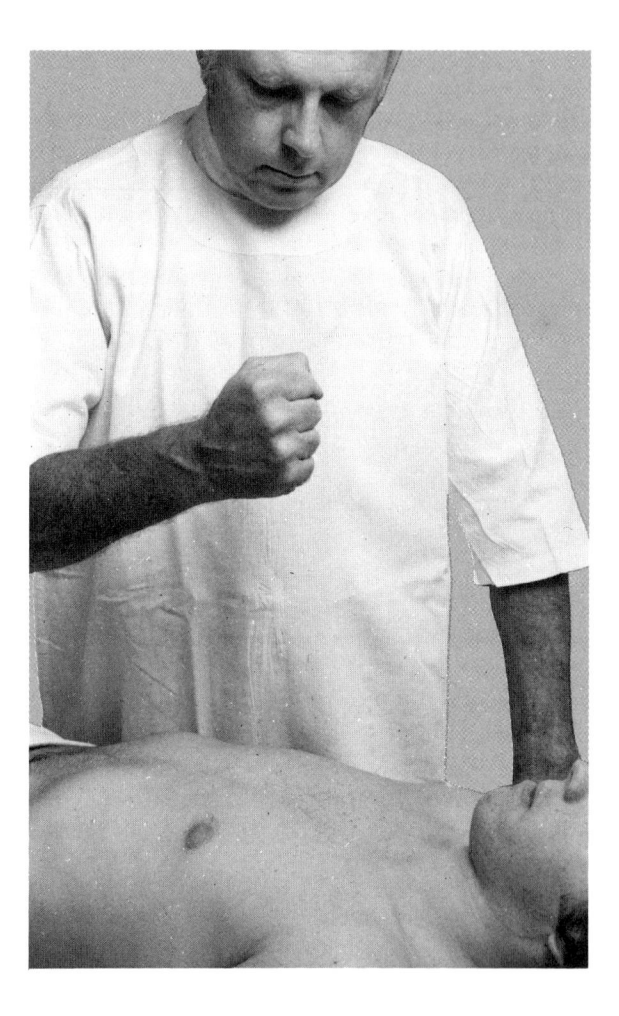

ADULTS. For adults, the point at which external cardiac massage is applied is the junction of the middle and lower thirds of the sternum. Pressure should be applied with the heel of the hand with one hand positioned over the other and the fingers interlocked, though this is not mandatory.

The fingers should *not* touch the chest wall, to minimize the chance of damage to the rib cage. Pressure too low on the sternum or over the xiphoid cartilage may cause injury to the liver. When performing external cardiac compression, stand directly over the patient with the elbows in extension. With this method, the force of compression is generated by the upper trunk and shoulders rather than the arms. This technique is much less tiring and provides more effective compression. The cardiac compressions should be regular, and at an effective rate of 80 per minute. After each compression, pressure on the sternum should be relieved momentarily to allow for better cardiac filling. The sternum should be depressed 1/2 to 2 inches.

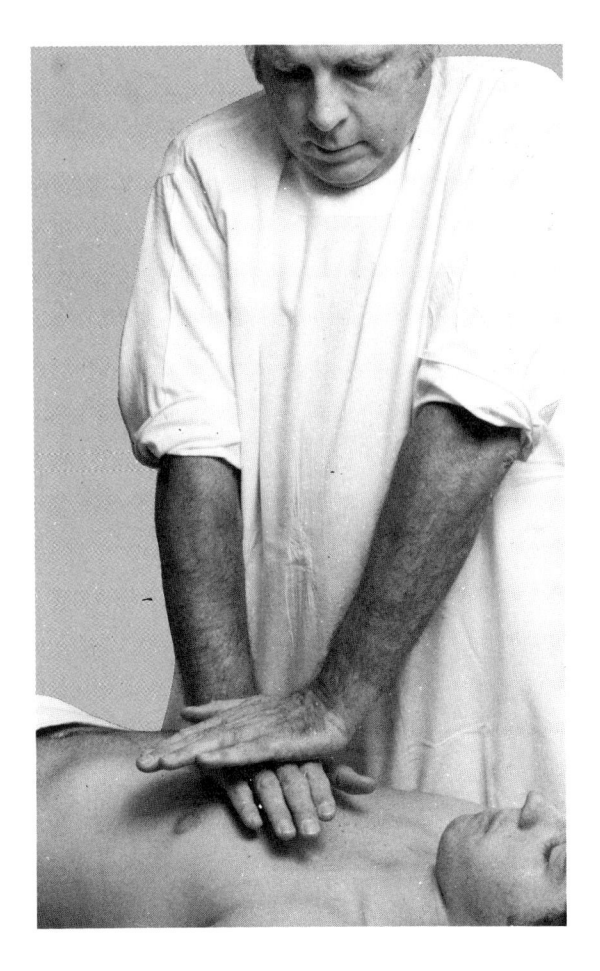

Cardiac compression must be coordinated with artificial ventilation. After five chest compressions, one breath is given. This format should be continued until spontaneous cardiorespiratory activity begins or the patient is considered unsalvagable.

INFANTS. In infants, the entire chest should be grasped in both hands. The body is held with the head toward the operator with the thumbs placed one atop the other over the midsternum. Pressure is applied to depress the sternum 1/2 to 3/4 inches and then released rapidly to allow cardiac filling.

The peripheral circulation may be monitored by palpation of the femoral pulse.

Cardiac compression should be at a rate of 60 to 80 per minute.

CHILDREN. In smaller children the tips of the index and middle fingers may be used to exert pressure over the junction of the middle and lower thirds of the sternum.

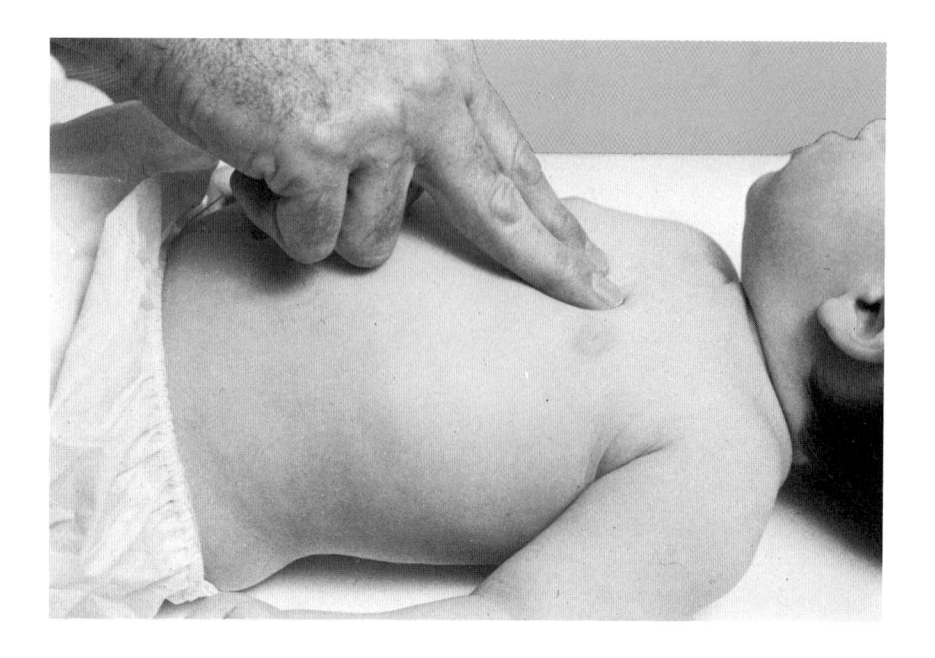

In larger children the heel of one hand may be used at the same level.

The sternum should be depressed 1 to 1½ inches at a rate of 60 to 80 per minute.

A palpable femoral pulse indicates proper cardiac compression.

ADJUNCT MEASURES

While external cardiac compression and artificial ventilation continues, a large bore needle or catheter should be placed in the extremity vein. This is an ideal site for it causes no interference with the vital life support measures. Once the veinway is established, begin an infusion of Ringer's lactate or 5% glucose in 0.2% saline. This will serve as a pathway for injection of specific cardiac drugs for more definitive therapy.

At the same time, electrocardiographic limb electrodes should be attached and the patient's heart rate and rhythm monitored.

DEFIBRILLATION

If ventricular fibrillation is present, electrical countershock is given. The amount of electrical energy delivered in an average adult should be 400 watt-seconds. In extremely obese or large persons, a stronger current may be required. Conversely, in children and infants considerably lower amounts of electrical energy are satisfactory. Indeed the larger dose may be harmful. For infants and children countershock should begin as low as 25 watt-seconds and increase to 400 watt-seconds for a fully grown adolescent.

Monitor-defibrillator equipment is available with the electrocardiographic leads in the paddles. This device is ideal for initial evaluation of cardiac rhythm, to determine whether standstill or fibrillation is present, before the skin electrodes are attached.

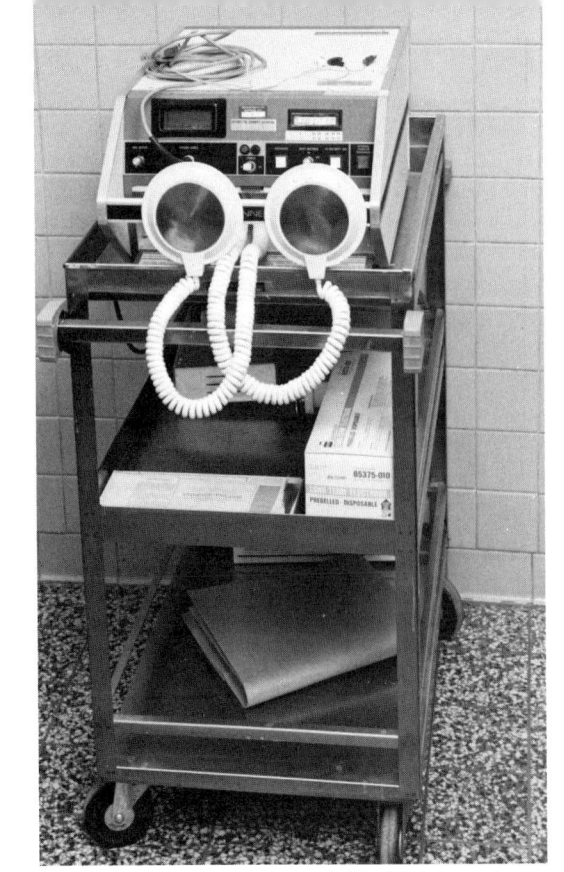

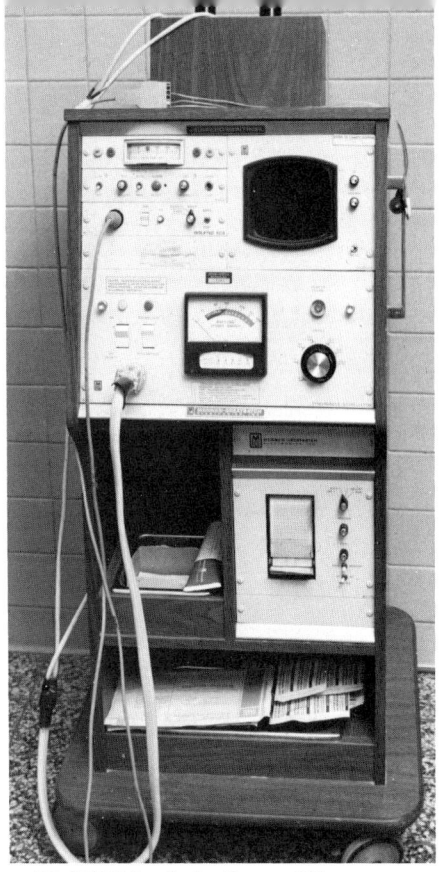

Portable monitor-defibrillator equipment with ECG leads in the paddles.

amounts of electrical energy for cardiac defibrillation

25 to 50 watt-seconds for infants
100 watt-seconds for children 12 to 25 kg.
200 watt-seconds for children 25 to 50 kg.
400 watt-seconds for fully grown adolescents and adults

Electrical countershock may be repeated as necessary. Its effect is lessened by acidosis; therefore, sodium bicarbonate should be given very early in the course of resuscitation to lessen or correct the acidotic state.

POSITION OF THE ELECTRODES. Positioning the electrodes for defibrillation is important. The standard electrode position is to place one to the right of the upper sternum just below the clavicle, the other to the left of the cardiac apex or left nipple line.

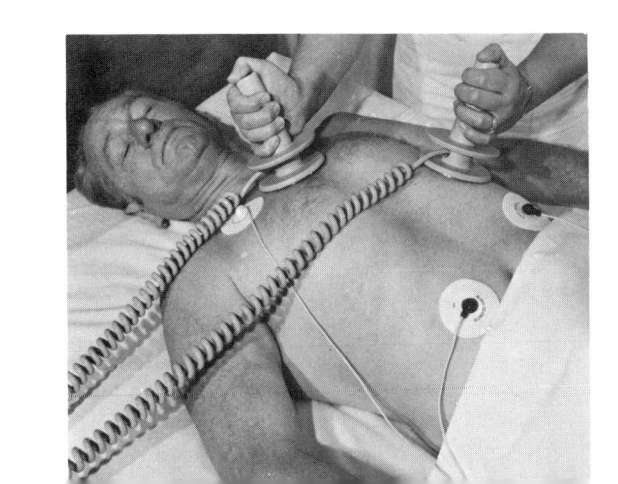

The defibrillation electrodes (paddles) should be well lubricated with electrically conductive jelly, or disposable prelubricated pads may be used (Defib Pads).

When the shock is given, *all* personnel should be warned to move away from the bed.

DRUG THERAPY

A number of drugs may be of value in the treatment of a patient being given CPR. In general these drugs are used to correct metabolic acidosis or have an effect on the myocardium, cardiac conduction system, or peripheral vascular system. They fall into two categories, essential and useful. When stocking a cardiac emergency cart, it is best to supply the most frequently used drugs in prefilled syringes when available. Those currently in use include sodium bicarbonate, epinephrine, atropine, and lidocaine.

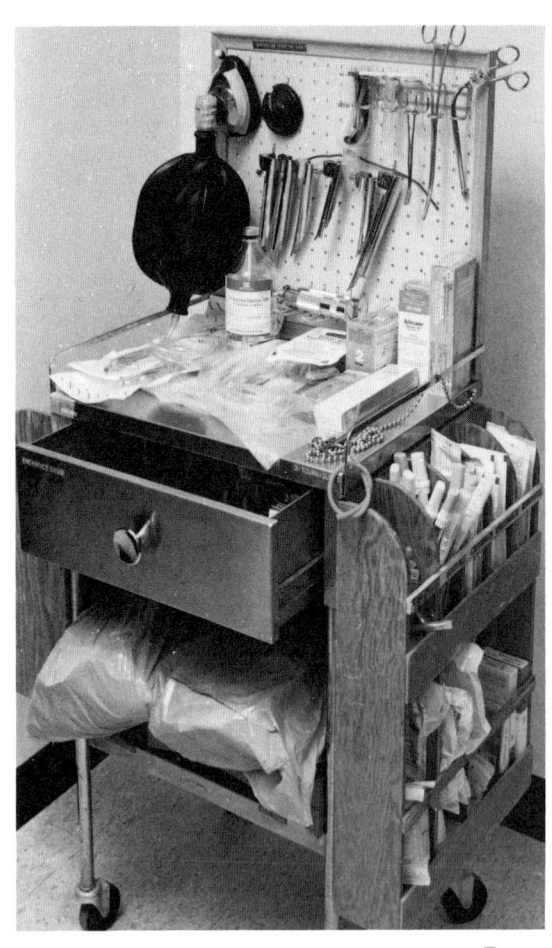

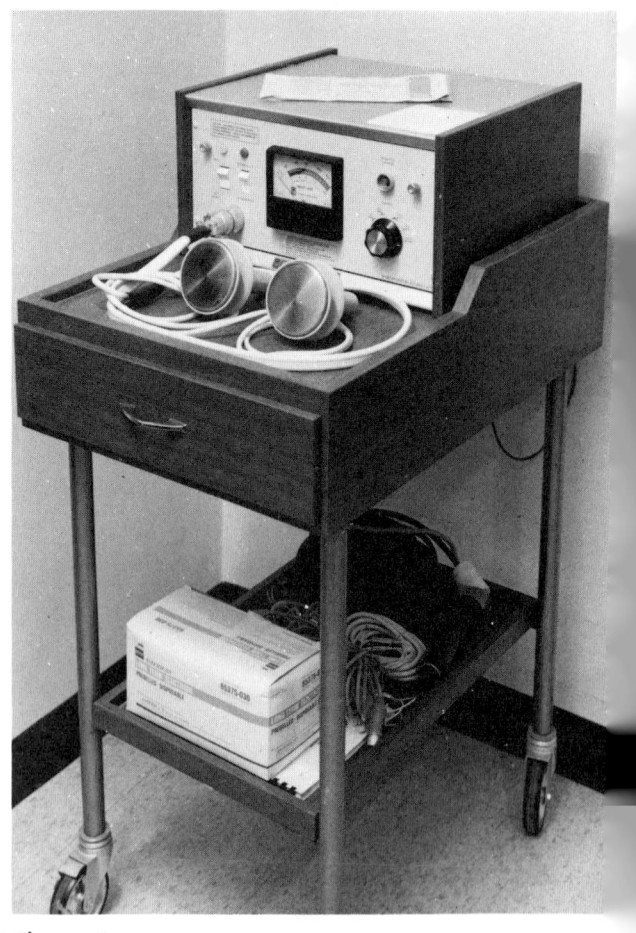

Resuscitation cart
Airway equipment   Defibrillator
Drug supplies
Infusion equipment

Drug therapy plays an essential role in the management of patients with cardiac problems. It is imperative that an intravenous line be inserted early to permit intermittent or continuous rapid administration of drugs and fluids necessary to support a stable cardiac rhythm and adequate circulation. Any one of several intravenous solutions can be used as the vehicle to transmit the drugs. The most common solutions are 5% dextrose in water, 5% dextrose in 0.2% normal saline or Ringer's lactate. A "cut-down" or "long line" (usually a large indwelling catheter) should not be established as the initial intravenous route, as it usually takes longer to insert; yet, a line of this type is indicated as soon as feasible, for maintaining an open line for further drug therapy. It is important to note that the CVP line, when inserted, should not be used for drug administration as well since it will not lend itself to a continuous accurate inflow of drug while taking frequent CVP readings.

Close monitoring of the patient's cardiac status, blood electrolytes, and arterial blood gases is essential to determine appropriate drugs and dosages. The following tables present a list of drugs which should be available in any cardiac emergency situation, and summarize recommended dosages most commonly used for both adults and children in this situation.

drugs used in adult cardiac emergencies

DRUG	SUGGESTED DOSE AND ROUTE OF ADMINISTRATION	REMARKS
Sodium bicarbonate	I.V. bolus or continuous infusion. Initial dose, 1 mEq/kg. Repeat, then monitor according to blood gases.	Repeat dose following blood pH results if base deficit.
Calcium chloride (10%)	I.V. bolus, 2.5-5 cc every 10 min.	If digitalized, watch carefully following administration. Check calcium blood levels frequently, as high levels are detrimental. Don't mix with sodium bicarbonate.
Epinephrine	I.V. bolus, 0.5 cc of 1:1,000 solution diluted to 10 cc.	Note dilution. (Dilution for child is 1:10,000)
Lidocaine	I.V. bolus, 50-100 mg, may repeat. I.V. drip, 1-3 mg/min. Mix I.V. bottle 500 mg/500 cc D5W (yields 1 mg/cc).	Do not exceed 4 mg/min. in adults.
Atropine	I.V. bolus, 0.5 mg. Repeat every 5 min. until pulse is greater than 60.	Adult: Total dose not to exceed 2 mg (except in third-degree block).
Levarterenol	I.V. bolus, 2-5 mg every 5-10 min. I.V. drip, 0.4 mg/min. in D5W	Don't use in endotoxic shock or renal shutdown. Titrate for desired blood pressure.
Metaraminol	I.V. drip, 0.5 mg in 500 cc D5W.	Titrate for desired blood pressure.
Isoproterenol	I.V. drip, 1 mg in 500 cc D5W.	Titrate for desired effect.

commonly used drugs for cpr in infants and children

DRUG	SUGGESTED DOSE	REMARKS
Atropine sulfate	0.01 mg/kg, I.V.	
Calcium gluconate (10% solution)	0.1-0.2 ml/kg, I.V.	Give slowly and watch for bradycardia. Use with caution in digitalized children.
Diphenylhydantoin	2.0-5.0 mg/kg, I.V.	Give slowly.
Epinephrine hydrochloride	0.1 ml/kg of 1:10,000 dilution, I.V. Same, intracardiac.	Intracardiac route is used as a last resort, since coronary arteries may be damaged. Note dilution.
Isoproterenol hydrochloride	1.0-5.0 mg/500 ml of 5% dextrose/water, I.V. drip.	Titrate to desired effect.
Levarterenol bitartrate	0.1-1.0 ug/kg/min., I.V. drip.	1 ml. of 0.2% solution diluted in 250 ml of solution equals 4 ug/ml. Not to be used in endotoxic shock or in renal shutdown.
Lidocaine, 2%	0.5-2.0 mg/kg, I.V.	Give slowly. Do not exceed 100 mg/hr. Excess amount may cause convulsions.
Metaraminol bitartrate	0.3-2.0 mg/kg, I.V. drip.	Titrate to desired effect.
Propranolol	0.1-0.2 mg/kg, I.V.	May repeat dose in 2 min., if necessary.
Sodium bicarbonate	3.0-5.0 mEq/kg, I.V.	Repeat dose after pH obtained and base deficit calculated.

Following emergency drug therapy, most patients will require the continued use of drugs in either antiarrhythmia, adrenergic vasopressor, or corticosteroid categories. These drugs are not discussed in detail in this text, as the particular drugs used vary from facility to facility and physician to physician. It is recommended that the physician and nurse become familiar with the drugs provided on the emergency cardiac cart. Actions, side effects, and normal dosages should become a part of orientation to the usual drugs prescribed in cardiac emergencies.

ACTIONS OF COMMONLY USED DRUGS

SODIUM BICARBONATE

Sodium bicarbonate is used to combat metabolic acidosis or reverse acidosis caused by anoxia. An acidotic heart cannot be resuscitated; therefore, it becomes imperative that an intravenous infusion of sodium bicarbonate (1 mEq/kg of body weight) be given every 5 minutes until blood gas results are available in the absence of cardiac and respiratory activity. Ventilation must accompany sodium bicarbonate administration to remove the carbon dioxide from arterial blood. After spontaneous circulation is restored, the use of sodium bicarbonate is not indicated and may be harmful, as it could cause metabolic alkalosis.

The administration of sodium bicarbonate should be titrated in accordance with arterial blood gas results. It should not be given alone in cases of cardiac standstill or in persistent ventricular fibrillation. Cardiopulmonary resuscitation accompanied by sodium bicarbonate and adrenalin or calcium chloride should increase the effectiveness of the countershock as well as improve the status of the myocardium.

EPINEPHRINE

Epinephrine is either given intravenously or injected directly into the heart through an intracardiac needle if an intravenous route is unavailable. Used intracardially, it may overcome asystole and stimulate spontaneous beating if the myocardium is simultaneously massaged to force the epinephrine through the coronary circulation.

Epinephrine is used to 1) increase contractility of the myocardium, 2) increase coronary blood flow, 3) increase cardiac rate, 4) elevate perfusion pressure, and 5) lower defibrillation threshold. It is important to note that epinephrine can produce ventricular fibrillation; however, this can usually be converted by defibrillation. It should be administered every 5 minutes during cardiopulmonary resuscitation. The usual dosage is 0.5 ml of a 1:1,000 solution diluted to 10 ml.

ATROPINE SULFATE

Atropine sulfate is used to counteract arrhythmias caused by excessive vagal action on the sinoatrial (S-A) and atrioventricular (A-V) nodes. It results in an increase in heart rate, making it a very useful drug in counteracting bradycardia. Atropine sulfate prevents cardiac arrest in profound bradycardia secondary to myocardial infarction, particularly where hypotension is also present. It is necessary to increase the heart rate to 60 to 80 beats per minute to improve the cardiac output and reduce the incidence of premature ventricular contractions and ventricular fibrillation.

Atropine is administered intravenously as a bolus of 0.5 mg and repeated at 5-minute intervals until the heart rate is greater than 60 beats per minute in cases of sinus bradycardia, accompanied by premature ventricular contractions or a systolic blood pressure of less than 90 mm Hg. Atropine is useless in ventricular ectopic bradycardia in the absence of atrial activity and in cardiac bradycardias caused by hypoxia or acid-base and electrolyte imbalances. The total dose of atropine sulfate should not exceed 2 mg except in cases of third-degree atrioventricular block.

LIDOCAINE

Lidocaine stabilizes the cell membrane of the heart muscle and nerve fibers. The arterial blood pressure is not affected. It also reduces cardiac excitability and conductivity; therefore, it is useful in the treatment of acute multifocal ventricular arrhythmias and episodes of ventricular tachycardia. It is not useful in asystole.

A bolus of 50 to 100 mg is administered intravenously, or the drug can be continuously infused, slowly, at a rate of 1 to 3 mg per minute. Lidocaine should not be given in excess of 4 mg per minute. If it is to be administered over a period of time, it is useful to mix a solution of 500 mg lidocaine to 500 cc 5% dextrose in water, which provides a 1 mg per ml solution.

CALCIUM CHLORIDE

Calcium chloride increases myocardial contractility, prolongs systole, and enhances ventricular excitability. Sudden death can result following rapid intravenous injection, particularly if the patient is fully digitalized. Calcium chloride is used in profound cardiovascular collapse.

The usual dose is 2.5 to 5 ml of a 10% solution. It should be given as a bolus at intervals of 10 minutes. It is important to monitor blood levels of calcium, as repeated large doses may elevate the calcium level of the blood and have negative effects.

Calcium cannot be mixed in the same I. V. or given through the same tubing as sodium bicarbonate, since they precipitate. If calcium gluconate is used, the dose should be increased to 10 ml of a 10% solution, as it provides less ionizable calcium per unit volume.

MORPHINE SULFATE

Morphine sulfate is not used in cardiac arrest, but it is a very important and essential drug in the treatment of the patient with myocardial infarction. It is used to tranquilize the patient as well as to relieve apprehension. It can produce periods of restful sleep.

Morphine in 3 to 4.5 mg doses, I. V., may be needed as often as every 5 to 30 minutes for relief of pain. The use of frequent small doses of the drug has proven more effective in reducing pain as well as avoiding respiratory distress than less frequent larger doses.

TERMINATION OF CPR

CPR should be terminated when the patient assumes spontaneous cardiac activity, or when it is apparent that the resuscitative effort is unsuccessful, as indicated by failure to resume spontaneous cardiac activity or widely dilated, nonreactive pupils indicative of irreversible brain damage.

CONTRAINDICATION TO CPR

CPR is a procedure which should not be taken lightly and should not be initiated in all patients who suffer cardiorespiratory arrest. A patient who has been dead (totally nonresponsive and areflexic) for an extended period of time, or one who has widely dilated nonreactive pupils should not be resuscitated. Similarly a patient known to be in a terminal phase of an incurable disease is best not resuscitated.

BIBLIOGRAPHY

Cosgriff, J. H., Jr. and Anderson, D. M. The Practice of Emergency Nursing. Philadelphia: J. B. Lippincott Co., 1975.

Goldring, D., Hernandez, A., Jr. and Hartmann, A. F., Jr. Cardiovascular emergencies in infants and children. Hosp. Med. 12:20, 1976.

Houser, D.: Emergency cardiac care. Nurs. Clin. N. Am. 8:401, 1973.

Shapter, R. K. and the members of the National Committee for Emergency Coronary Care. Clin. Symp. 25:7, 1974.

Standards for cardiopulmonary resuscitation and emergency cardiac care. Supplement to JAMA 227:837, 1974.

Williams, W. G. and Brummitt, W. M. Cardiac Arrest in Care of the Injured Child Baltimore: Williams & Wilkins, 1975.

20 TEMPORARY EMERGENCY TRANSVENOUS PACEMAKER

In patients with an acute myocardial infarction complicated by varying degrees of block and/or complete heart block, or in patients with syncope from Stokes-Adams attacks, effective electrical control of heart rate may be achieved by inserting a pacing electrode via a peripheral vein into the right ventricle and attaching this to an external pulse generator. This method is to be used primarily for short-term pacing and has been used successfully for two to six weeks. If long-term pacing is required, an implantable pacemaker may be considered once the patient's condition is stable.

INDICATIONS
1. Acute myocardial infarction with complete heart block or varying degrees of heart block that do not satisfactorily respond to medication (atropine or isoproterenol).
2. Stokes-Adams disease with syncope.

EQUIPMENT
1. Venous cutdown tray (see page 71)
2. Bipolar catheter electrode (a number are available commercially)
3. Sterile alligator clip leads
4. Povidone-iodine
5. 3-0 catgut on needle
6. 4-0 silk on needle
7. Small curved hemostat
8. External demand pulse generator with variable output and rate capability. For utmost safety, a battery-powered generator should be used.

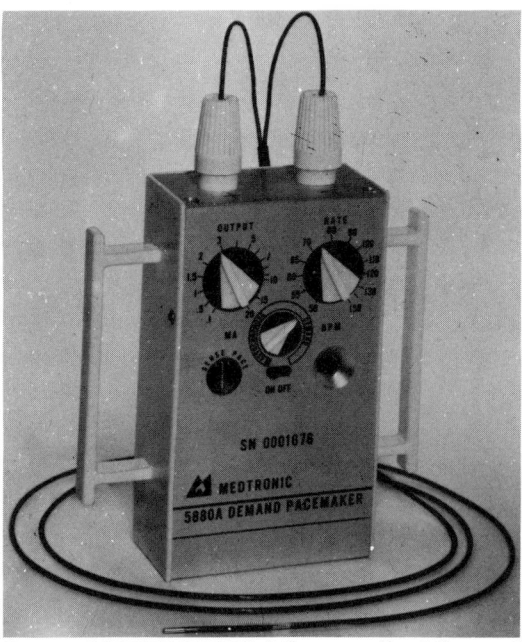

Source: MEDTRONICS, Minneapolis, Minnesota

ANATOMICAL CONSIDERATIONS

1. Electrical stimulation of the heart is achieved by a catheter electrode placed in the right ventricle.
2. Access to the right heart may be via the jugular, brachial, subclavian, or femoral veins. The left brachial vein is the approach most commonly used.
3. The patient should be on a cardiac monitor throughout the procedure. A defibrillator should be plugged in and on stand-by. An intravenous line should be in place and medications such as isoproterenol and lidocaine immediately available.

PROCEDURE

1. Choose the vein for passage of the catheter.
2. Prep the skin of the selected site with povidone-iodine.
3. Using the field block technique (pages 185-187) anesthetize the skin in the selected area.
4. Make a 1 to 2 cm incision through the skin over the vein.
5. Mobilize a 2 cm length of vein and place a tie of 3-0 chromic catgut about the lowermost portion of the mobilized segment. Place a loose tie about the upper end of the vein.
6. Make a small transverse incision in the vein between the sutures.
7. Put slight traction on the proximal suture to control bleeding from obscuring the field.
8. Dilate the venotomy with the tip of a small curved hemostat.
9. Insert the electrode catheter into the vein and advance it into the right ventricle. The position of the catheter is checked by fluoroscopy or by elec-

trocardiogram. If the EKG is used, take care to avoid the use of other 60-cycle electrical equipment attached to the patient simultaneously. Accidental discharge of small quantities of 60-cycle current can occur through the electrodes, when two or more pieces of electrical equipment that do not have a common ground are attached to the patient. A 60-cycle current as low as 150 microamperes (ma) can induce ventricular fibrillation when making direct contact with the myocardium.

10. Once the catheter is properly positioned in the ventricle, suture it to the skin.
11. Close the skin incision with 4-0 silk.
12. Apply povidone-iodine ointment to the skin incision and cover with a sterile dressing.
13. Set the pulse generator at a low effective current using 2 to 4 ma with the rate adjusted to between 70 to 80 a minute, or higher if it is necessary to suppress multifocal premature beats.

NOTE: When an endocardiac electrode catheter is placed, anticoagulant medication is not required. Systemic antibiotic therapy should be initiated to lessen the possibility of sepsis. Continuous EKG monitoring is advisable to identify any pacemaker dysfunction or ectopic cardiac rhythm.

BIBLIOGRAPHY

DeSantis, R. W. Short-term use of intravenous electrode in heart block. JAMA 184:544, 1963.

Federico, A. J.: Personal communications.

Furman, S., Schwedel, J. B., Robinson, G., and Hurwit, E. Use of an intracardiac pacemaker in the control of heart block. Surgery 49:98, 1961.

Parsonnet, V., Zucker, R., Gilbert, L., and Asa, M. M. An intracardiac bipolar electrode for interim treatment of complete heart block. Am. J. Cardiol. 10:261, 1962.

Schnedel, J. B. and Escher, D. J. W. Transvenous electrical stimulation of the heart. Ann. N.Y. Acad. Sci. 111:972, 1964.

Solomon, N. and Escher, D. J. W. A rapid method for insertion of the pacemaker catheter electrode. Am. Heart J. 66:717, 1963.

Weale, F. E. Cardiac resuscitation via jugular vein. Lancet 2:73, 1959.

21 ANTISHOCK SUIT

This device serves only as an adjunct in the management of patients with massive blood loss secondary to injury or bleeding lesions in the abdomen, pelvis, or lower extremities. It should not be used in patients with major injuries above the diaphragm, and its use is also contraindicated in patients with pulmonary edema or congestive heart failure.

INDICATIONS

1. Hypovolemic shock associated with massive injuries to the lower limbs.
2. Hypovolemic shock associated with severe pelvic fracture and major blood loss.
3. Hypovolemic shock due to penetrating wounds of the abdomen with damage to the major vessels.
4. Hypovolemic shock due to a ruptured abdominal aortic aneurysm.

EQUIPMENT

Currently available equipment includes a number of commercial devices, most of which are made in styles for adults and children. The variations in style refer to the chambers in the suit, which number from one to three. The three-chambered suit consists of one chamber for each extremity and one for the abdomen. Whichever device is used, caution must be taken that it is not overinflated.

The pressure suit is used in both the prehospital and the initial hospital care of the acutely ill or injured patient. The three-chambered suit is used principally in hospitals. The three chambers are pressurized with a single pump, while any one of the chambers may be closed off by a stopcock. An individual chamber is deflated by opening the stopcock.

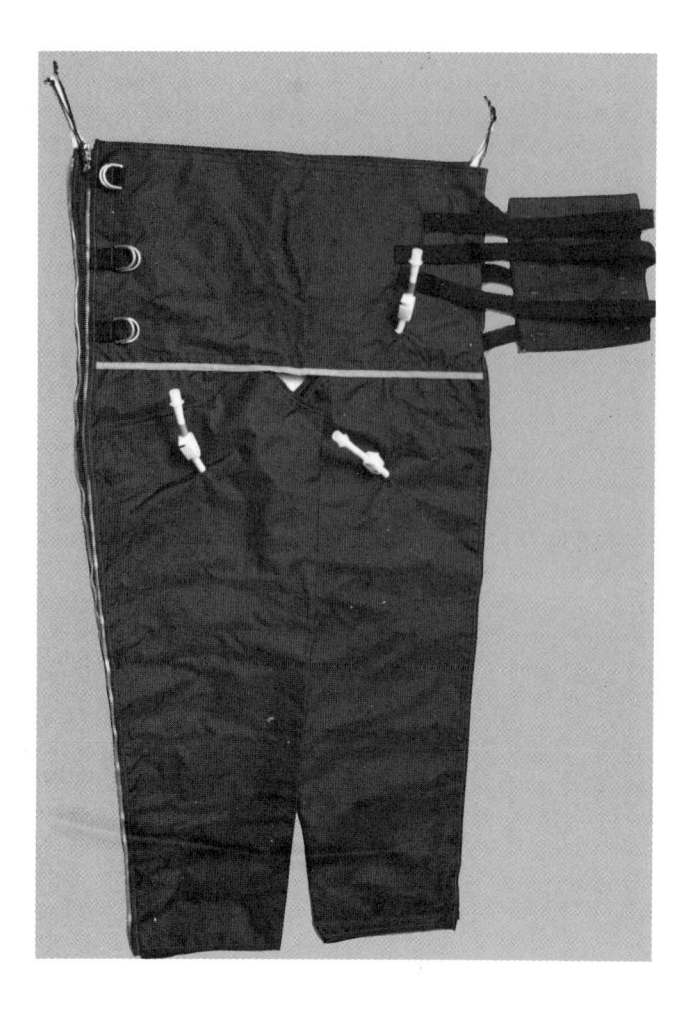

Pediatric units are also available commercially. These units will fit children between 46 to 58 inches in height and 40 and 100 pounds in weight.

Each unit is inflated by a foot pump which is attached to the apparatus.

ANATOMICAL CONSIDERATIONS

1. The suit should extend from the lower margin of the rib cage to the ankles.
2. It fits around each leg and the torso.
3. Pressure should not be exerted on the chest.

PROCEDURE

1. Place the patient in a supine position.
2. Do a complete evaluation of the abdomen and lower extremities before applying the suit.
3. Fold the front half of the legs inward and the anterior abdominal flap downward.

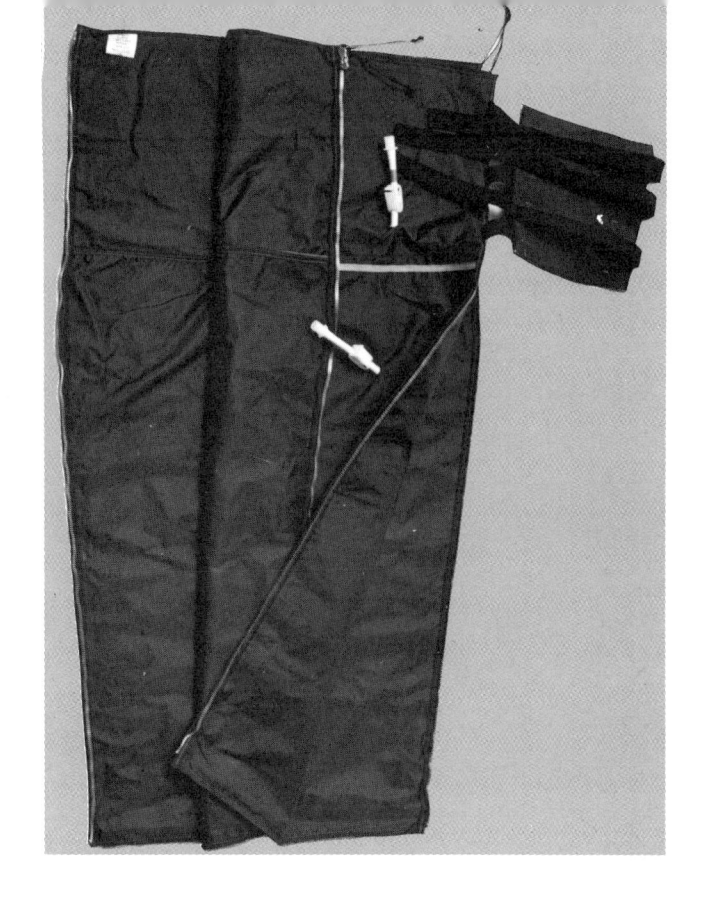

4. Place the suit under the patient. Fit the crotch of the suit to the patient's perineum.

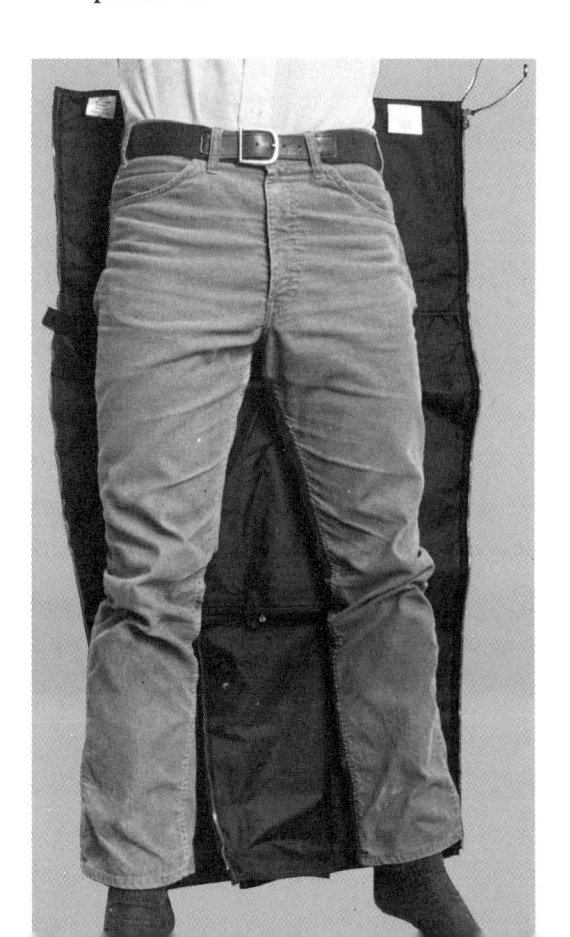

5. Splints or dressings may be used to immobilize fractures or seal wounds as indicated. A uretheral catheter may also be placed in the patient.
6. Wrap the device around the trunk and each leg and fix in place with fasteners.

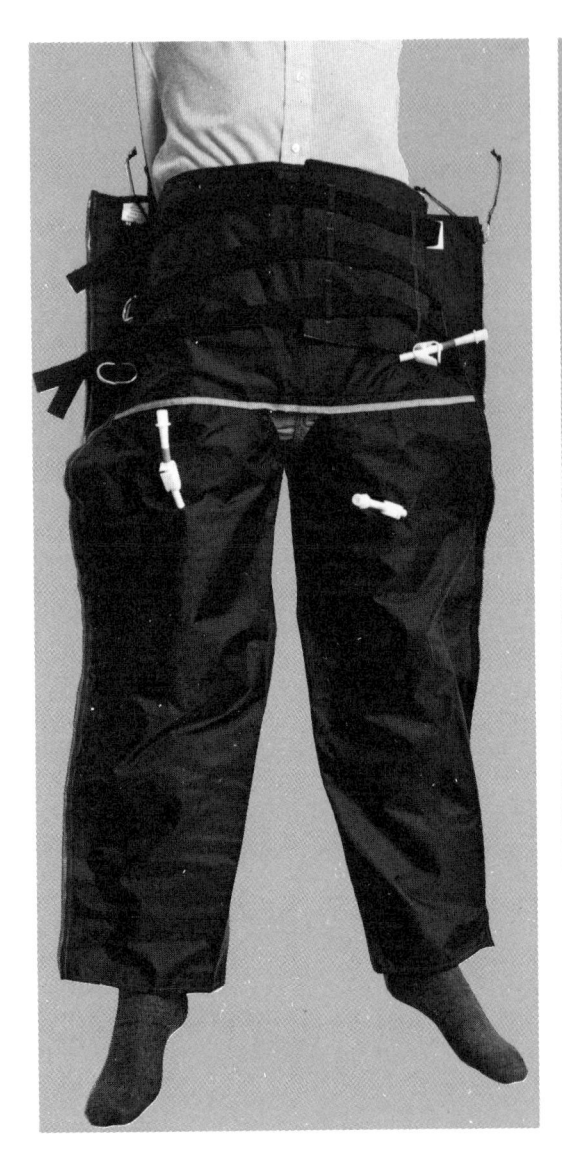

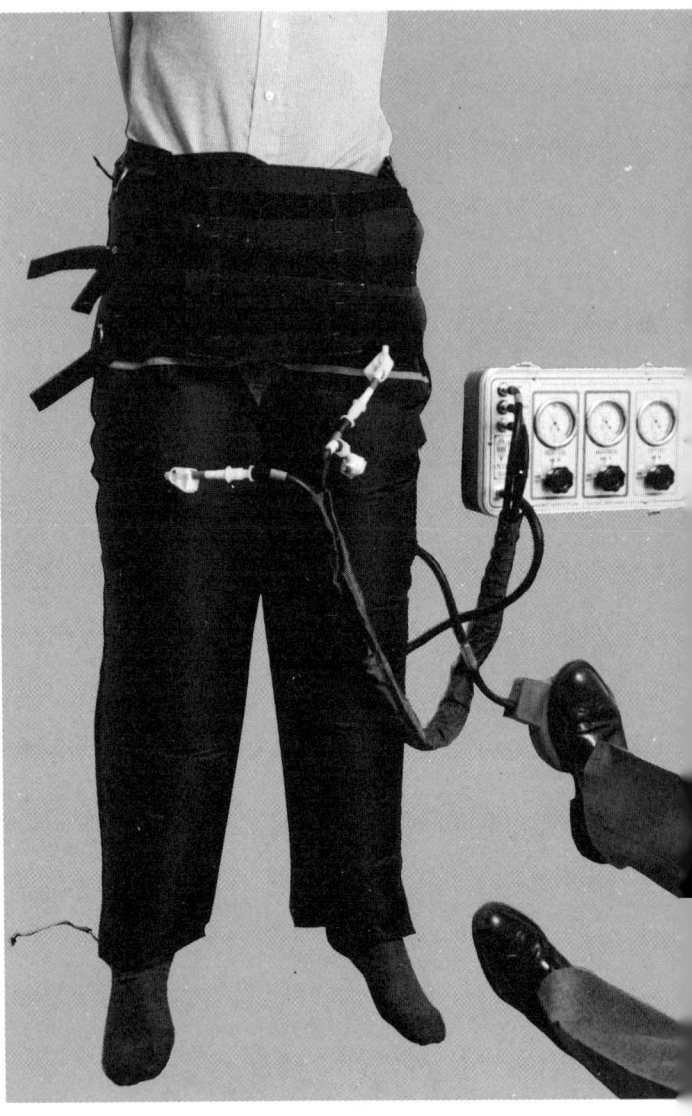

7. Inflate the device to 20 to 30 mm Hg and check vital signs including blood pressure.
8. Continue to inflate the antishock suit until the patient's blood pressure approaches normal.
9. Attach a blow-off valve to the system to prevent undue pressure.
10. Leave the suit in place 24 to 48 hours or less if the patient's pressure stabilizes. However, it is best to initiate blood volume replacement as early as possible.

REMOVING THE SUIT

1. Do not remove the suit until the patient's condition is stable.
2. Release the pressure slowly, taking care to observe vital signs. If there is any sign of deterioration of the patient's condition, reinflate the suit immediately.
3. Once the pressure in the suit has dropped to zero, leave the suit in place for a time while assessing the patient further. If necessary the patient may be taken to the operating room with the suit in place.
4. Unfasten the suit only after adequate fluid and blood replacement is underway.

BIBLIOGRAPHY

Batalden, D. J., Wickstrom, P. H., Ruiz, E., and Gustilo, R. B. Value of the G-suit in patients with severe pelvic fracture controlling hemorrhagil shock. Arch. Surg. 109:326-328, 1974.

Cutler, B. S. and Daggett, W. M. Application of the G-suit to the control of hemorrhage in massive trauma. Ann. Surg. 173:511-514, 1971.

Gardner, W. J. Circumferential pneumatic compression. JAMA 196:491-3, 1966.

Gardner, W. J. and Storer, J. The use of the G-suit in control of intra-abdominal bleeding. SG & O 123:792-8, 1966.

———. Personal communication.

Kaplan, B. C., Civetta, J. M., Nagel, E. L., Jussenfield, S. R., and Hirschman, J. C. The military anti-shock trouser in civilian pre-hospital emergency care. J. Trauma 13:843-8, 1973.

22 CENTRAL VENOUS CATHETERIZATION

Central venous catheterization (CVC) may be defined as the introduction of a satisfactory veinway (catheter) into the superior vena cava or inlet of the right atrium. It has become an integral part in the management of the critically ill or injured patient. When used in conjunction with other modalities, CVC is helpful in monitoring the patient's progress and as a pathway for fluid replacement and medication.

When it originally came into use, CVC was performed primarily for central venous pressure monitoring which was viewed as an accurate method of assessing cardiac function. Experience has shown that this is not the case. Rather, the central venous pressure directly reflects effective cardiac filling pressure and in the absence of cardiopulmonary problems may provide an index of functional intravascular volume. It has proven of value in infants and adults. Many other uses of CVC have evolved, these include:

1. A pathway for rapid infusion of fluids, including electrolyte solutions, and blood.
2. A pathway for administering medication.
3. A pathway for long-term parenteral hyperalimentation.

At present, this parameter is also used in conjunction with an intra-arterial catheter for blood pressure monitoring and/or a balloon flotation catheter (Swan-Ganz) which directly measures pulmonary artery and pulmonary wedge pressures.

NORMAL VALUES AND METHODS OF CENTRAL VENOUS PRESSURE MEASUREMENT

At least three methods are used to measure baseline central venous pressure (CVP).

When the measurement is taken, the patient should be supine and the base of the CVP manometer at the line of the right atrium. This is the point of controversy. The level of the right atrium is considered by different clinicians to be as follows:

1. 10 cm above the dorsal spine.
2. 5 cm below the sternal notch.
3. One-half the anteroposterior diameter of the chest at the fourth intercostal space adjacent to the sternum.

Perhaps the best method to use is the one applicable to both children and adults, a point 5 cm below the sternal notch.

The normal CVP may vary from -2 to $+10$ cm of water in children and adults. More important than actual isolated pressure measurements is the relative change which occurs in CVP during the course of treatment. Hence, accurate charting of serial CVP values is vital.

ROUTES OF ACCESS FOR CVC

The central vein is usually catheterized via a peripheral vein. A number of pathways may be used for CVC. Any active clinician who treats critically ill patients should become familiar with each. In infants and small children, a venous cutdown may be necessary to insert the catheter, while in adults percutaneous puncture is usually accomplished without difficulty. The peripheral veins most commonly used are the brachial or cephalic at the antecubital fossa, the subclavian, the external or internal jugular veins.

The method of choice depends on the clinician and the patient. The author favors the infraclavicular approach to the subclavian vein.

PROCEDURE

Since this is an invasive procedure, strict aseptic technique is mandatory. While some do not use gloves, sterile towels, and so on, most, including the author, strongly favor the use of all safeguards since sepsis is a major complication of this procedure.

Whatever method is used, once the catheter is in place, a sterile dressing with antibiotic ointment should be placed over the puncture site and changed every 24 or 48 hours.

EQUIPMENT

While a number of indwelling devices are available commercially, they may be classed into one of two major groups, catheter-over-needle or catheter-through-needle. The equipment is sterilized by the manufacturer. Each package contains all the necessary material for insertion of the particular style catheter-needle assembly. For pressure measurements additional connector tubing, a 3-way stopcock, and manometer are needed to complete the setup. All the equipment in use today is disposable.

COMPLICATIONS

The frequency of complications seem to be inversely related to the training and experience of the operator.

Complications common to all the methods of CVC are local inflammation of the puncture site, injury to the vein wall, phlebitis, venous thrombosis, and septicemia.

In addition, CVC via the subclavian route may be complicated by pneumothorax, tension pneumothorax, hemothorax, subcutaneous emphysema, air embolism and injury to the thoracic duct.

Strict adherence to the details of the procedure will lead to a minimum number of complications.

SUMMARY

Central venous catheterization has been proved to be an integral part of the care of the critically ill or injured. It can serve a number of functions. A variety of pathways are available for CVC. The methods described subsequently are those most commonly used today. Any active clinician should be familiar with the procedure. While complications do occur, they can be minimized by careful attention to details of technique and asepsis.

BIBLIOGRAPHY

Bower, E. B. Choosing a catheter for central venous catheterization. Surg. Clin. N. A. 53:639, 1973.

Christensen, K. H., Nerstrom, B., and Baden, H. Complications of percutaneous catheterization of the subclavian vein in 129 cases. Acta. Chir. Scand. 133:615, 1967.

Daly, B. D. T. Jr., Berger, R. L. Antecubital approach for intravascular monitoring. Surg. Gynec. & Obstet. 135:434, 1972.

Dudrick, S. J., Wilmore, D. W., Vars, H. M., et al: Can intravenous feeding as the sole means of nutrition support growth in a child and restore weight loss in an adult: An affirmative answer. Ann. Surg. 199:974, 1969.

Gallitano, A. L., Kondi, E. S., Deckers, P. J. A safe approach to the subclavian vein. Surg. Gynec. & Obstet. 135:96, 1972.

Gassaniga, A. B., Byrd, C. L., Stewart, D. R., O'Connor, N. E. Evaluation of central venous pressure as a guide to volume replacement in children following cardiopulmonary bypass. Ann. Thor. Surg. 13:148, 1972.

Gowan, G. F. Interpretation of central venous pressure. Surg. Clin. N. A. 53:649, 1973.

Hoshal, V. L., Jr. Total intravenous nutrition with peripherally inserted silicone elastomer central venous catheters. Arch. Surg. 110:644, 1975.

Jernigan, W. R., Gardner, W. C., Mahr, M. H., Milburn, J. L. Use of the internal jugular vein for placement of CVP. Surg. Gynec. & Obstet. 130:520, 1970.

McDonough, J. J. and Altemeter, W. A. Subclavian venous thrombosis secondary to indwelling catheters. Surg. Gynec. & Obstet. 133:397, 1971.

Schapira, M. and Stern, W. Z. Hazards of subclavian vein cannulation for central venous pressure monitoring. JAMA 201:327, 1967.

Sullivan, R. and Pomerantz, M. Central venous pressure monitoring. Surg. Clin. N. A. 49:1489, 1969.

Talbert, J. L. Intraoperative & postoperative monitoring of infants. Surg. Clin. N. A. 50:787, 1970.

Wilmore, D. and Dudrick, S. Safe long-term venous catheterization. Arch. Surg. 98:256, 1969.

Wilson, J. N., Grow, J. B., Deming, C. V., Prevedel, A. E., and Owens, J. C. Central venous pressure in optimal blood replacement. Arch. Surg. 85:563, 1962.

23 CENTRAL VENOUS CATHETER ANTECUBITAL APPROACH

INDICATIONS

1. To monitor central venous pressure.
2. To give hyperalimentation fluid.
3. If unable to use subclavian approach.
4. To serve as a guide in early recognition of congestive heart failure.
5. To indicate status of patient in shock or response to treatment.
6. To permit withdrawal of blood for blood samples and/or phlebotomy.

NOTE: This is not the approach of choice in the author's opinion.

EQUIPMENT

1. Central venous pressure catheter set, 26-inch length (Jelco)*
2. Manometer set (for central venous pressure only)
3. Intravenous set
4. Local set (see page 181)

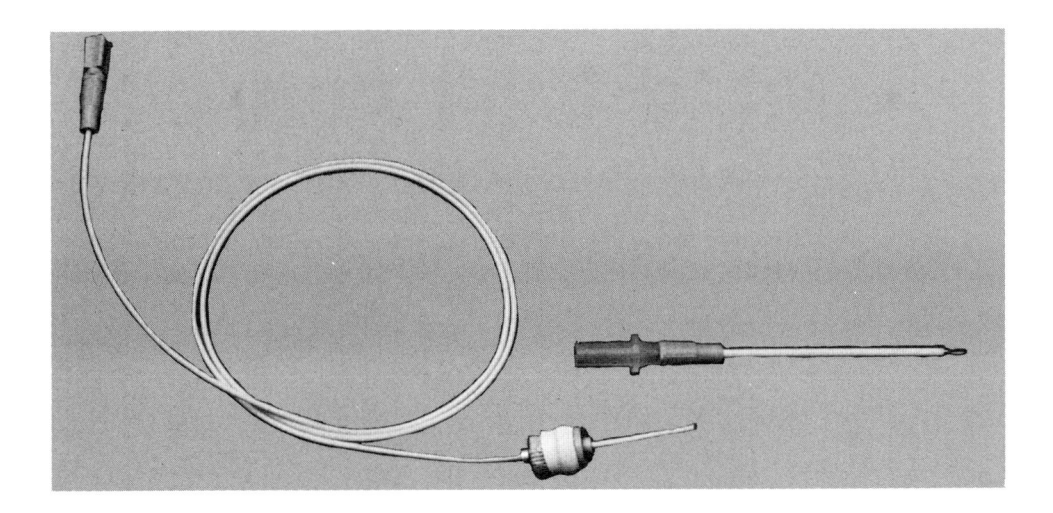

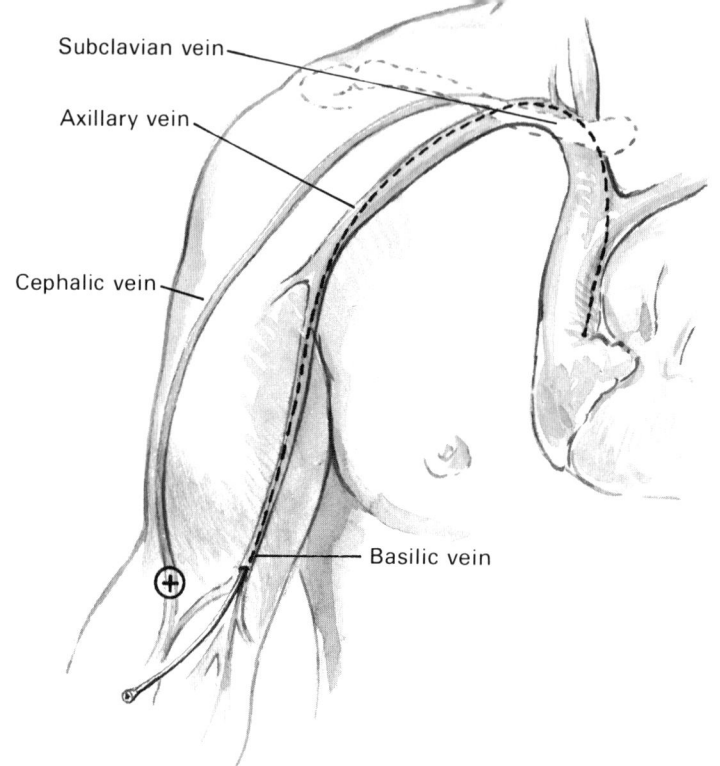

ANATOMICAL CONSIDERATIONS

1. Access to the large central vein via a peripheral vein may be accomplished in the upper extremity.
2. The basilic or cephalic vein may be cannulated in the antecubital space of the elbow. Each empties into axillary vein.
3. This approach has the disadvantage of transgressing the flexion crease of the arm since the catheter can be kinked by prolonged flexion of the elbow.
4. Access via the saphenous or femoral veins is usually contraindicated.

PROCEDURE

1. Prep the antecubital space widely with povidone-iodine.
2. Apply a tourniquet to the upper arm.
3. Using the catheter-over-needle assembly, perform a venipuncture in the antecubital space.
4. Once blood is returned into the flash chamber, remove the tourniquet.
5. Hold the catheter-needle assembly in place by digital pressure and remove the needle leaving the catheter in the vein.
6. Connect the Luer-Lock fitting to the catheter leaving the plastic wrapping on the long catheter.
7. Leaving the stylet-catheter intact introduce it into the catheter in position in the vein and advance it into the vein until the superior vena cava is reached.
8. Remove the stylet and the clear plastic sleeve from the Luer-Lock fitting.
9. Attach the intravenous set to the catheter.
10. Apply a sterile gauze dressing with povidone-iodine ointment and secure in place with adhesive tape to prevent movement of the catheter.
11. Check the location of the tip of the catheter by x-ray examination of the chest. It should be in the lower end of the superior vena cava at the level of the interspace between the seventh and eighth thoracic vertebrae.

24 CENTRAL VENOUS CATHETER EXTERNAL JUGULAR APPROACH

INDICATIONS

1. To monitor central venous pressure.
2. To administer hyperalimentation fluid.
3. If unable to use subclavian approach.
4. To serve as a guide in early recognition of congestive heart failure.
5. To indicate status of patient in shock or response to treatment.
6. To permit withdrawal of blood for blood samples and for phlebotomy.

NOTE: This approach to the central venous system is used infrequently.

EQUIPMENT

1. Central venous pressure catheter set. (Deseret 775 or Jelco 12-inch catheter
2. Manometer set (for CVP only)
3. Local set (see page 181)

ANATOMICAL CONSIDERATIONS

1. The external jugular vein may be of sufficient size to cannulate, particularly in adults.
2. The external jugular vein is found on the lateral aspect of the neck by drawing an imaginary line from a point midway between the angle of the jaw and the earlobe to the midpoint of the clavicle.
3. The external jugular vein enters the subclavian vein at an acute angle to the midline which may prevent the catheter from passing medially into the subclavian vein.
4. Because of this acute angle, this approach is the least favorable.

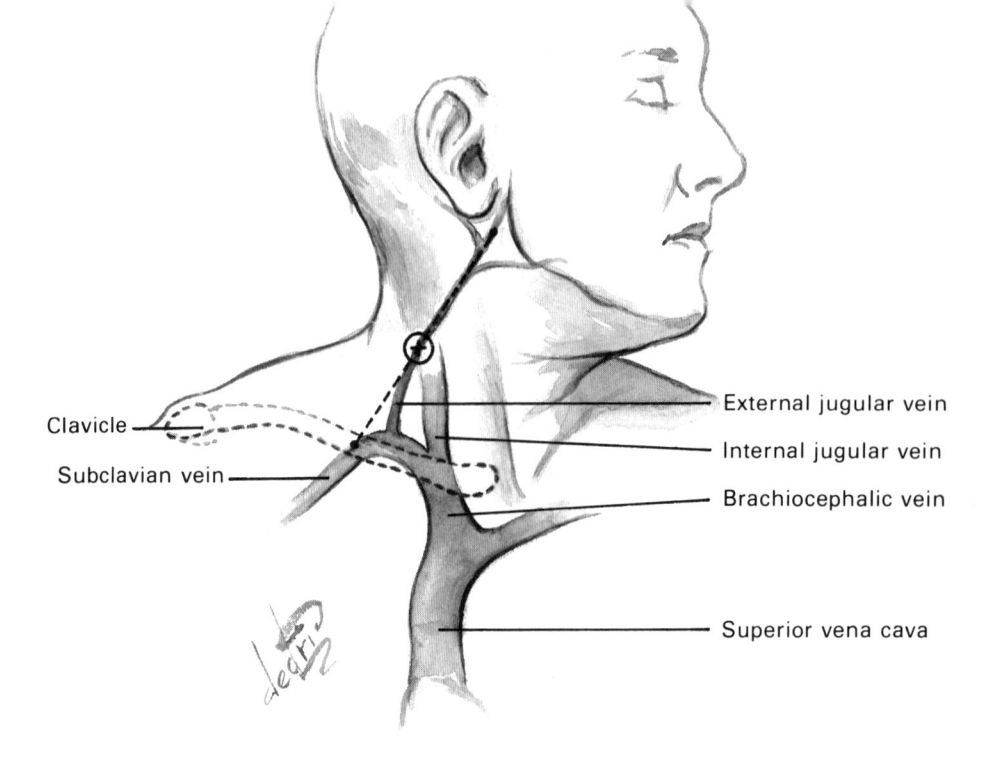

PROCEDURE

1. Place the patient in a slight Trendelenburg's position to fill the external jugular vein. Rotate the patient's head away from the side to be catheterized.
2. Prep the neck with povidone-iodine and drape.
3. Identify the external jugular vein: entry should be made midway along its length.
4. Raise a skin wheal with 0.5% lidocaine.
5. Introduce the needle using the syringe-and-needle assembly through the skin wheal just posterior and parallel to the vein.
6. Then angle the needle forward and penetrate the vein wall. Aspirate gently and a free flow of blood indicates the needle is in the proper position.
7. Detach the syringe and insert the catheter the desired distance which is approximately 8 inches. (The catheters for this procedure are usually 12 inches in length.)
8. Advance the catheter carefully. When the right subclavian vein is being catheterized, *tilting* (not rotating) the patient's head slightly to the right shoulder may decrease the angle of entry into the subclavian vein. Do *not* advance the catheter forcefully at any time since it may penetrate the subclavian vein.
9. If the catheter passes easily, advance it to the desired distance and carefully withdraw the needle-over-the-catheter, taking care not to angle the bevel of the needle into the catheter.
10. Place the blunt needle into the catheter and secure it to the catheter support which is then sutured to the skin.
11. Apply a gauze pad with povidone-iodine ointment over the site of skin puncture.
12. At the completion of the procedure, an x-ray examination of the chest should be taken to check the position of the catheter. The lower end of the superior vena cava is at the level of the interspace between the seventh and eighth thoracic vertebrae.

25 CENTRAL VENOUS CATHETER INTERNAL JUGULAR APPROACH

INDICATIONS
1. Need for monitoring central venous pressure.
2. Need for administering hyperalimentation fluid.
3. A guide for early recognition of congestive heart failure.
4. Need for indicating the status of the patient in shock or response to treatment.
5. Need for permitting withdrawal of blood for blood samples and/or phlebotomy.

EQUIPMENT
1. Central venous catheter set (Deseret 775 or Jelco catheter, 12-inch length)
2. Manometer set (for central venous pressure only)
3. Intravenous set
4. Local set

ANATOMICAL CONSIDERATIONS
1. The internal jugular vein runs vertically down the side of the neck. Throughout its course it lies lateral to the carotid artery.

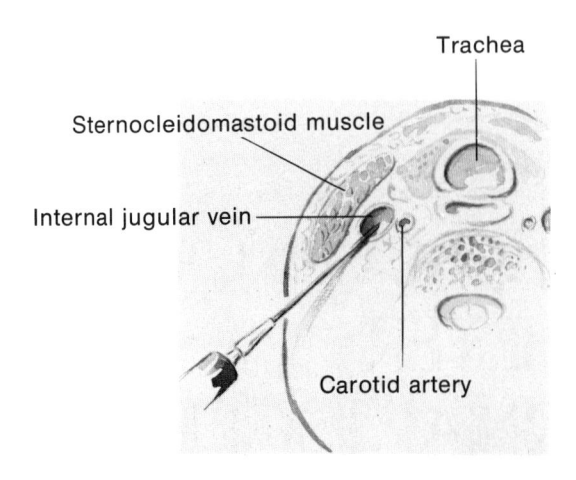

Trachea
Sternocleidomastoid muscle
Internal jugular vein
Carotid artery

2. At its lower end before emptying into the subclavian vein is a dilated segment, the inferior bulb.
3. Proximal to the bulb, about 2.5 cm above the termination of the vein, is a valve.
4. Overlying the vein in the lower half of the neck is the sternocleidomastoid muscle.
5. With the patient in the Trendelenburg's position, performing a Valsalva's maneuver, the vein may enlarge to a diameter of 1 inch.

PROCEDURE

1. Place the patient in Trendelenburg's position to enlarge the vein and minimize the chance of air embolization.
2. Rotate the patient's head 90 degrees to the opposite side.

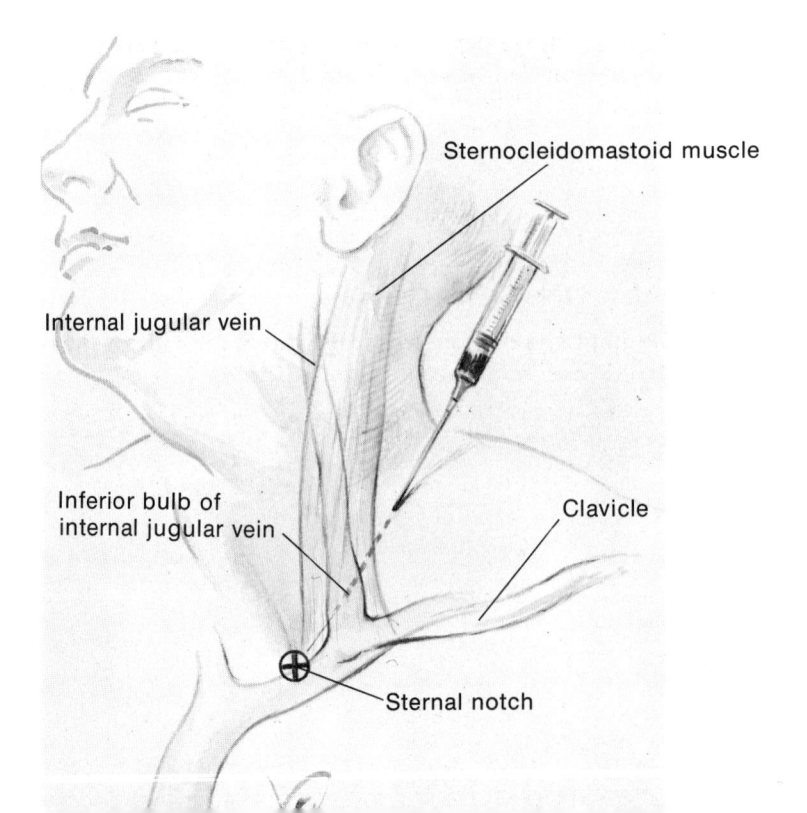

Sternocleidomastoid muscle
Internal jugular vein
Inferior bulb of internal jugular vein
Clavicle
Sternal notch

3. Prep the entire side of the neck, beyond the midline and below the clavicle and sternal notch, then drape.
4. Identify a point approximately 3.5 to 4 cm above the clavicle, at the lateral border of the sternocleidomastoid muscle and raise a skin wheal with 0.5% lidocaine.
5. With the needle and syringe assembly, introduce the needle through the wheal with a sharp jabbing motion.
6. Place the index finger of the opposite hand in the suprasternal notch and direct the needle toward it, keeping behind the posterior edge of the sternocleidomastoid muscle.
7. The vein lies posterior to the midpoint of the breadth of the sternocleidomastoid muscle at this level.
8. When the needle is at this depth, aspirate gently. Entry into the internal jugular vein will allow a free return of venous blood.
9. Once the needle is in the vein, remove the syringe carefully and immediately cover the needle hub with the gloved finger.
10. Insert the catheter through the needle the desired distance. Once the catheter has passed beyond the point of the needle, do not advance the needle since the bevel may cut through the catheter.
11. Carefully withdraw the needle, straight over the catheter.
12. Place the blunt needle and hub on the free end of the catheter and attach the intravenous line and manometer set.
13. Suture the catheter to the skin and apply a sterile dressing with povidone-iodine ointment.
14. Tape the free end of the catheter attached to the intravenous tubing to the cheek or frontal area. (In infants and small children a small incision may be made in the neck and the catheter placed in the subcutaneous space and brought out through another incision just behind the ear.)
15. When the procedure is completed, check the position of the catheter by an x-ray film of the chest. The lower end of the superior cava is at the interspace between the seventh and eighth thoracic vertebrae.

26 CENTRAL VENOUS CATHETER SUBCLAVIAN APPROACH

INDICATIONS
1. Need for monitoring central venous pressure.
2. Need for administering hyperalimentation fluid.
3. A guide for early recognition of congestive heart failure.
4. Need for indicating the status of the patient in shock or response to treatment.
5. Need for permitting withdrawal of blood for blood samples and/or phlebotomy.

EQUIPMENT
1. Subclavian catheter set (Deseret #775 or Jelco catheter, 12-inch length)
2. Manometer set (includes tubing)
3. Intravenous set
4. Local set

ANATOMICAL CONSIDERATIONS
1. The subclavian vein courses anterior to the scalene muscles and over the first rib. It joins the internal jugular vein near the medial border of the anterior scalene muscle and forms the innominate vein.
2. The vein lies anterior and inferior to the subclavian artery.

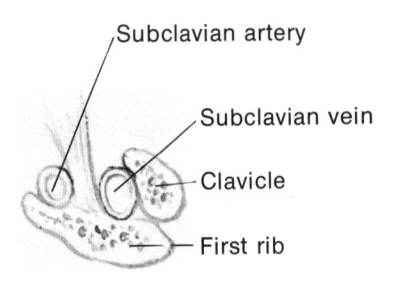

Subclavian artery
Subclavian vein
Clavicle
First rib

3. The apex of the pleura extends to the neck of the first rib close to the origin of the innominate vein.
4. Either subclavian vein may be cannulated.

PROCEDURE

1. Place the patient flat or in slight Trendelenburg's position to increase the pressure in the subclavian vein and minimize the chance of air embolization.
2. Rotate the patient's head 90 degrees to the opposite side.
3. Prep an area 8 to 10 inches square centered at the midpoint of the clavicle with povidone-iodine and drape.
4. Raise a skin wheal with 0.5% lidocaine one fingerbreadth below the inferior border of the midpoint of the clavicle.
5. Introduce the needle using the needle and syringe assembly into the skin wheal.
6. Place the index or middle finger of the opposite hand in the suprasternal notch as a target, and slowly advance the needle and syringe assembly toward the suprasternal notch. The syringe is approximately parallel to the line of the lateral one-half of the clavicle. The angle of penetration is parallel to the skin.

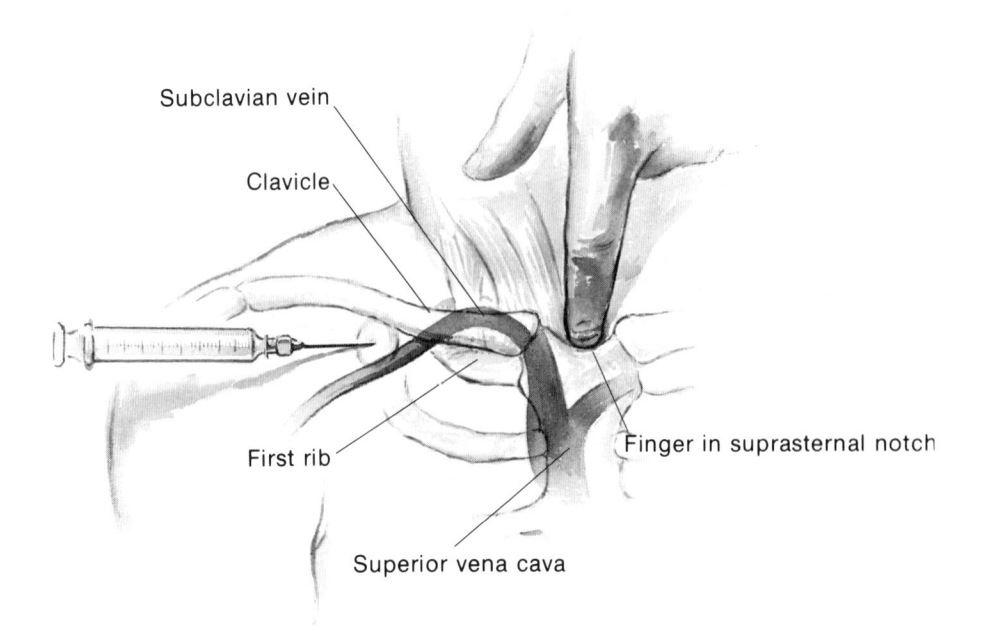

Subclavian vein
Clavicle
First rib
Finger in suprasternal notch
Superior vena cava

7. Advance the needle deep to the clavicle but above the first rib. If the rib is encountered, carefully withdraw the needle and redirect it until it can be passed just above the superior border of the rib.
8. Once the needle passes the rib, aspirate gently. A free return of venous blood indicates the needle is properly placed in the subclavian vein.
9. If blood is not recovered, advance the needle a few millimeters and re-aspirate. Continue to do so until blood is drawn into the syringe.
10. Carefully detach the syringe and immediately cover the needle hub with the gloved finger. Insert the catheter through the needle the desired distance. Once the catheter has passed beyond the point of the needle, do not advance the needle for the bevel may cut the catheter.
11. After inserting the catheter, hold it in position and carefully withdraw the needle over the catheter, taking care not to angle the bevel into the catheter.
12. Place the blunt needle into the catheter and secure it to the catheter support which can then be sutured to the skin.
13. Apply a dressing over the site using a gauze pad with povidone-iodine ointment.
14. At the completion of the procedure, take an x-ray film of the chest to check the position of the catheter in the superior vena cava and to rule out the presence of a pneumothorax. The lower end of the superior cava is at the level of the interspace between the seventh and eighth thoracic vertebrae.

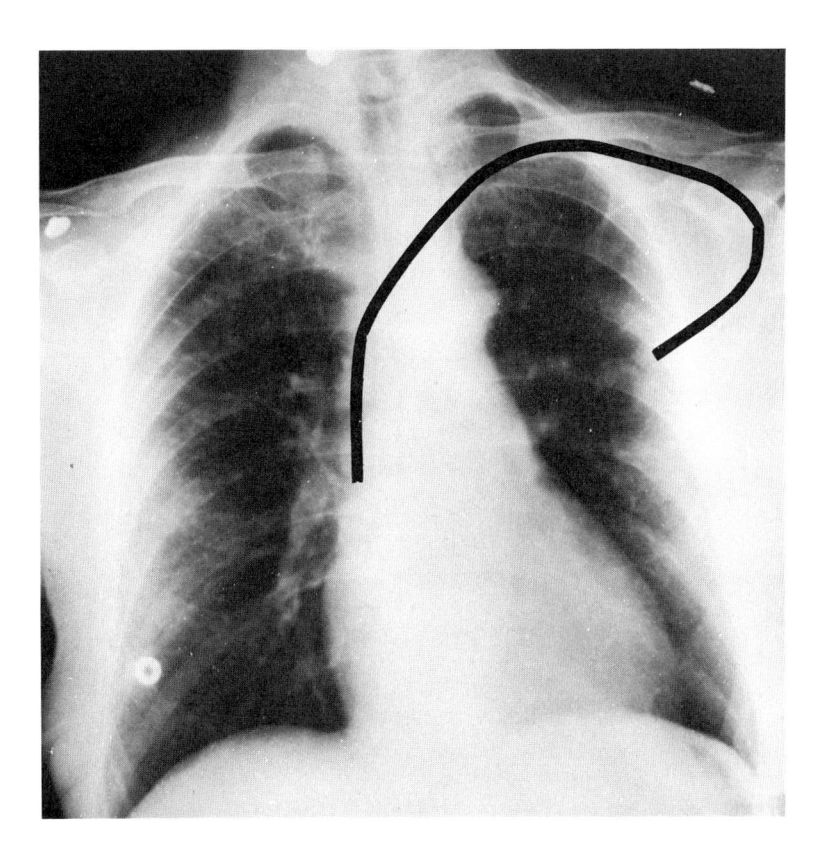

NOTE: A rare complication of the subclavian approach is tension pneumothorax.

27 EVERSION OF THE UPPER EYELID

INDICATIONS
1. Examination of the undersurface of the upper lid.
2. Examination of the upper portion of the globe (eyeball).
3. Removal of a foreign body from the eye or lid.

EQUIPMENT
1. Cotton-tip applicator stick

PROCEDURE
1. Ask the patient to gaze downward, toward the feet.

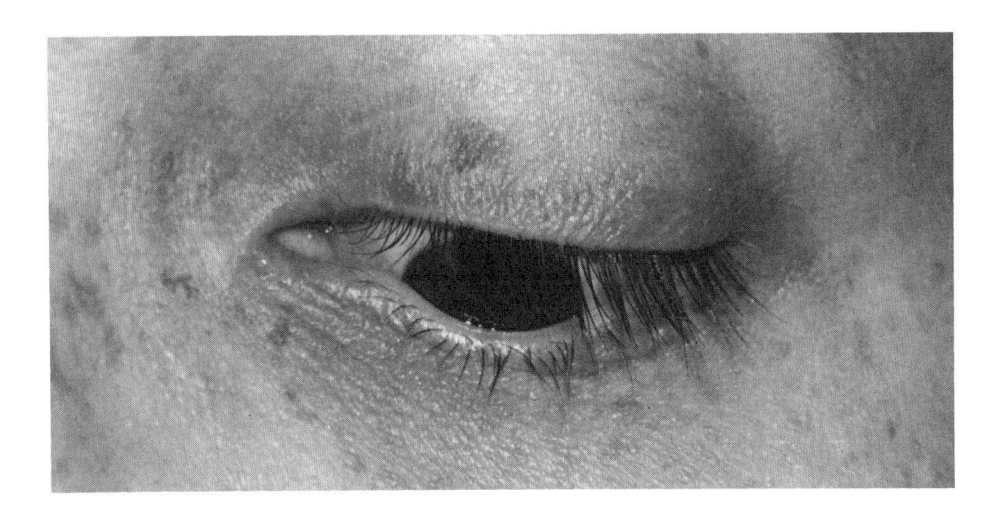

2. Grasp the eyelashes of the upper lid and gently pull the lid down and away from the globe.

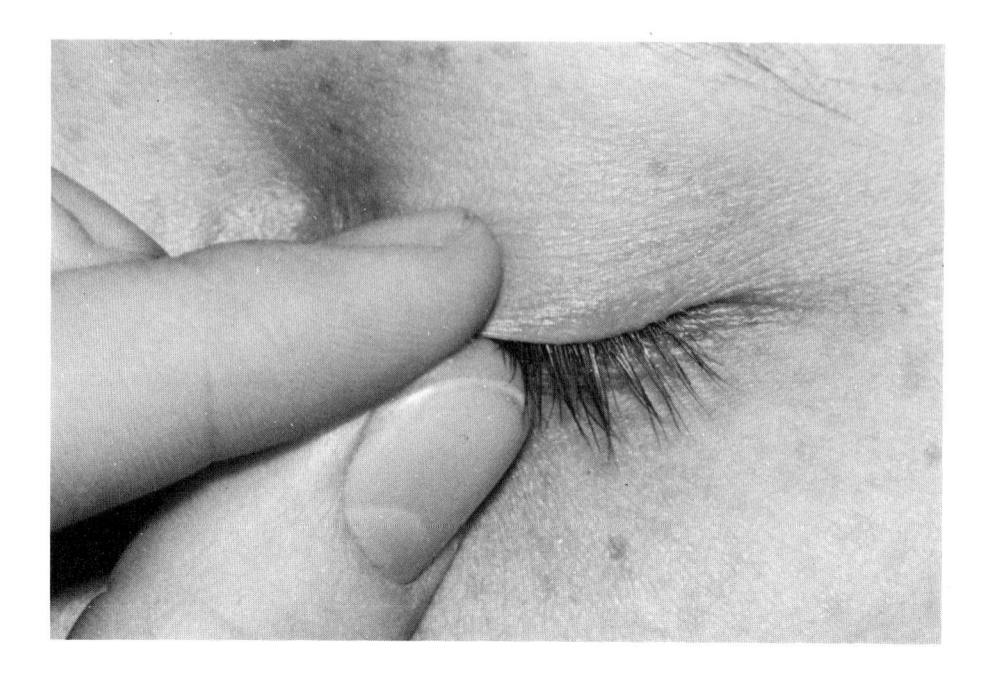

3. At the same time, apply pressure to the skin of the lid, 8 to 10 mm above the lid margin, using a cotton-tip applicator.

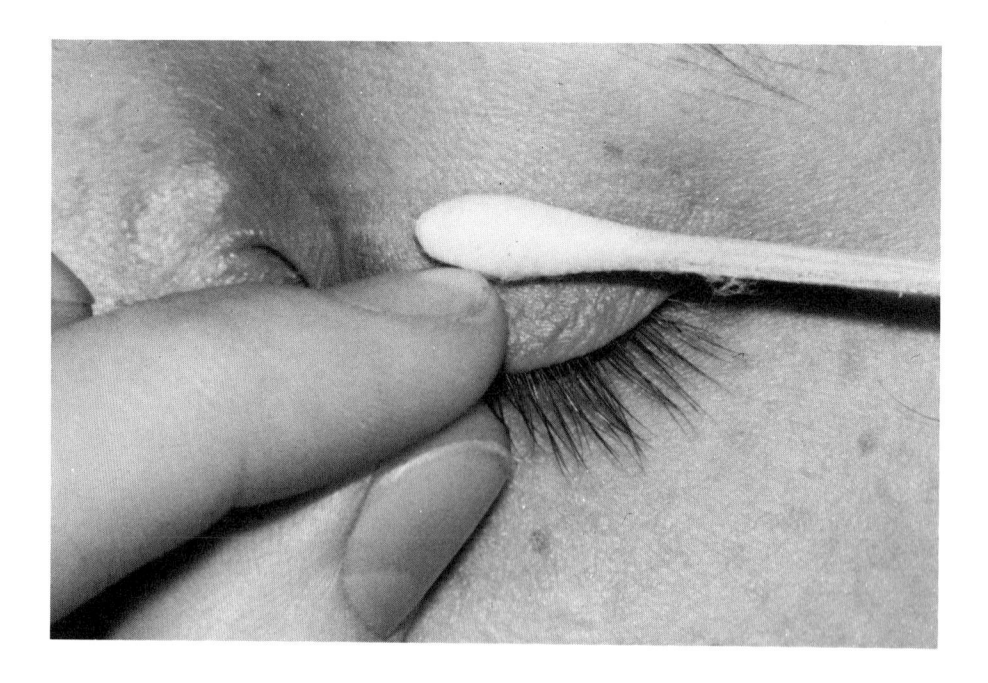

4. Gently pull the eyelashes upward and over the applicator. The lid will evert easily.

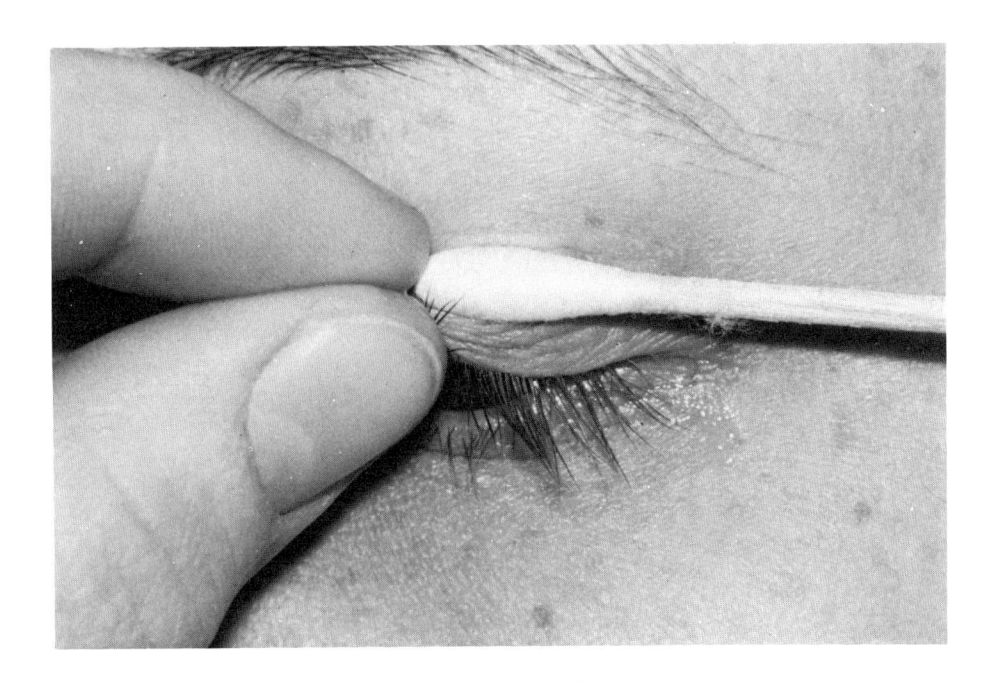

5. After the examination is completed, release the eyelashes and ask the patient to gaze upward. The lid will easily flip back into its normal position.

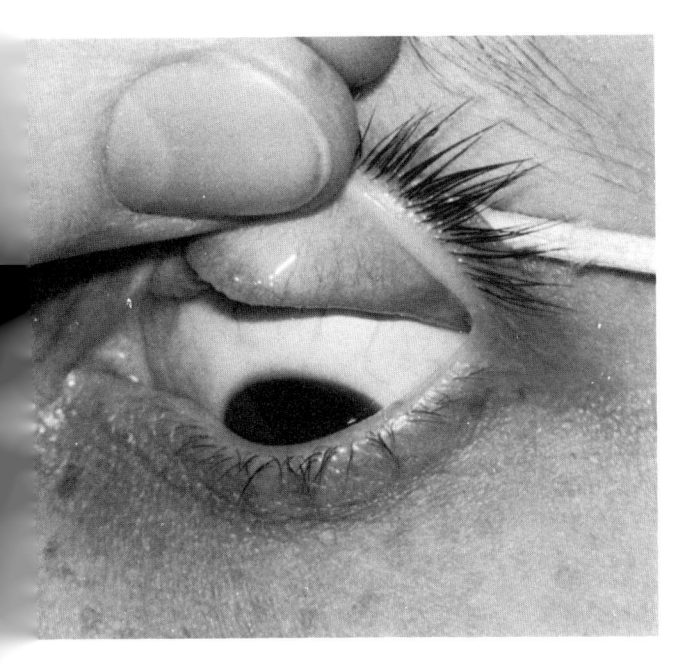

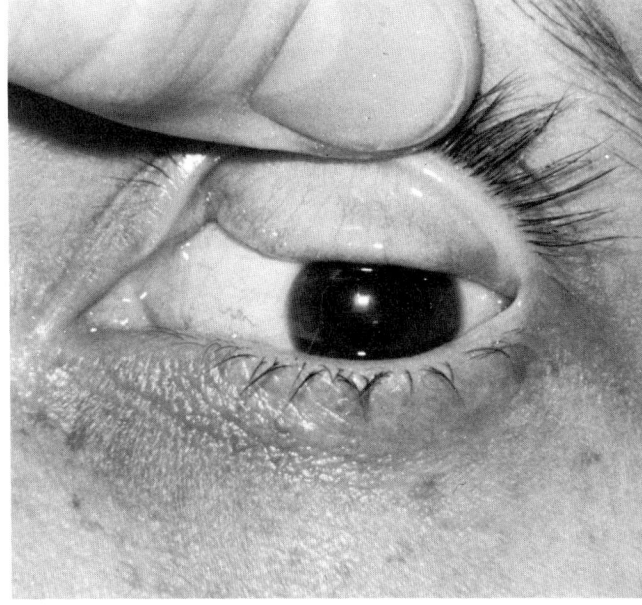

139

28 REMOVAL OF HARD CORNEAL (CONTACT) LENS

INDICATIONS

1. Removal of lenses in an unconscious patient.
2. Removal of lenses if the patient is unable to do so.
3. Thorough examination of the globe (eyeball).

EQUIPMENT

1. Small vacuum rubber lens remover. (A new suction-type lens remover is

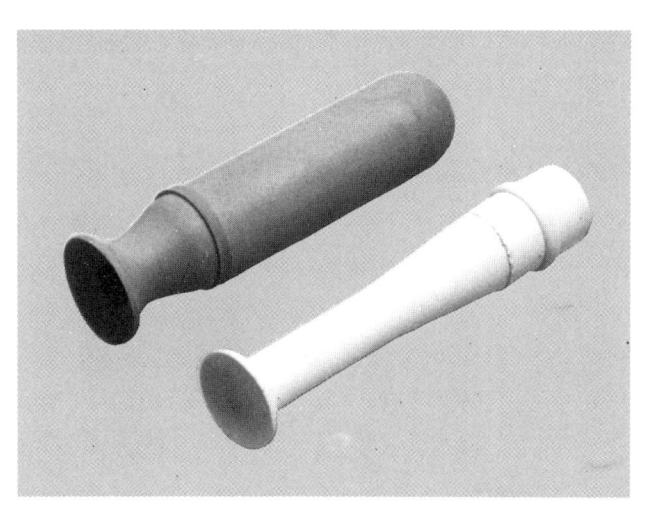

(Top) Vacuum remover
(Bottom) Suction remover

available which requires no squeezing. It has a solid stem. When the tip is moistened, sufficient suction is developed to remove the lens.)
2. Sterile isotonic irrigating fluid
3. Good light source

ANATOMICAL CONSIDERATIONS

1. The corneal lens is correctly placed directly on the cornea.
2. The lens may become displaced from the cornea and lie on the medial or lateral scleral portion of the globe.

PROCEDURE

1. Examine the eye gently, carefully, and completely to ascertain that a lens is present on the globe. This will require a good light source.
2. Moisten the tip of the vacuum cup with sterile isotonic fluid.
3. Gently spread the lids apart with the thumb and index fingers of the left hand to expose the edges of the contact lens.
4. Squeeze the vacuum device and apply its tip to the contact lens, with a minimum of pressure to get a seal on the lens.

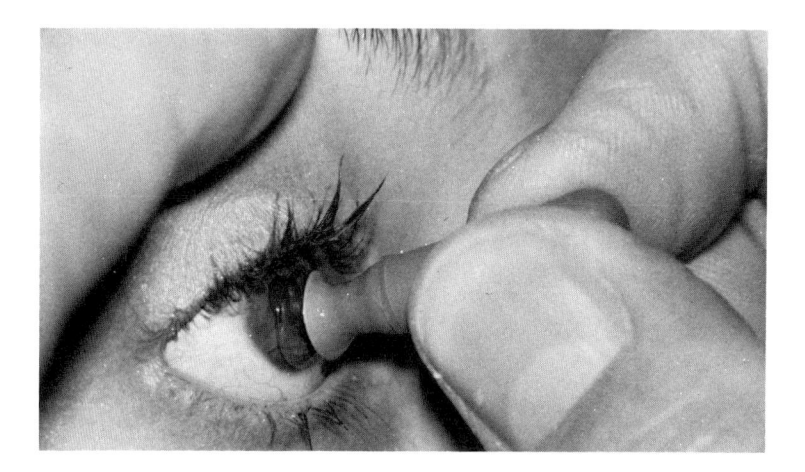

5. Release the pressure on the vacuum device and carefully remove the lens from the cornea.

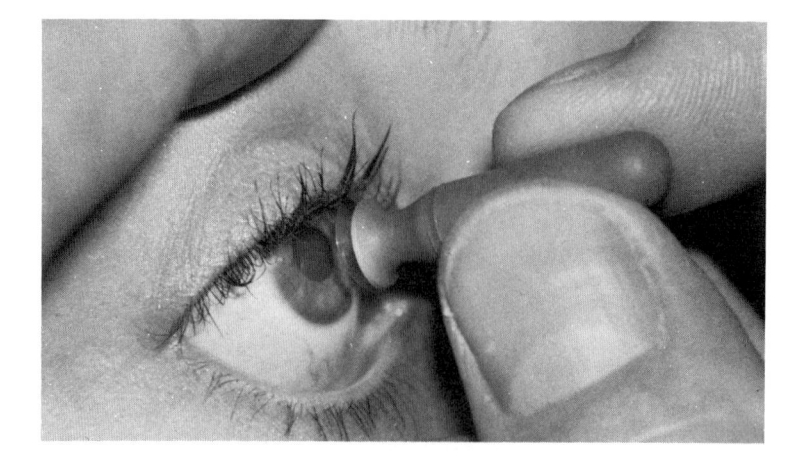

6. Place the lens in a container with isotonic saline and label with the patient's name for safe-keeping.

29 REMOVAL OF SOFT CORNEAL (CONTACT) LENS

Arthur J. Schaefer, M. D.

INDICATIONS
1. Removal of lenses in an unconscious patient.
2. Removal of lenses if the patient is unable to do so.
3. Thorough examination of the globe.

EQUIPMENT
Sterile isotonic irrigating fluid

ANATOMICAL CONSIDERATIONS
1. The soft lens is larger than the cornea and is correctly worn directly on the cornea.
2. The lens may be displaced from the cornea and lie over the lateral portion of the sclera.

PROCEDURE
1. Examine the eye gently, carefully, and completely to determine where the lens is on the globe. This will require a good light source.
2. Moisten the lens well with sterile irrigating fluid.

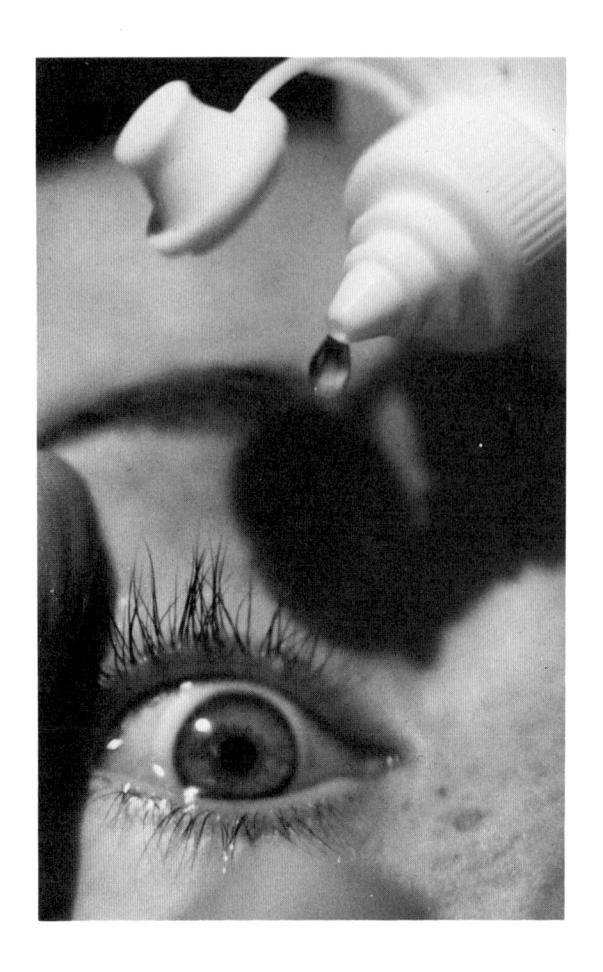

3. Ask the patient to turn the eye medially. If the patient is unconscious omit this step.

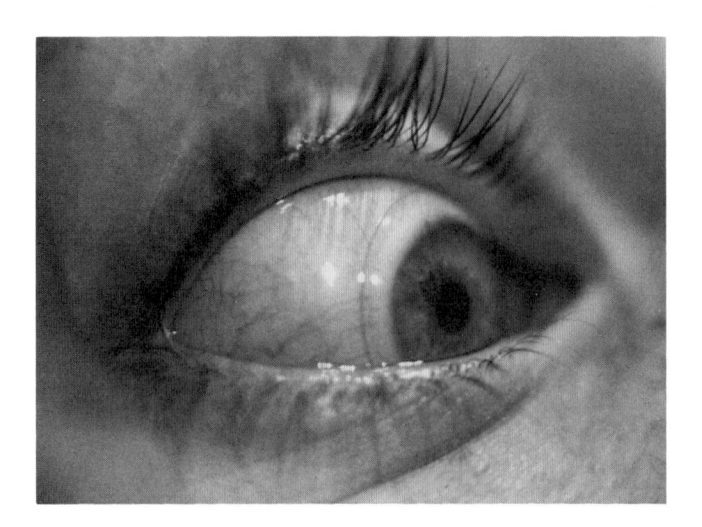

4. Slide the lens from the cornea onto the lateral portion of the sclera using the index finger.

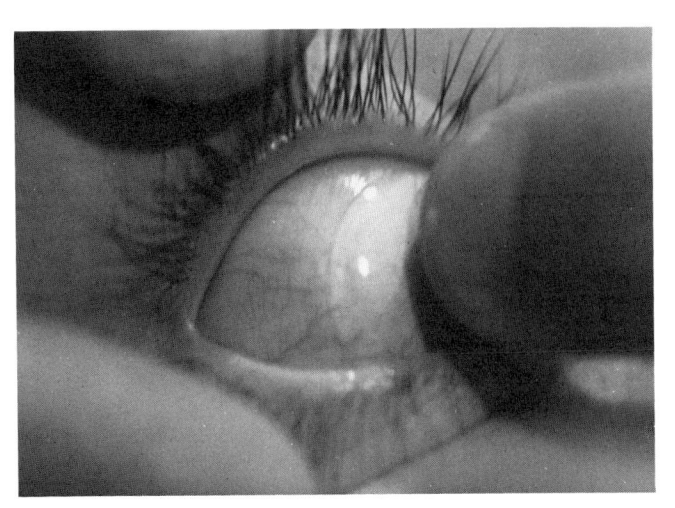

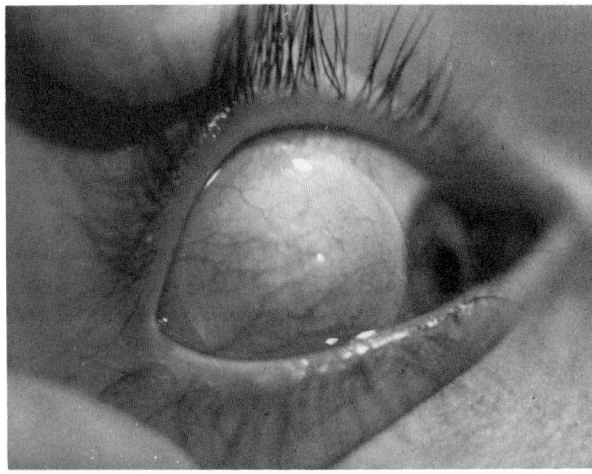

5. Squeeze the lens between the thumb and index finger and it will easily come off the sclera.

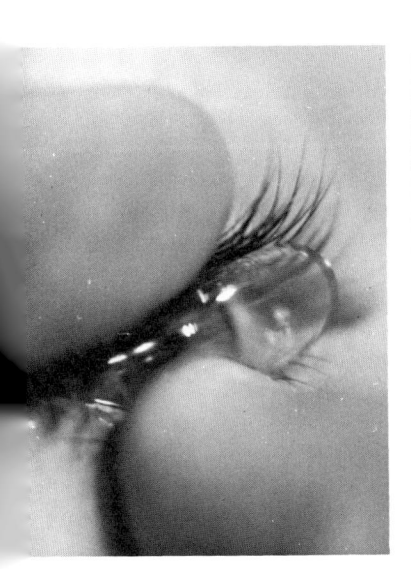

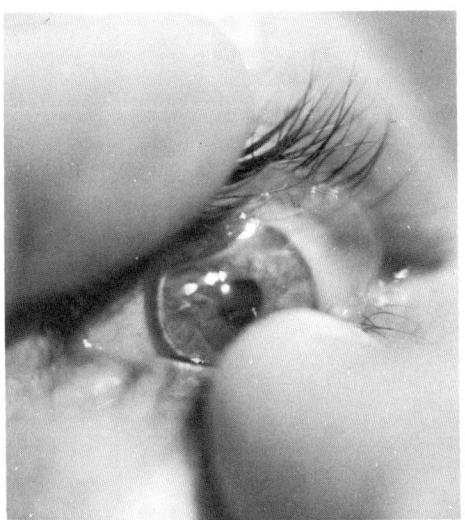

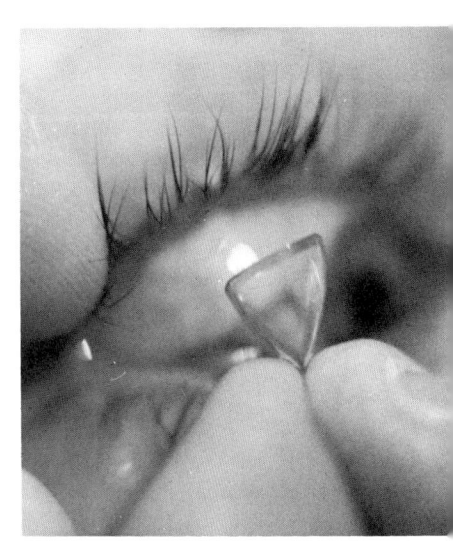

NOTE: If the lens does not easily slide from the cornea onto the sclera, drop more irrigating solution onto the lens. After removal place the lens in isotonic solution to protect them from damage.

30 DRAINAGE OF FELON

INDICATION
Drainage of abscess of the pulp space of a finger.

EQUIPMENT
1. Local set
2. 1% lidocaine
3. #3 scalpel handle and #11 blade
4. Small curved hemostat
5. Small rubber tissue drain or rubber band

ANATOMICAL CONSIDERATIONS
1. A felon is an infection of the pulp space of a finger. This portion of the finger contains numerous fibrous septa which extend volarward from the distal portion of the terminal phalanx. These septa divide the volar space into a number of closed spaces. If not properly drained, the felon may invade the bone, causing osteomyelitis.
2. The incision to drain a felon must divide all the fibrous bands in the pulp space. It should be properly placed to avoid the flexor tendon and the neurovascular bundles of the finger.
3. The incision should be placed approximately at the midpoint of the length of the nail bed, midway between the anterior aspect of the phalanx and the volar skin.
4. The incision should extend through the skin of both sides of the finger to insure complete division of the fascial septa and adequate drainage.

PROCEDURE

1. Prep the finger with povidone-iodine.
2. Block the digital nerves near the metacarpophalangeal joint.
3. Identify the appropriate point for the incision.

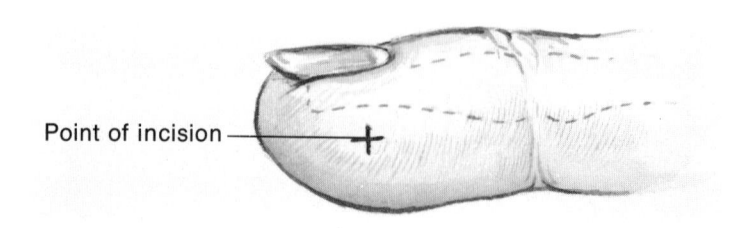

Point of incision

4. Incise the skin on the side of the terminal phalanx using a #11 knife blade, and pass the blade across the entire width of the finger, penetrating the opposite side.

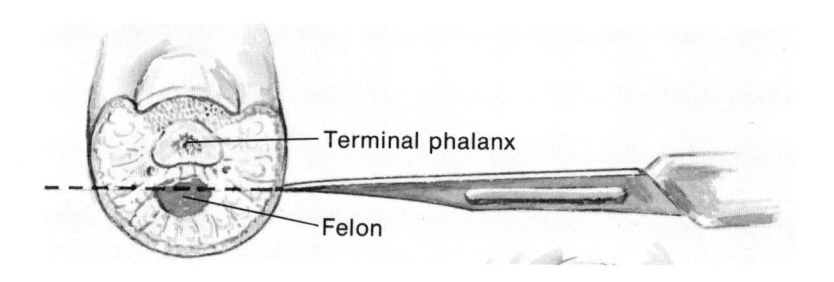

Terminal phalanx

Felon

5. Withdraw the knife blade.
6. Insert a small curved hemostat through the entire length of incision and spread it gently to open the incision.
7. Grasp a sterile rubber band or small rubber tissue drain with the hemostat and pull it through the wound until it protrudes from either side.

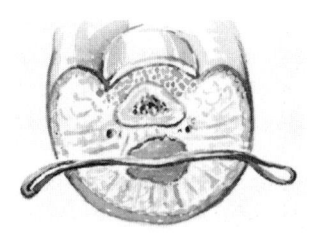

8. Apply firm pressure for five minutes to control bleeding.
9. Apply a dry sterile dressing.

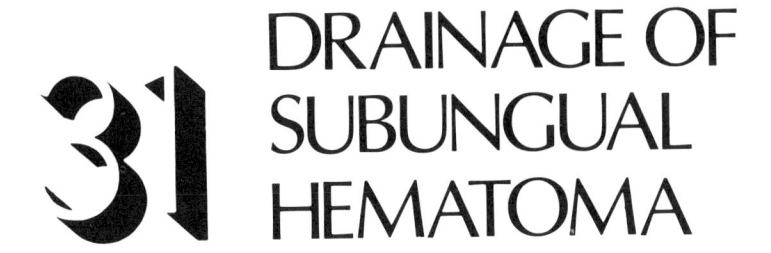

31 DRAINAGE OF SUBUNGUAL HEMATOMA

INDICATION
Subungual hematoma

EQUIPMENT
1. Hand-operated dental drill (battery-operated drill optional)

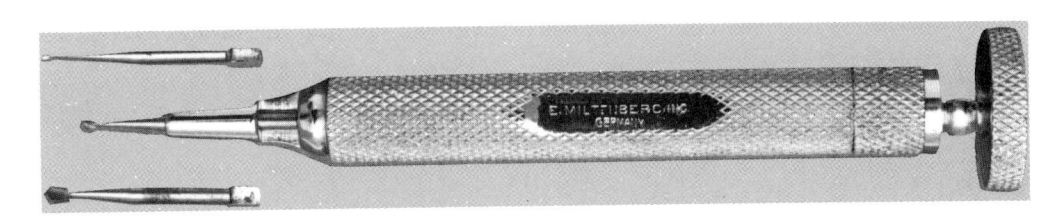

2. #11 scapel blade with handle

PROCEDURE
This condition is very painful due to the pressure built up by the hematoma in the closed space between the nail and its bed. The treatment is evacuation of the hematoma. The patient's comfort is improved by making every effort to avoid removing any portion of the nail ordinarily in contact with the nail bed. The preferred method of evacuation depends on the size of the hematoma and its relation to the distal tip of the nail bed.

HEMATOMA OF THE PROXIMAL PORTION OF THE NAIL BED
1. No anesthesia is necessary. Place the patient's finger on a firm base, such as a table.
2. Use a hand drill or a battery-operated drill with a dental drill tip, or a #11 scalpel blade with handle.

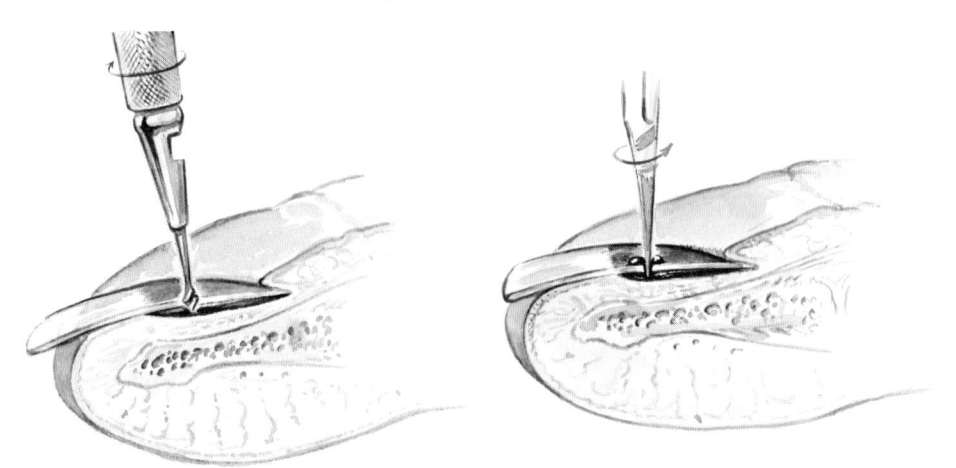

3. Prep the finger with povidone-iodine.
4. Apply firm, but gentle, pressure to the nail, over the hematoma.
5. As the drill penetrates the nail, the pressure should be decreased to avoid plunging the drill tip into the nail bed. As soon as the nail is perforated the blood will spontaneously evacuate.
6. Two or three holes should be drilled to allow for complete evacuation of the hematoma and lessen the likelihood of its reformation.
7. Apply an adhesive dressing over the nail.

HEMATOMA OF THE DISTAL PORTION OF THE NAIL BED

1. No anesthesia is necessary. Place the patient's finger on a firm base.
2. Prep the finger with povidone-iodine.
3. Carefully insert a #11 scalpel blade with handle under the nail into the hematoma, keeping the blade in contact with the undersurface of the nail. This maneuver can be accomplished without discomfort to the patient.

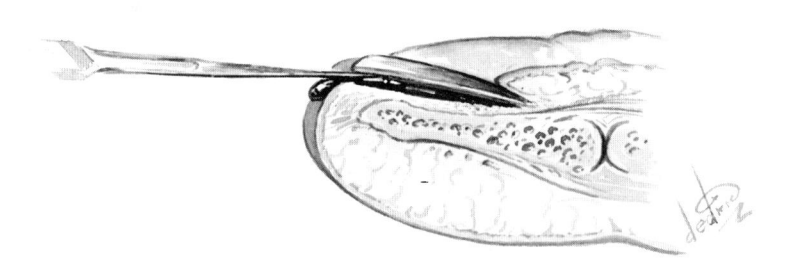

4. Completely evacuate the hematoma.
5. Apply an adhesive dressing.

NOTE: A subungual hematoma is often associated with a fracture of the terminal phalanx. X-ray examination of the finger is indicated to determine if a fracture is present. If so, the digit should be immobilized with a simple padded metal splint or some other appropriate device.

32 REMOVAL OF FINGER RING

INDICATION

Injuries to the arm, hand, or ring-bearing fingers which may cause swelling of the finger. These include fractures, burns, lacerations, bites, or crush injuries.

NOTE: Anticipation of secondary swelling with early removal of the ring is desirable, since once swelling has developed, the procedure is more difficult.

After the ring has been removed, it should be given to the patient or his family and a suitable note placed in the hospital record.

EQUIPMENT

1. Ring cutter
2. Curved hemostat
3. Umbilical tape
4. Lubricating jelly

ANATOMICAL CONSIDERATIONS

1. Removal of a finger ring may be hindered by swelling of the digit, particularly of the proximal interphalangeal joint.
2. When removing the ring, caution must be taken to avoid further damage to the injured digit.
3. If the chosen method of removal is the ring cutter, the cutter should be placed

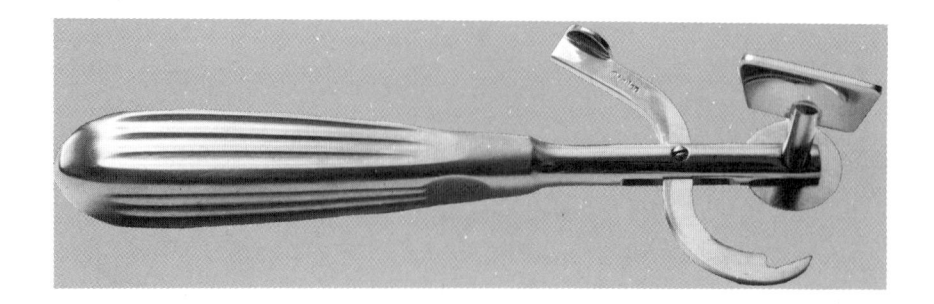

on the circumference of the band opposite the face, or setting, of the ring. This is the usual location of the weld of a fitted ring. Cutting the ring in this area will do no damage that cannot be repaired. Every effort should be made to avoid unnecessary damage to the ring.
4. If the ring-bearing finger is extensively damaged, the ring cutter method is the one of choice.

PROCEDURE

RING-CUTTER METHOD
1. Select the site on the ring to be cut. Rotate this side to the palmar aspect of the finger, or away from the site of injury if it happens to be on the volar side of the digit.
2. Slip the curved tip of the ring cutter under the ring at the chosen site and rotate the cutting wheel until the metal is completely cut.

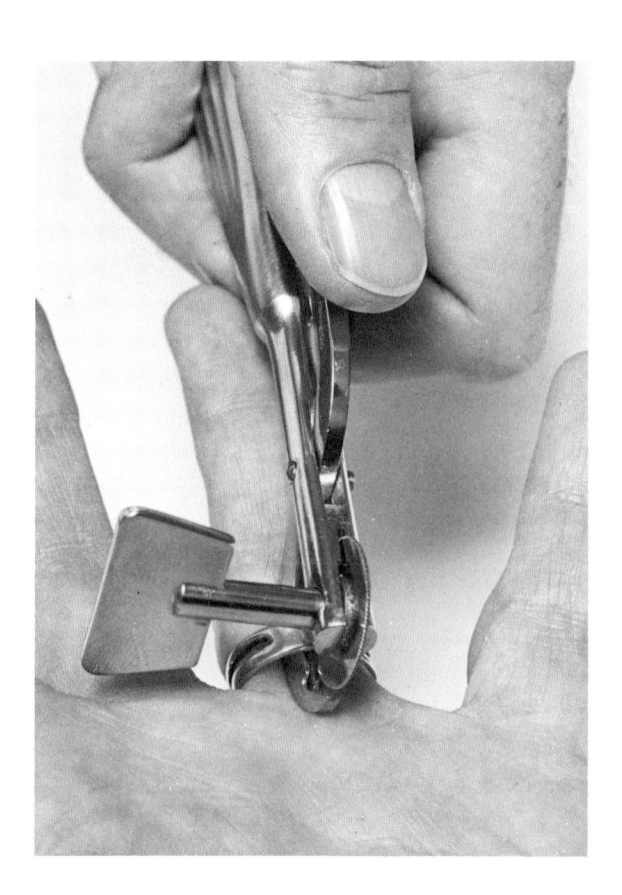

3. Spread the opening made in the ring.
4. Lubricate the finger.
5. Slide the opened ring off the finger.

SUTURE METHOD

1. Slip one end of the umbilical tape under the ring from the distal side until a 1½- to 2-inch tail of tape is drawn proximally.
2. Hold the tail of the tape.
3. Take the longer end of the tape and wrap this snugly about the distal finger to a point beyond the proximal interphalangeal joint and hold this in place.

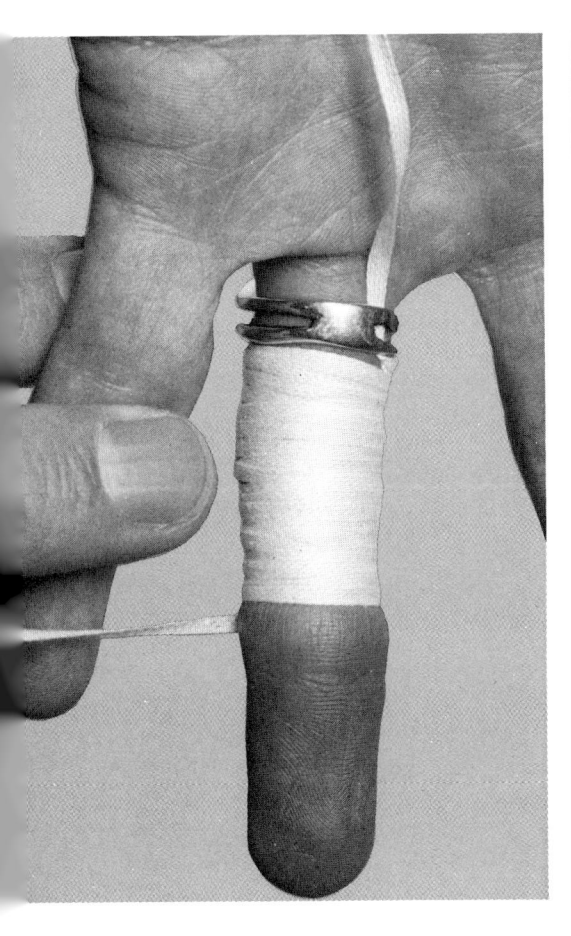

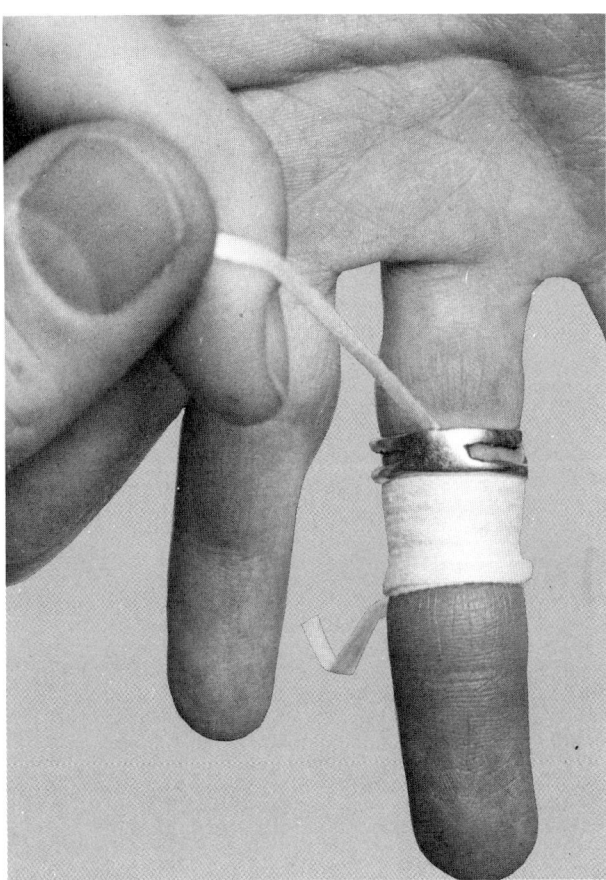

4. Grasp the short proximal tail of the tape, pull this over the ring, and begin to unwind this toward the distal end of the finger.
5. As the tape unwinds, the ring will begin to slide distally and usually will pass easily over the proximal interphalangeal joint and slip off.

33 REMOVAL OF AN IMBEDDED FISH HOOK

INDICATION

Fish hook imbedded in soft tissue.

ANATOMICAL CONSIDERATIONS

1. The end of the fish hook may be imbedded in the subcutaneous tissue or may be protruding through the skin.

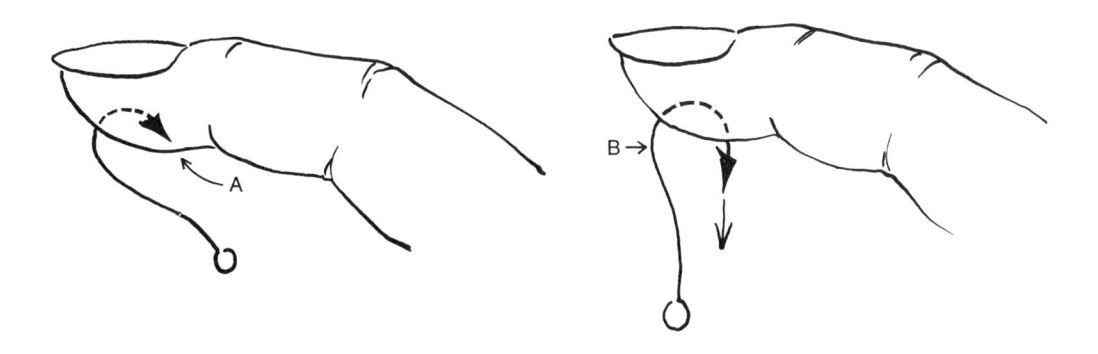

2. The barb on the end of the hook makes it impossible to remove by "backing" it out. The hook must be cut in two pieces and each segment removed separately.

155

EQUIPMENT

1. Local set
2. 0.5% lidocaine
3. Wire cutter
4. Small hemostat

PROCEDURE

FISH HOOK IMBEDDED IN THE SOFT TISSUE (A)

1. Prep the part with povidone-iodine.
2. Anesthetize the part by local field block or peripheral nerve block technique.
3. Advance the hook so that the barbed end protrudes through the skin.
4. Cut the barbed end off the hook with the wire cutter.
5. Withdraw the remainder of the hook back through the point of entry.
6. Apply a sterile dressing with povidone-iodine ointment.

FISH HOOK PROTRUDING THROUGH THE SKIN (B)

1. Prep the part with povidone-iodine.
2. Anesthetize the part by local field block or peripheral nerve block technique.
3. Cut the fish hook flush with the skin at the point of entry, using the wire cutter.
4. Grasp the barbed end with a small hemostat and draw this fragment from the subcutaneous tissue.
5. Apply a sterile dressing with povidone-iodine ointment.

34 GASTROINTESTINAL TUBES

A number of tube devices are available for insertion into the gastrointestinal tract, depending on specific indications and the requirements of the patient. These tubes vary from a simple urethral catheter used for gastric decompression in an infant to the Blakemore-Sengstaken tube for the control of bleeding from esophageal varices.

Generally, these tubes are used in the emergency setting for the following purposes:
1. Decompression,
2. Lavage (irrigation),
3. Local pressure in the esophagus and fundus of the stomach.

While there are a number of other uses for these tubes in hospitalized patients (i.e., duodenal drainage collection, gavage, and so on), these procedures rarely are done in the emergency setting and thus are omitted from discussion in this volume.

EQUIPMENT

Generally, the tubes described in this section vary in diameter from 10 to 18 Fr. and in length up to 9 feet. The smaller sizes are used primarily in children, the larger ones in adults. In infants, a Robinson urethral catheter is of sufficient length to extend from the nose to the stomach and may adequately serve this size patient.

NASOGASTRIC TUBE

There are two types of nasogastric tubes in common usage, the single-lumen tube (Levin) and the double-lumen variety (Salem-sump). Both types

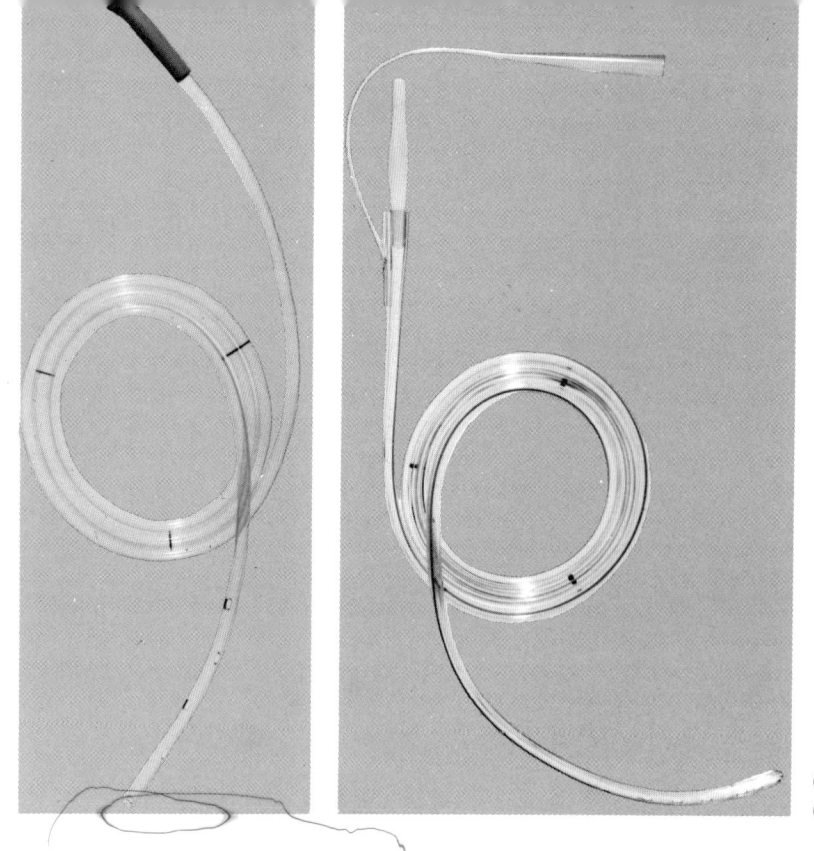

(Left) Levin tube
(Right) Salem-sump tube

contain radiopaque markings so that the position of the tube in the gastrointestinal tract can be accurately determined.

The single-lumen tube is best for decompression, although it can be used for gastric lavage. The double-lumen sump tube also may be used for decompression, but serves admirably for continuous lavage or irrigation of the stomach. This is described in detail on pages 163-165. Each tube is 48 inches long with markings at 4-inch intervals from 18 to 30 inches from the distal end.

INTESTINAL TUBE

The devices used for passage into the small intestine are the Cantor tube and the Miller-Abbott tube. Each is approximately 9 feet long and is appropriately marked at intervals so that the position of the tube in the gastrointestinal tract can be seen.

The Cantor tube is a single-lumen tube with a rubber balloon fastened to its tip. When used, the balloon is partially filled with mercury which eases passage into the stomach by gravity. When the patient is properly positioned, gravity again helps the tube to enter the duodenum and finally pass the duodeno-jejunal flexure, from which point peristaltic activity will carry the tube further into the small bowel.

The Miller-Abbott tube is a double-lumen device. One lumen is used for aspiration, while the other connects with a balloon attached to the distal end of the tube. Once the tube has entered the small bowel, the balloon is inflated and acts as a propellant to cause peristalsis to pass the tube into the distal small bowel.

Selection of one of these two intestinal decompression tubes is usually a matter of the physician's personal choice.

Before using either of these tubes, the balloon should be checked.

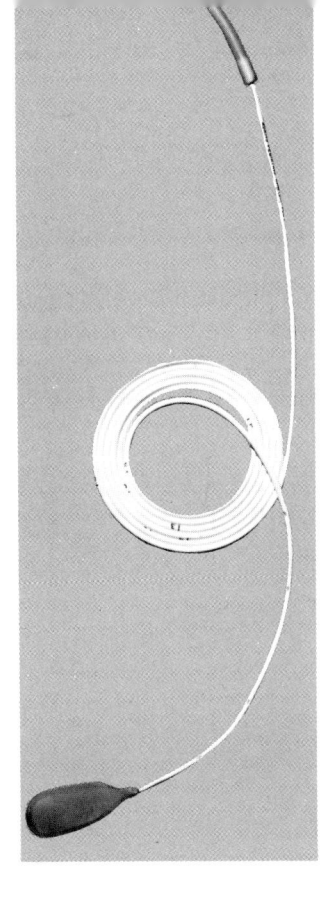

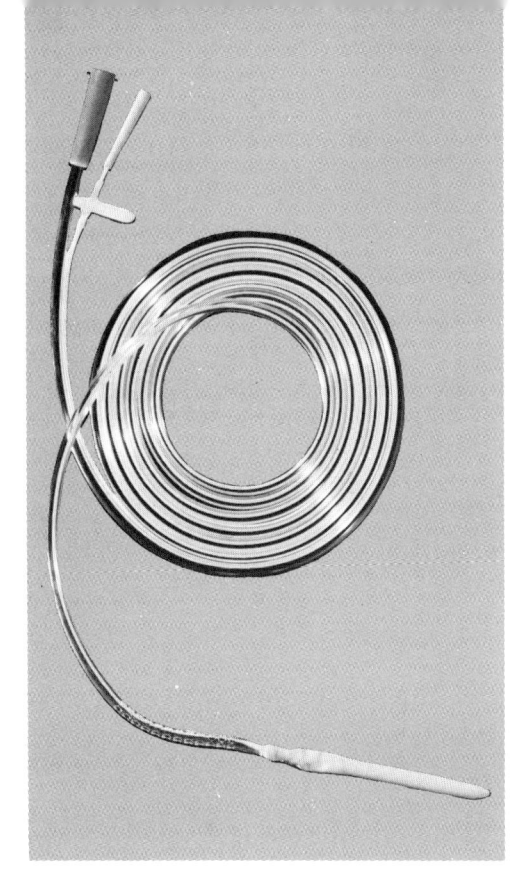

The operator should tug firmly on the Cantor tube to assure it is attached to the balloon. With the Miller-Abbott tube, the balloon should be inflated with air before use, to make certain it does not leak.

The drainage holes are located only in the distal end of these intestinal tubes; thus, when the tube is in proper position in the small bowel, it is possible for the stomach to be distended with air and/or fluid. In such a patient, a nasogastric tube may be passed through the other nostril for decompression of the stomach.

BLAKEMORE-SENGSTAKEN TUBE

This is a triple-lumen, double-balloon tube which is used exclusively for control of bleeding esophageal varices by tamponade.

The balloons are located near the distal end of the tube. The proximal balloon is long, roughly sausage-shaped, when inflated and conforms to the configuration of the esophagus. When properly positioned it lies in the distal half of the esophagus. The distal balloon is globular in shape and when inflated fills the fundus of the stomach and the area of the cardio-esophageal junction.

The tip of the tube extending beyond the gastric balloon is perforated to aspirate gastric contents. Thus, one of the lumens is used for gastric decompression, while each of the other lumens is used to inflate each balloon.

This tube must be maintained in position with traction which enhances the tamponade effect of the gastric balloon. However, pressure from the tube must not bear on the skin of the nares because ulceration will result with permanent deformity. Several methods are available to lessen the occurrence of this complication. A 2-inch cube of sponge or foam rubber may be fixed about the tube as it exits from the nares, keeping pressure off the skin. Or, the tube may be fixed to a device similar to a football helmet, with the tube attached to a point similar to a face mask, thus maintaining traction but lessening pressure on the ala nasi.

As with other balloon tubes, the balloons should be inflated to determine integrity before insertion.

With the tube in place and the balloons inflated, the esophagus is occluded. Hence, the patient cannot swallow his own saliva. A second tube may have to be passed through the nose into the esophagus to remove these secretions and prevent aspiration into the airway. A Robinson urethral catheter may serve this purpose.

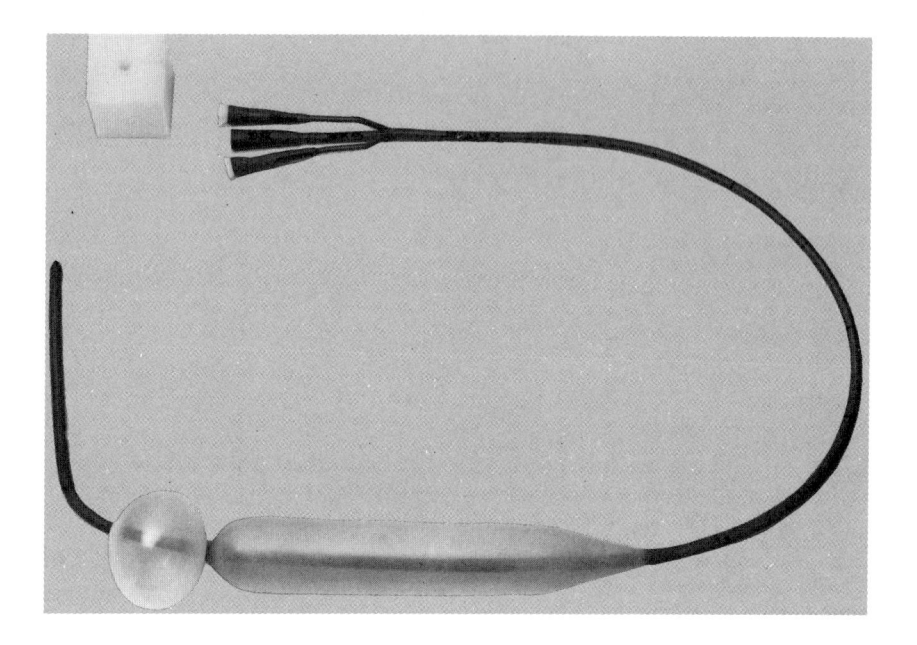

PLACING THE TUBE

Passing a tube through the nostril into the gastrointestinal tract can be a terrifying and an uncomfortable ordeal for the patient. A tube should not be used without specific indications. At the same time, it should not be withheld merely as a convenience to the patient. The tube should be well lubricated with a water-soluble jelly and passed along the floor of the nose to minimize trauma to the turbinates. The operator should ask if the patient has had any nasal problems in the past, such as fracture, deviated septum, prior surgery, and make every effort to avoid an injured area.

Use of a topical anesthetic spray, such as 4% lidocaine applied to the nasal passage via an atomizer, may lessen discomfort to the patient. This is particularly true when a balloon tube is necessary.

Calm reassurance to the patient, while the tube is being placed will make the procedure easier for both patient and operator.

Once the tube is in the pharynx, passage may be made smoother by giving the patient small sips of water through a straw or small portions (about a teaspoon at a time) of ice chips.

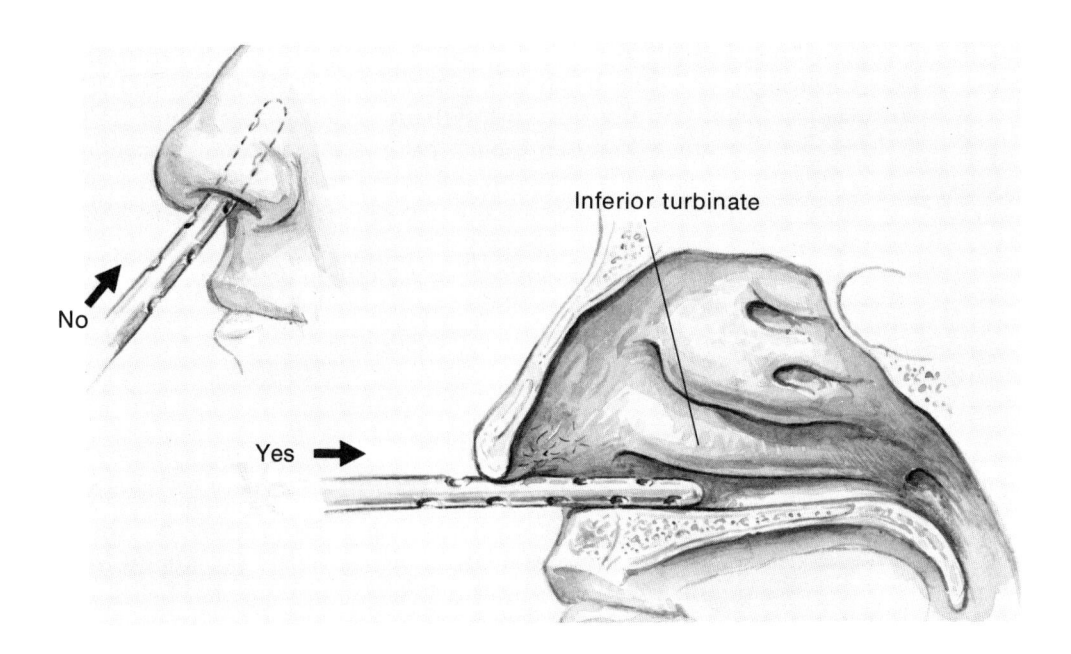

Each time the patient swallows, the tube is advanced several inches. It will proceed surprisingly well with this maneuver.

Once the tube is in the desired position, it is taped to the nostril. It should also be fixed to the patient's face or gown so that as the patient turns or moves about, the tube will not be pulled at the point of exit from the nose.

While the tube is being inserted, the operator should proceed slowly but deliberately. On occasion, the tube may inadvertently be passed into the glottis provoking a coughing spasm. If this occurs, the tube should be withdrawn quickly and repositioned. If the tube is inserted too rapidly, it may provoke a gag reflex with vomiting. In this circumstance, the tube can be expelled through the mouth and must be withdrawn and repositioned.

OTHER CONSIDERATIONS

Any nasogastrointestinal tube is an irritant to the pharynx and nose. It may cause local swelling in the nostril with occlusion of the ostium of a paranasal sinus. It may cause an increase in secretions in the nose and pharynx which can be aspirated into the airway, particularly in elderly or debilitated patients.

The tube is especially irritating to the pharynx and epiglottis and may interfere with the swallowing mechanism. This is magnified by the fact that the patient may change from a "nose-breather" to a "mouth-breather" once the tube is in place, resulting in drying and further irritation to the mucosa of the pharynx and epiglottis. This can be lessened to some extent by keeping the patient properly hydrated and prescribing anesthetic throat discs or lozenges to be dissolved in the mouth. These candies contain benzocaine or a similar topical anesthetic agent and serve to alleviate, albeit not completely, the annoyance of the tube.

For the reasons just mentioned, good oral care must be given to any patient with an indwelling nasogastrointestinal tube.

Accurate measurement and a description of the tube aspirate is a sine qua non of good care. The type and amount of parenteral replacement fluid is based to some extent on the aspirate and the patient's general condition.

In a critically ill or injured emergency patient, appropriate replacement depends on an evaluation of many parameters, including urine output, tube output, arterial pressure, central venous pressure, arterial blood gases, cardiac function, particularly as measured by pulmonary artery, and pulmonary wedge pressures.

Baseline determinations of blood count, blood electrolytes, and urinalysis are minimum laboratory determinations made on any patient who requires an indwelling gastrointestinal drainage tube.

SUMMARY

Nasogastrointestinal tubes are used most commonly in the emergency for the following purposes: decompression, lavage, local pressure.

They cause varying degrees of discomfort in patients and can lead to a significant number of complications, minor and major.

Their use should be confined to specific indications, and marked by concern for the patient. All physicians and nurses who have occasion to order and insert such tubes in patients would benefit greatly from the personal experience of nasogastric intubation.

BIBLIOGRAPHY

Boyce, H. W. Jr. Modification of the Sengstaken-Blakemore tube. New Eng. J. Med. 267:195, 1962.

Malt, R. A. Control of massive upper gastrointestinal hemorrhage. New Eng. J. Med. 286:1043, 1972.

———. Emergency and elective operations for bleeding esophageal varices. Surg. Clin. N. Am. 54:561, 1974.

35 LEVIN AND SALEM-SUMP TUBE

INDICATIONS

1. Gastric or upper intestinal decompression.
2. Pyloric obstruction.
3. Intestinal obstruction.
4. Lavage of stomach in patient suspected of drug overdose.
5. Lavage of stomach in patient with upper gastrointestinal hemorrhage, with or without iced saline lavage.
6. Prevention of emesis.
7. Gastric decompression or lavage of stomach in unconscious patient.

EQUIPMENT

There are two types of nasogastric suction tubes in common use. One is the Levin tube which is 48 inches long. It is a straight rubber or plastic tube with a perforated tip and four or five side holes in the distal end for aspiration of gastric content. The other is the Salem-sump tube which is a double-lumen tube, the smaller lumen serving as an air intake. It is 48 inches long.

Both tubes vary in external diameter from 10 to 18 Fr. The smaller sizes are used in pediatric patients. In infants, a straight Robinson urethral catheter, 10 to 12 Fr. in diameter, may be used for gastric decompression.

1. Levin or Salem-sump tube
2. Water-soluble lubricating jelly
3. Topical anesthetic spray (optional)
4. Glass of water and straw
5. Asepto syringe
6. Adapter
7. Decompression machine

To suction machine

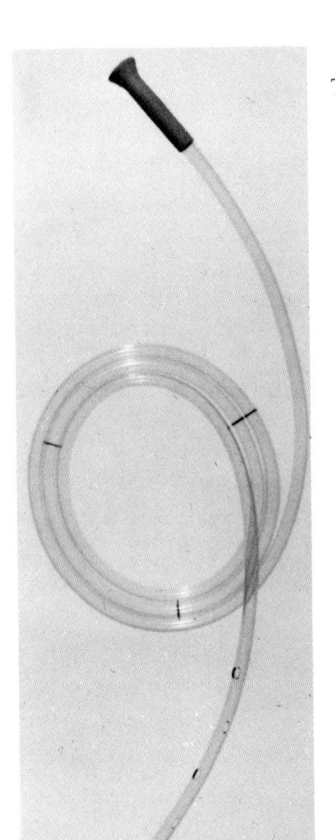

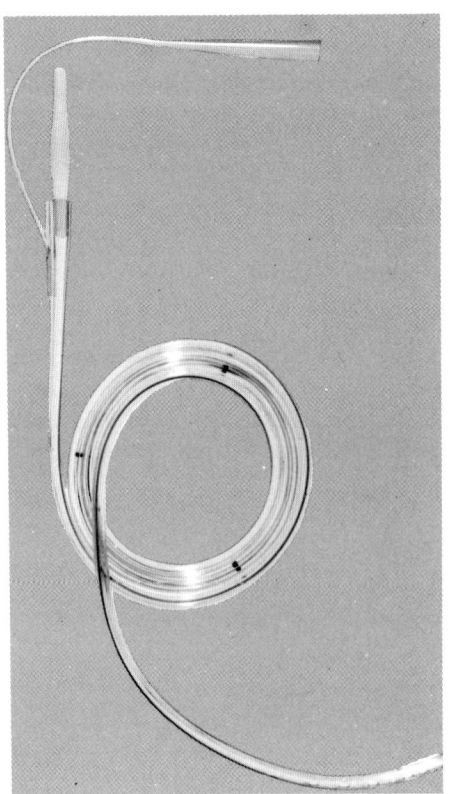

(Left) To suction machine (Right) Sump intake

ANATOMICAL CONSIDERATION

Insert the tube along the floor of the nose to avoid trauma to the turbinates.

PROCEDURE

1. If patient is conscious, ask if there is any nasal deformity. Avoid trauma to the nasal passage.
2. Elevate the head of the bed 30 to 40 degrees. Ask the patient not to extend his neck.
3. Lubricate the distal 3 or 4 inches of the tube with water-soluble jelly. Spray the nasal membrane with lidocaine if desired.
4. Gently insert the tube along the floor of the nasal passageway. As the tube nears the posterior nares, the tip of the tube may abut against the lower tip of the inferior turbinate. Maintain gentle pressure which usually will allow the tube to enter the nasopharynx.
5. Once the tube has been passed into the pharynx, have the patient swallow small amounts of water. With each swallow, gently advance the tube 2 to 3 inches.
6. In the average adult, the tube should be inserted to the third mark which is 26 inches from the tip. This generally allows the tip of the tube to be in the pars media of the stomach.
7. Aspirate the gastric content to be sure the tube is properly placed.
8. Further actions will depend on patient's need. The gastric aspirate may be tested for free acid, blood, or toxicology, as the patient's condition indicates.
9. In patients suspected of overdose, the stomach should be thoroughly lavaged with measured amounts of saline.
10. In patients with massive upper gastrointestinal bleeding, the stomach may be lavaged with measured amounts of iced saline.
11. Following evacuation and/or lavage of the stomach, the tube should be attached to an intermittent decompression machine.

FOR CONTINUOUS GASTRIC LAVAGE

1. This may be done only with the Salem-sump tube.
2. After the tube is in position in the stomach, attach the tube to continuous suction.
3. Place container of irrigating solution (saline or Ringer's lactate) in an ice-water bath above the patient.
4. Connect the container to a straight infusion set and attach the lower end to the tube drain (blue tip).
5. Adjust the rate of flow of the lavage fluid by setting the crimp roller at the desired level.
6. Measure and record the amount of lavage fluid and include this in the patient's intake and output record.
7. With this method, lavage may be continued indefinitely.

36 CANTOR TUBE

The Cantor tube is a single-lumen tube which has a balloon attached to its tip. The balloon is partially filled with liquid mercury and facilitates passage of the tube along the intestinal tract. Proximal to the tip, the tube contains multiple perforations through which intestinal contents are aspirated. The tube is marked at intervals, S (stomach), P (pylorus), D (duodenum), then every 12 inches to 6 or 9 feet. The mercury-filled bag functions to ease passage of the tube by gravity and intestinal peristalsis. This tube is approximately 225 cm in length and 12 Fr. (pediatric) or 300 cm in length and 16 Fr. (adult).

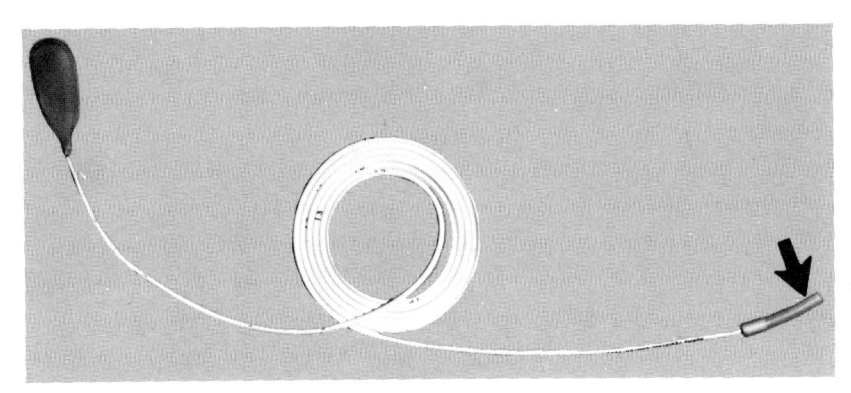

To suction machine

INDICATIONS
1. Intestinal obstruction.
2. Paralytic ileus.

EQUIPMENT

1. 16 Fr. Cantor tube (pediatric size — 12 Fr.)
2. 10 cc mercury
3. 5 cc syringe with 21-gauge needle
4. Water-soluble lubricating jelly
5. Bayonet forceps (optional)
6. Asepto syringe
7. Topical anesthetic spray (4% lidocaine)
8. Glass of water and straw
9. Plastic adapter
10. Decompression machine

ANATOMICAL CONSIDERATION

The tube should be inserted along the floor of the nasal passage to avoid trauma to the turbinates.

PROCEDURE

1. Ask if the patient has any nasal deformity, such as a deviated septum, or has had any prior injury. Make every effort to avoid these.
2. Test the attachment of the rubber bag to the Cantor tube. It should not be used if the bag is not firmly attached.
3. Draw up 5 cc of mercury into the syringe.
4. Using a 21-gauge needle, inject the mercury into the midportion of the bag.

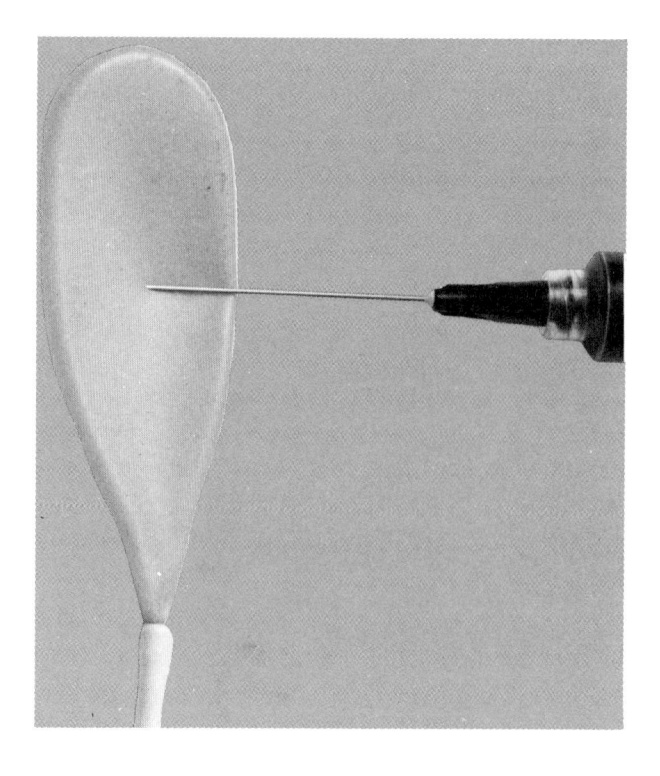

5. Before withdrawing the needle, aspirate all the air from the bag.
6. Lubricate the bag and 6 or 8 inches of the tube with jelly.
7. Spray the nasal passage with 4% lidocaine.
8. Keep patient semirecumbent with the neck slightly hyperextended to maintain the floor of the nose in a perpendicular direction.
9. Hold the bag by its tip and let the mercury fall into the neck of the bag.
10. Fold the bag lengthwise and pinch it in its midportion to keep the mercury in the neck of the bag.

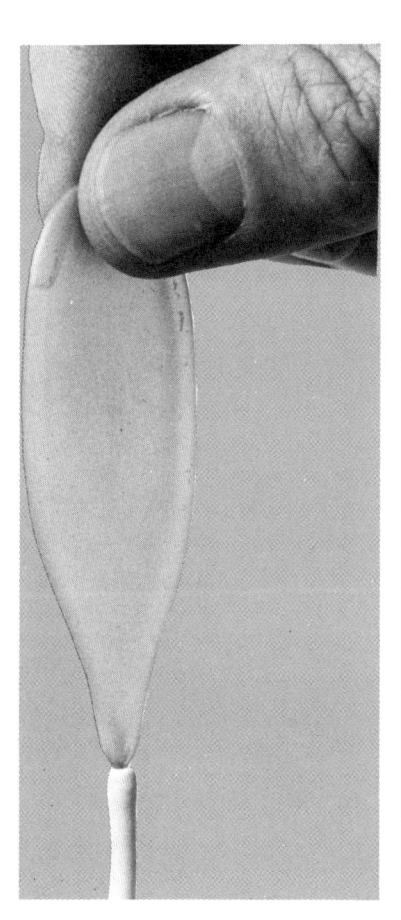

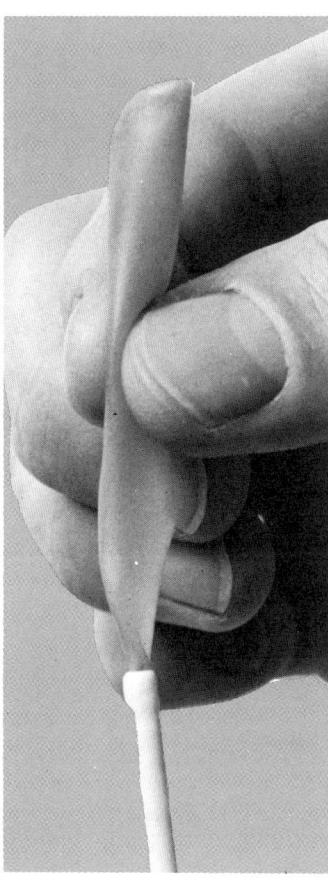

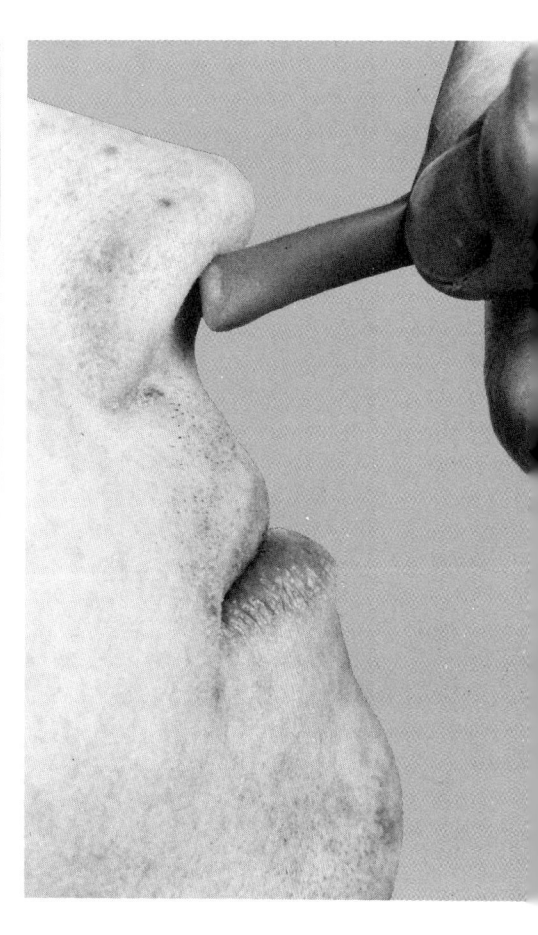

11. Insert the folded tip of the bag into the nose. As the bag is released, the mercury will fall into the tip of the bag and carry it by gravity into the nasopharynx. If the bag becomes lodged in the nasal passage, it may be advanced by gently pushing it with a cotton applicator stick or bayonet forceps.
12. Once the bag is in the oropharynx, give the patient a sip of water and the bag should pass along the esophagus into the stomach. At the same time gently feed the tube into the nose until the letter S is at the external nares. At this point, the tube should be in the stomach.
13. Aspirate the stomach contents.
14. Advance the tube to P and have the patient turn on his right side to allow gravity to advance the bag into the duodenum.

169

15. Do NOT tape the tube to the nose.
16. Place the tube on low intermittent suction.
17. Advance the tube 2 inches an hour. Intestinal peristalsis and gravity should carry the tube down the intestinal tract.
18. Take an x-ray film of the abdomen in 2 hours to check the position of the tip of the tube.

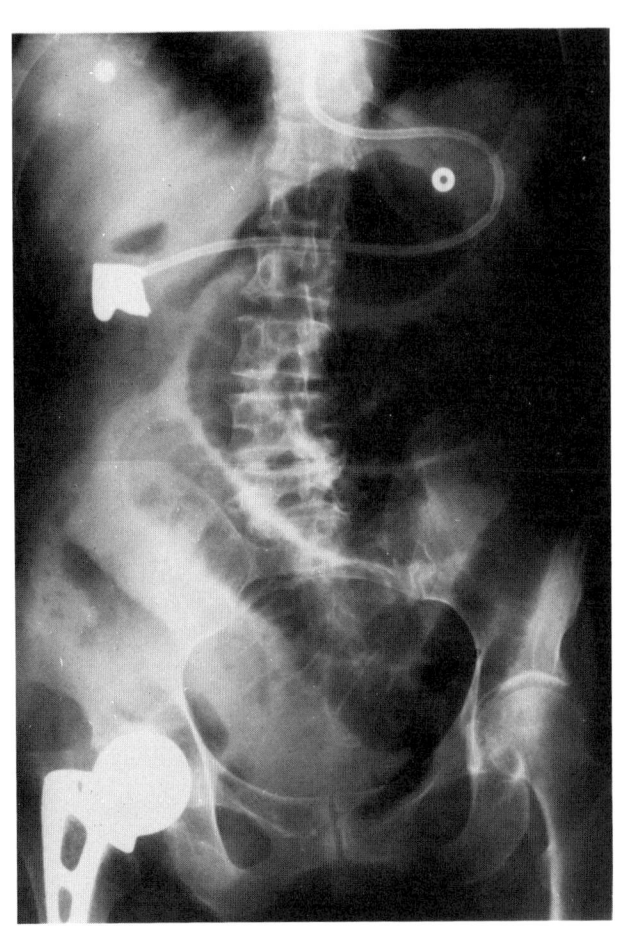

Tip of tube in duodenum

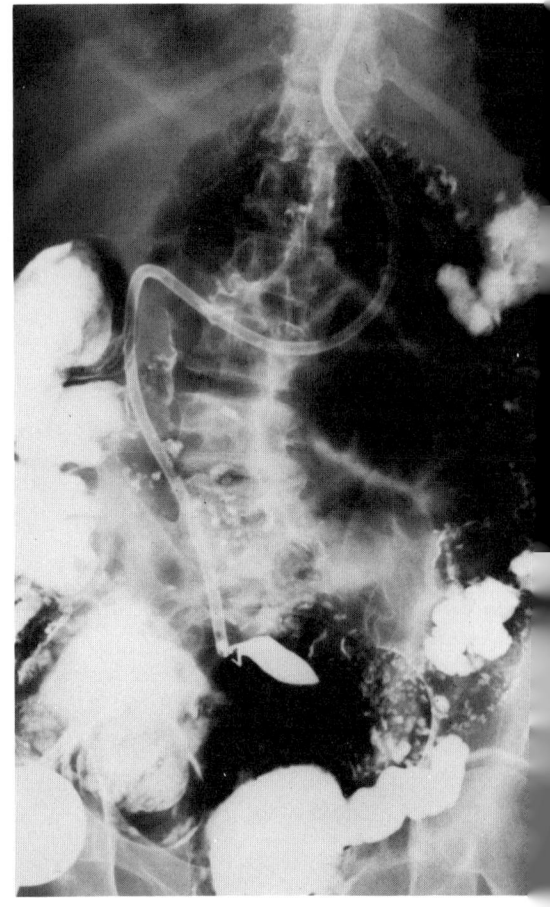

Tip of tube in small bowel

37 MILLER-ABBOTT TUBE

The Miller-Abbott tube is a double-lumen device containing a balloon which, when inflated, facilitates passage of the tube along the intestine. One lumen is used to inflate the balloon, the other to aspirate intestinal contents. The distal end of the tube has the balloon attached. Proximal to the tip are a number of perforations for aspiration. The proximal end of the tube is fitted with a Y-shaped metal connector which joins with each of the two lumens. One of the tips of the connector is used to inflate the balloon and is marked "air." The other is marked "suction" and is used to aspirate intestinal contents. The tube is approximately 240 cm long and 18 Fr. in diameter. The one shown below has markings at 65 and 75 cm, then at every 25 cm until 200 cm is reached.

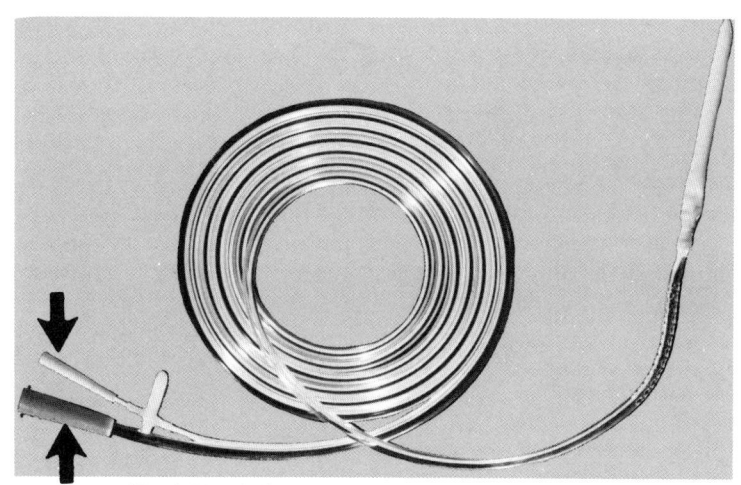

(Top) To air bag (Bottom) To suction machine

INDICATIONS

1. Intestinal obstruction
2. Ileus

EQUIPMENT

1. Miller-Abbott tube
2. 20 cc syringe
3. Water-soluble lubricating jelly
4. Topical anesthetic spray (4% lidocaine)
5. Glass of water and straw
6. Decompression machine
7. 3 cc mercury

ANATOMICAL CONSIDERATIONS

The tube is passed along the floor of the nasal passage to minimize trauma to the turbinates.

PROCEDURE

1. Determine whether the patient has any deformity of the nasal passage and select the nasal passage without narrowing or prior injury.
2. Inflate the balloon with air to insure there are no leaks, then deflate.
3. Spray the selected nasal passage for intubation with 4% lidocaine.
4. Lubricate the tip of the tube including the balloon.
5. Have the head of the cart or bed elevated 30 to 45 degrees.
6. Gently insert the tube into the lowermost portion of the nasal passage, parallel to the floor of the nose. Some resistance may be encountered near the posterior end of the inferior turbinate, but this can usually be overcome without difficulty.
7. Once the tube has entered the oropharynx, allow the patient to take small sips of water through a straw. Advance the tube 2 to 3 inches with each swallow.
8. When the tube has advanced to the stomach (65 cm mark), aspirate to check for gastric contents and empty the stomach. If necessary, lavage the stomach with measured amounts of saline.
9. Inflate the balloon with 5 to 10 cc air.
10. Inject 2 to 3 cc mercury and allow it to gravitate into the balloon. Then deflate the balloon of air.

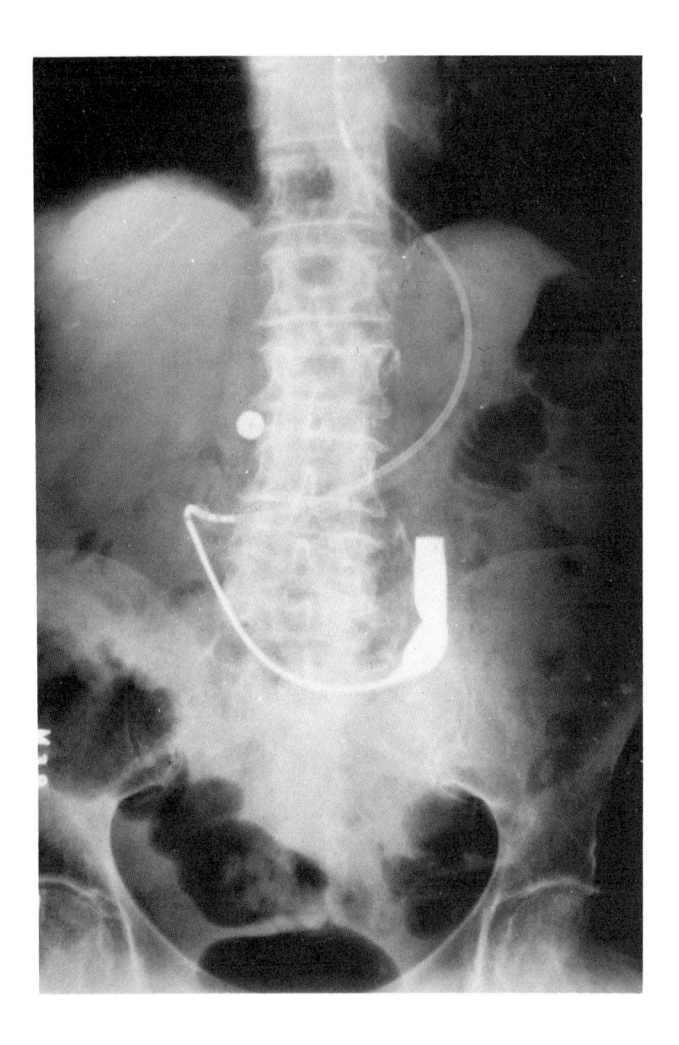

11. Rotate the patient to the right lateral position which should place the tip of the tube near the pylorus.
12. The tube should pass through the pylorus and, once it is in the duodenum, bile-stained material will be recovered by aspiration. Continue to advance the tube slowly to the 75 cm mark.
13. Inflate the balloon with 10 cc air, clamp the air intake, and attach to intermittent suction.
14. When the tip has passed the ligament of Treitz, inflate the balloon with 20 to 30 cc of air and attach to intermittent suction.
15. Turn the patient onto his back.
16. Do NOT tape the tube to the patient's nose, but advance it 2 inches every 30 to 60 minutes.
17. With the ballon inflated, intestinal peristalsis should carry the tube lower

into the intestinal tract. Keep the first 4 to 5 inches protruding from the nose lubricated with water-soluble jelly to ease passage.
18. Check the position of the tube by x-ray film of the abdomen after two hours.

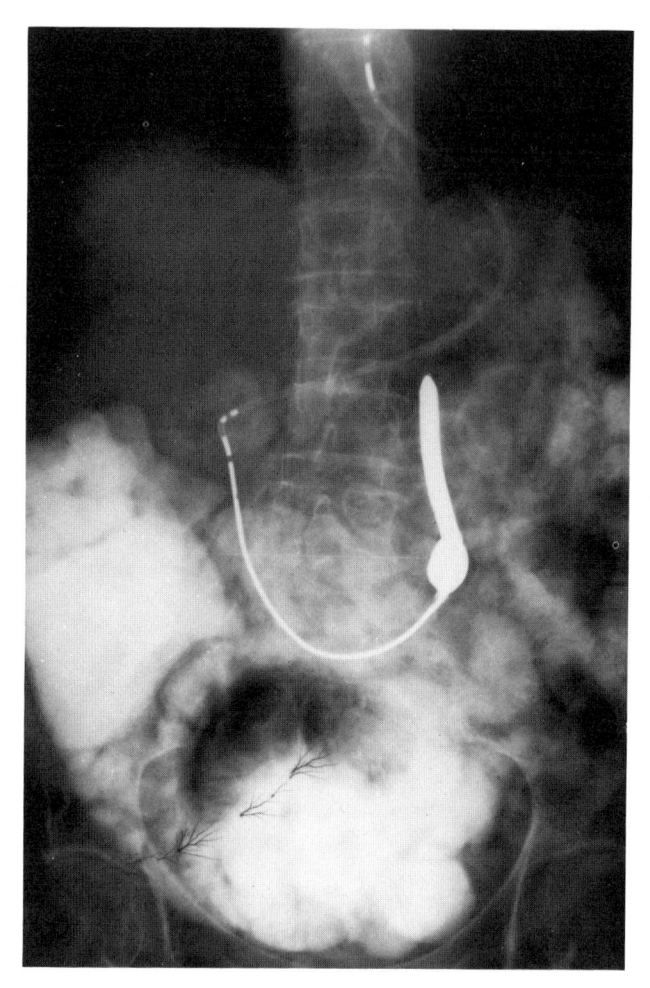

Tip of Miller-Abbott tube in distal duodenum

Irrigate the tube with measured amounts of normal saline every two hours.
19. Allow the tube to pass to the last mark.

38 BLAKEMORE-SENGSTAKEN TUBE

INDICATIONS
1. Need to arrest bleeding from esophageal varices.
2. At times need to distinguish between bleeding from esophageal varices and other upper gastrointestinal lesions.

EQUIPMENT
1. Blakemore-Sengstaken tube
2. Mercury or aneroid sphygmomanometer
3. Y-connector tube
4. 50 cc syringe and Brodie tip
5. Asepto syringe
6. Hemostat
7. Screw clamp
8. Lubricating jelly (lidocaine jelly)
9. Bayonet forceps
10. Plastic foam cube
11. Glass of water with straw
12. 4% lidocaine solution

PROCEDURE

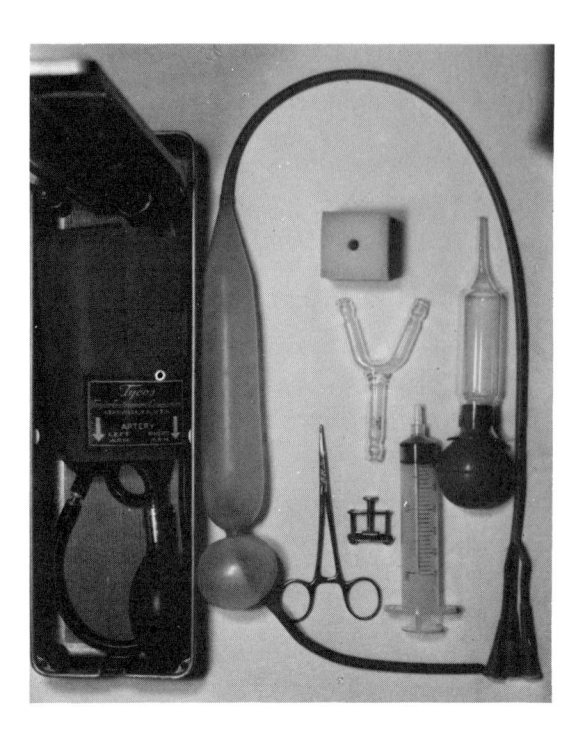

1. Before inserting the tube, inflate both the esophageal and gastric balloons to make certain they do not leak.
2. Spray the nasal membrane with lidocaine solution.
3. Grease the tube with lubricating jelly.
4. Gently insert the tube into the patient's nostril along the floor of the nose. Apply gentle pressure until the balloons have passed the posterior end of the turbinates.
5. Once the tube has entered the oropharynx, have the patient sip small amounts of water to facilitate its passage and advance the tube as each bolus of liquid is swallowed.
6. Pass the tube until the 50 cm mark is reached.
7. Inflate the gastric balloon with 150 to 200 cc of air and close the air intake with a screw clamp. Apply gentle traction until the gastric balloon is snugged against the cardia of the stomach. When this is reached, resistance will be felt.
8. Maintain the traction by placing the foam sponge about the tube as it exits from the nares and taping the tube and sponge in place. This device not only maintains traction, but prevents ulceration of the nasal skin and cartilage.
9. Inflate the esophageal balloon with a mercury or aneroid sphygmomanometer to a pressure of 40 mm Hg and clamp this outlet of the tube.

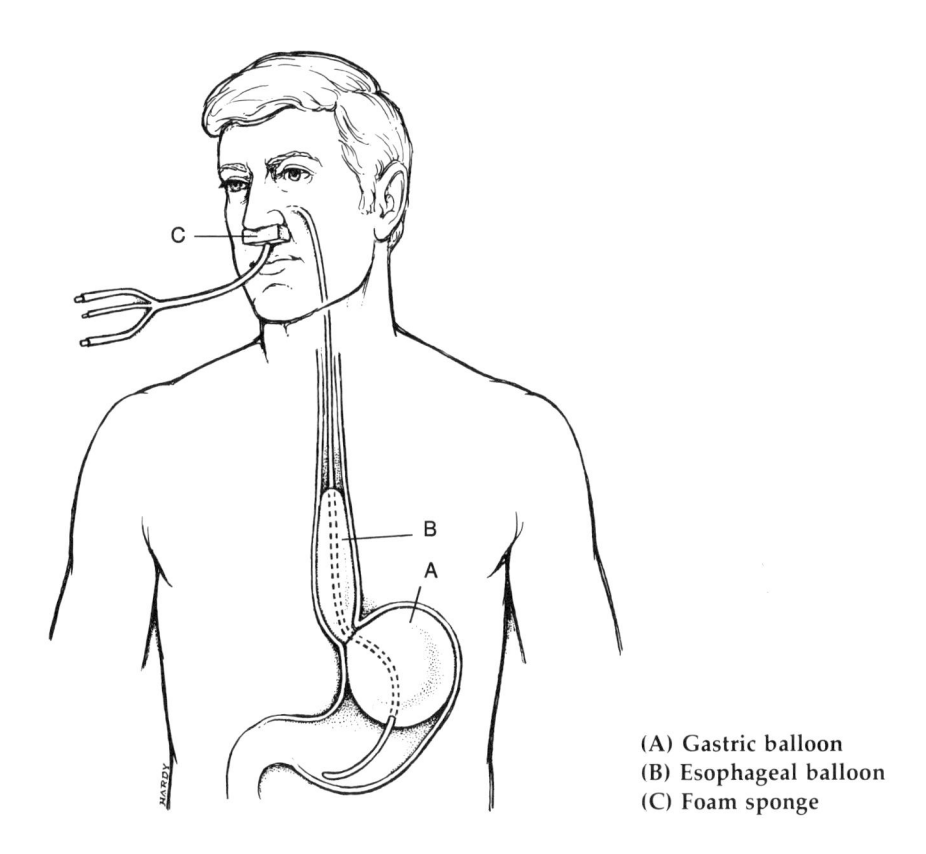

(A) Gastric balloon
(B) Esophageal balloon
(C) Foam sponge

10. Aspirate the gastric contents through the third outlet of the tube using an Asepto syringe.
11. After the stomach has been emptied in this manner, attach the third limb of the tube (that used for aspiration) to an intermittent suction machine.

NOTE: Remember that, once the tube has been inserted and the balloons inflated, the patient's esophagus is completely occluded; thus all oral intake is discontinued.

If the patient has excessive amounts of saliva, a nasogastric tube may be inserted through the opposite nostril into the upper esophagus and placed on intermittent suction to remove any secretions. This maneuver helps to prevent aspiration of these contents into the airway.

39 LOCAL ANESTHESIA

Local anesthesia is a wonderful tool available to emergency personnel. It may be used to relieve pain in conjunction with another procedure, for example, suture of a laceration or reduction of a fracture, or as an independent therapeutic modality to relieve pain, such as an intercostal nerve block for rib fracture(s).

To utilize local anesthesia to fullest advantage, personnel must be familiar with pharmacology and anatomy and possess the skill to perform the technical task of administering the agent properly.

Local anesthesia is effected by blocking the conduction of impulses along a peripheral nerve. A peripheral nerve may contain motor or sensory fibers, alone or in combination. Successful block of a peripheral nerve thus produces motor and/or sensory loss distal to the point of injection.

TYPES

Emergency personnel may employ a number of techniques to produce local anesthesia, depending on the needs of the patient and the procedure to be performed. The techniques which are most often used in the emergency setting are local infiltration, field block, or block of a specific nerve.

LOCAL INFILTRATION is a method of injecting the anesthetic agent directly into the wound or line of incision. It should be used primarily to drain an abscess but is to be avoided in dealing with an incised or open wound which requires accurate approximation, because it may distort the tissue. A FIELD BLOCK is accomplished by flooding the normal tissues around and deep to the lesion without injecting the lesion itself. This is the method that is used most frequently in the emergency department and produces little or no distortion of the tissues when properly employed. With a NERVE BLOCK, a specific peripheral nerve is injected at a point remote from the lesion, between the lesion and the spinal cord, and produces anesthesia in the area supplied by the nerve, distal to the block. This is perhaps the most difficult of the three techniques described, for it demands a familiarity with neuroanatomy. When successfully performed, it requires a minimal amount of anesthetic agent, usually much less than the field block technique, and produces anesthesia over a wider area than either of the other two methods.

RELATED FACTORS

Successful local anesthesia depends on a number of factors, including proper technique, nerve size (diameter), adequate concentration of anesthetic agent, and local tissue conditions. Obviously, to be effective, the anesthetic agent must be deposited near a nerve. This is particularly important when performing a nerve block.

Generally, the larger the cross-sectional diameter of a nerve is, the higher the concentration of anesthetic agent to effect a block must be. Tissue vascularity may affect diffusion and absorption of the drug. Drug dilution results from local tissue fluid and impairs or delays the action of the anesthetic agent. One other important factor is tissue pH. The concentration of anesthetic agent is directly proportional to pH. This is especially evident in patients with an infected lesion, such as a felon or paronychia, around which acid metabolites may collect producing a significant drop in pH which hinders the effects of digital nerve block.

ANESTHETIC AGENTS

A number of drugs are available for local anesthesia. It is unnecessary for a physician to become familiar with all such agents; rather, he should become well versed in the use of one or two agents for infiltration and a similar number for topical use. Only four of the more commonly used drugs will be mentioned. These are procaine, lidocaine, bupivacaine and mepivacaine which are used as a chloride or sulfate salt, and available in concentrations varying from 0.25 percent (2.5 mg per cc) to 2.0 percent (20 mg per cc). One should be aware of the total dosage of drug used and be guided by the principle of using the smallest concentration and smallest total dose required to achieve the maximal desired effect. The suggested maximum dosages of the agents listed above is shown in the following table. The dosages mentioned are for the mythical average 70 kg Human. Obviously, the total dose will be less in infants, children, and small adults and greater in a 100 to 125 kg man.

DRUG	DOSAGE	TOTAL DOSE	DURATION OF ACTION
Procaine	14 mg/kg	1000 mg	¾-1½ hrs.
Lidocaine	7 mg/kg	500 mg	1½-2 hrs.
Bupivacaine	3 mg/kg	200 mg	4-6 hrs.
Mepivacaine	7 mg/kg	500 mg	2-3 hrs.

Because of its vasoconstrictor effect, epinephrine may be added to the anesthetic solution to delay absorption, prolong the onset and extend the duration of the anesthesia, and lessen vascularity of the part. The anesthetic-vasoconstrictor combination is available commercially. Epinephrine is added in a 1:100,000 or 1:200,000 solution. This combination drug is particularly valuable for field block in highly vascular areas, such as the scalp, because it diminishes bleeding at the operative site. It should also be considered when prolonged anesthesia is needed because of the number and/or size of the lesion(s).

Epinephrine should be used with caution in patients with hypertensive or cardiac disease and in those receiving antidepressant medication, such as imipramine or protriptyline, or monoamine oxidase inhibitors. Even in normal patients, excessive amounts of epinephrine may produce tachycardia, hypertension, apprehension and precordial oppression. (See section on Adverse Reactions.) Under no circumstances should epinephrine-anesthetic drug combinations be used for digital nerve block for operative procedures on the fingers or toes. The vessels in these areas are end arteries with no significant collateral circulation. The vasoconstrictor can produce local vascular spasm with resulting gangrene of the digit(s).

EQUIPMENT

The local anesthesia procedures described in this section can be used in the emergency setting without any special equipment.

The local set used for each block consists of the following items:
1. 5 and 10 cc syringes
2. 25-gauge ⅝-inch needle
3. 22-gauge 1½-inch needle
4. Gauze sponges
5. Antiseptic skin prep
6. Sterile towels
7. Medicine glass

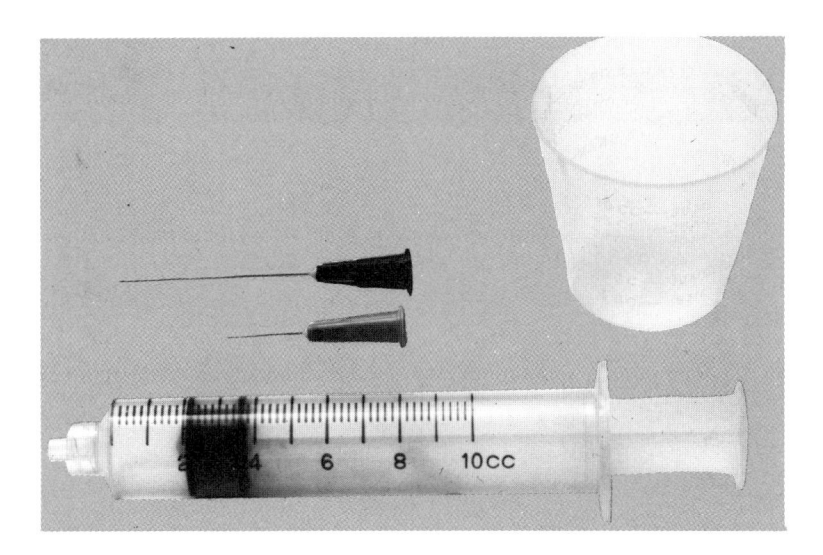

On occasion, when the depth of the tissue to be anesthetized is greater than the 1½-inch needle a 22-gauge 3½-inch spinal type needle can be used. The smallest gauge needle should be used to deliver the anesthetic drug to the operative site in order to minimize patient discomfort.

TECHNIQUE

Prior to initiating the anesthesia make an effort to allay anxiety in the patient by briefly explaining the procedure. In small children and apprehensive adults, some form of premedication is very helpful. For children give secobarbital 1 mg per kg of body weight intramuscularly 10 to 15 minutes before starting the procedure. In adults, diazepam 5 mg given slowly intravenously is extremely effective. Immobilize small children to prevent injury. A Papoose Board serves this purpose very well.

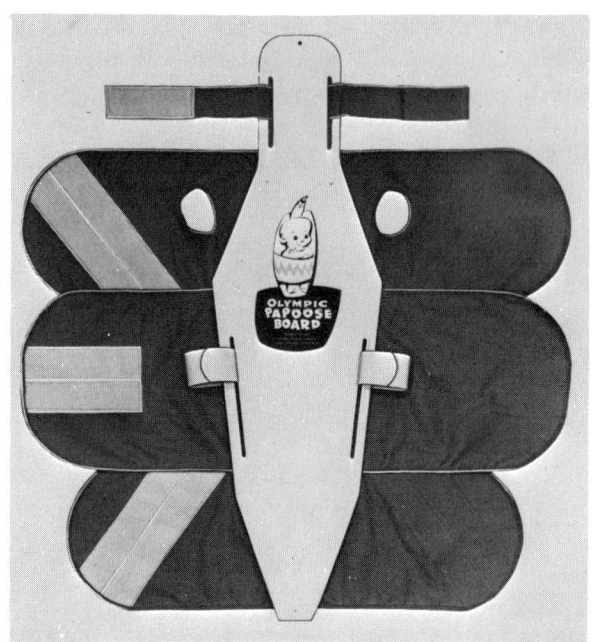

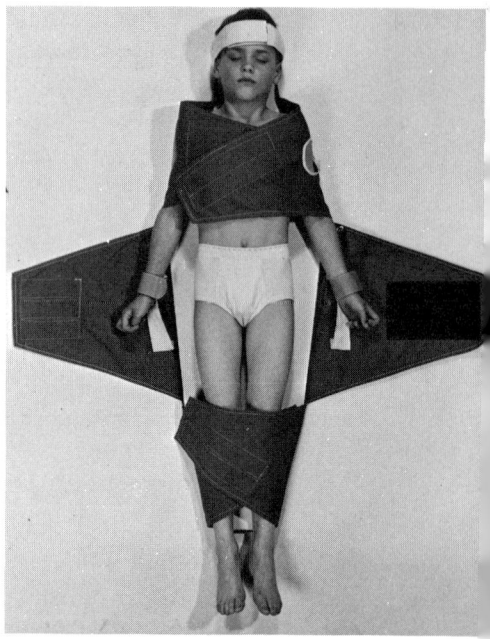

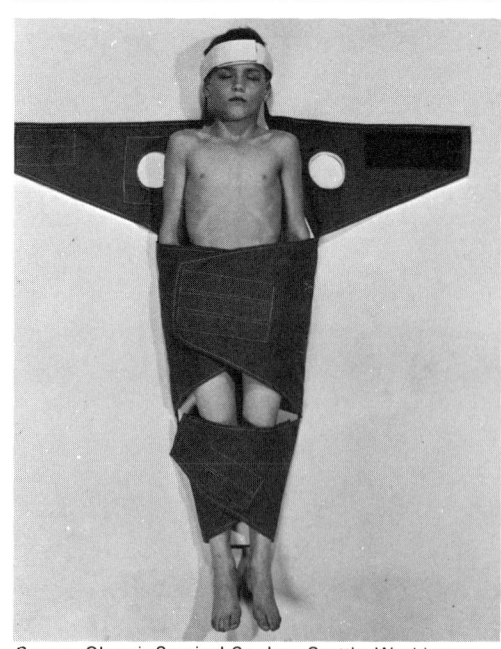

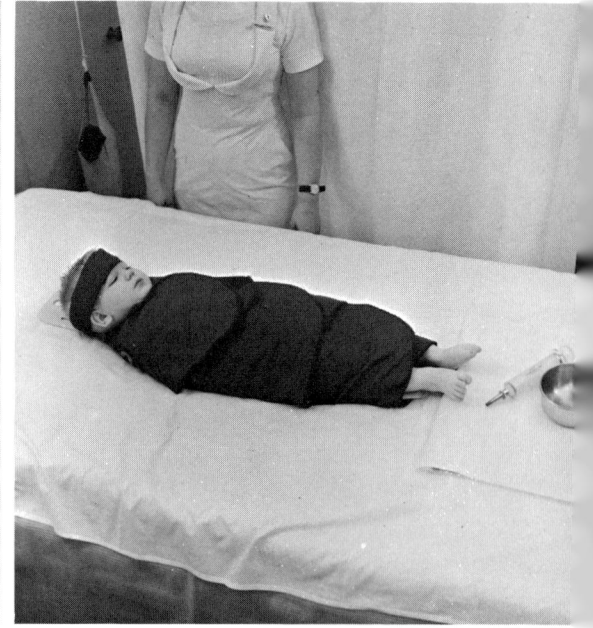

Source: Olympic Surgical Co., Inc., Seattle, Washington

Injection of drugs into the skin and deeper tissues initially causes local pain usually described as a burning sensation. Many blocks are initiated with a skin wheal using a 25-gauge ⁵/₈-inch needle to minimize pain. Introduce the larger 22-gauge 1¹/₂-inch needle through the wheal. Making the skin wheal itself produces a certain amount of pain. For this reason, in some of the block procedures described, the suggestion is made to omit this step.

Once the block procedure is completed, allow a minimum of three to five minutes to pass, then test the area for pin prick sensation. Do not start the operative procedure until complete anesthesia of the operative site has been achieved.

In many emergency departments, as an economy measure, the anesthetic solution is drawn from a multiple-dose vial prior to use. If more drug is needed, additional amounts are withdrawn during the course of the procedure. This technique is viewed by some as a violation of principles of surgical asepsis. A better method is to estimate the total amount of drug to be used and withdraw it by multiple aspirations as needed and place it in a sterile medicine glass on the set to be used as required.

The procedures described are not difficult. As one gains experience with each block, the advantages of this approach will be obvious. This section is not meant to be a comprehensive review of local anesthesia techniques. Rather, attention is paid to nerve blocks which, in the author's experience, are frequently used or of special value in the emergency setting.

ADVERSE REACTIONS

A patient may experience an adverse reaction to a local anesthetic agent for one of many reasons. The foremost is that the patient is known to have a history of hypersensitivity to it. This information should be elicited from the patient prior to injection of the drug.

Other causes of adverse reactions include a diminished tolerance to the drug or inordinately high plasma levels which may follow rapid absorption or accidental intravascular injection of the agent or excessive dosage of the drug.

Reactions are usually systemic and affect the central nervous and cardiorespiratory systems. Unrecognized or untreated, such reactions may be fatal. As a precaution, resuscitative equipment and appropriate drugs should be readily available whenever a local anesthetic agent is used.

The reader is referred to standard pharmacology tests for additional information.

BIBLIOGRAPHY

Adriani, J. Nerve Blocks. Springfield: Charles C Thomas, 1954.
Banks, S. W. and Laufman, H. L. An Atlas of Surgical Exposures of the Extremities. Philadelphia: W. B. Saunders Co., 1953.
Bunnell, S. Surgery of the Hand. Philadelphia: J. B. Lippincott Co., ed. 3, 1956.
Chase, R. A. Surgical Anatomy of the Hand. Surg. Clin. N. Am. 44:1349, 1964.
Henry, A. K. Extensile Exposure. Baltimore: The Williams & Wilkins Co., ed. 2, 1957.
de Jong, R. H. Physiology and Pharmacology of Local Anesthesia. Springfield: Charles C Thomas, 2nd Print., 1974.
Moore, D. C. Regional Block. Springfield: Charles C Thomas, ed. 2, 1957.

40 FIELD BLOCK

INDICATIONS
1. Anesthesia of the skin and underlying tissue for debridement and repair of accidental incised wounds (lacerations).
2. Removal of imbedded foreign bodies.
3. Elective excision of lesions of the skin or subcutaneous tissue.
4. Incision and drainage of an abscess.
5. Biopsy of the skin and underlying tissues.
6. Exploration of superficial wounds of the skin and underlying tissue.

EQUIPMENT
1. Local set (see page 181)
2. 1% anesthetic agent

ANATOMICAL CONSIDERATIONS
1. Regional anesthesia by field block is achieved by injecting the anesthetic agent on all sides and deep to the operative site, while avoiding injection of the lesion itself. Local infiltration implies the injection of the anesthetic directly into the line of incision of the wound itself.
2. An incised or open accidental wound should <u>not</u> be injected, especially when grossly contaminated, for contaminated tissue or materials may be introduced or forced into surrounding clean tissues, producing sepsis.
3. The operative site is identified and an imaginary triangle or diamond drawn about it to enclose the entire lesion.
4. To minimize pain or discomfort to the patient, a skin wheal should be raised at the points of the triangle or diamond using a 25-gauge needle. Once this is done, the larger bore, longer needle may be used to infiltrate the deeper tissues along imaginary lines connecting the skin wheals. The total area of

infiltration should include an area conforming roughly to the shape of an inverted pyramid, so that the anesthetic agent is deposited in the tissues surrounding and deep to the lesion.

5. Intravascular injection of the anesthetic agent is to be avoided at all times. This can be minimized to a great extent by gently aspirating the syringe before each injection. The aspiration is done in two planes. Once the injection site in the deeper tissues is entered, the plunger of the syringe is withdrawn. If no blood is recovered, the syringe is rotated 180 degrees clockwise and aspirated again. If no blood is recovered, the agent may be injected.

   If blood is recovered, the agent should <u>not</u> be injected. The needle is withdrawn a few millimeters and repositioned in the area to be infiltrated and the above maneuver repeated until no blood is aspirated.

PROCEDURE

1. Cleanse the wound or skin of the operative site with an antiseptic soap, such as povidone-iodine.
2. Shave any hair about the area with the exception of the eyebrow which may not regrow.
3. Prep the area with povidone-iodine and drape. The area thus prepared should measure at least 3 inches wide about the edges of the wound or planned incision.
4. Draw an imaginary triangle or diamond about the lesion and, using the 25-gauge needle attached to the syringe, raise a skin wheal at each point of the geometric figure. Introduce the needle quickly with the face of the bevel down into the dermis (the layer of the skin beneath the epidermis) and parallel to the surface of the skin.

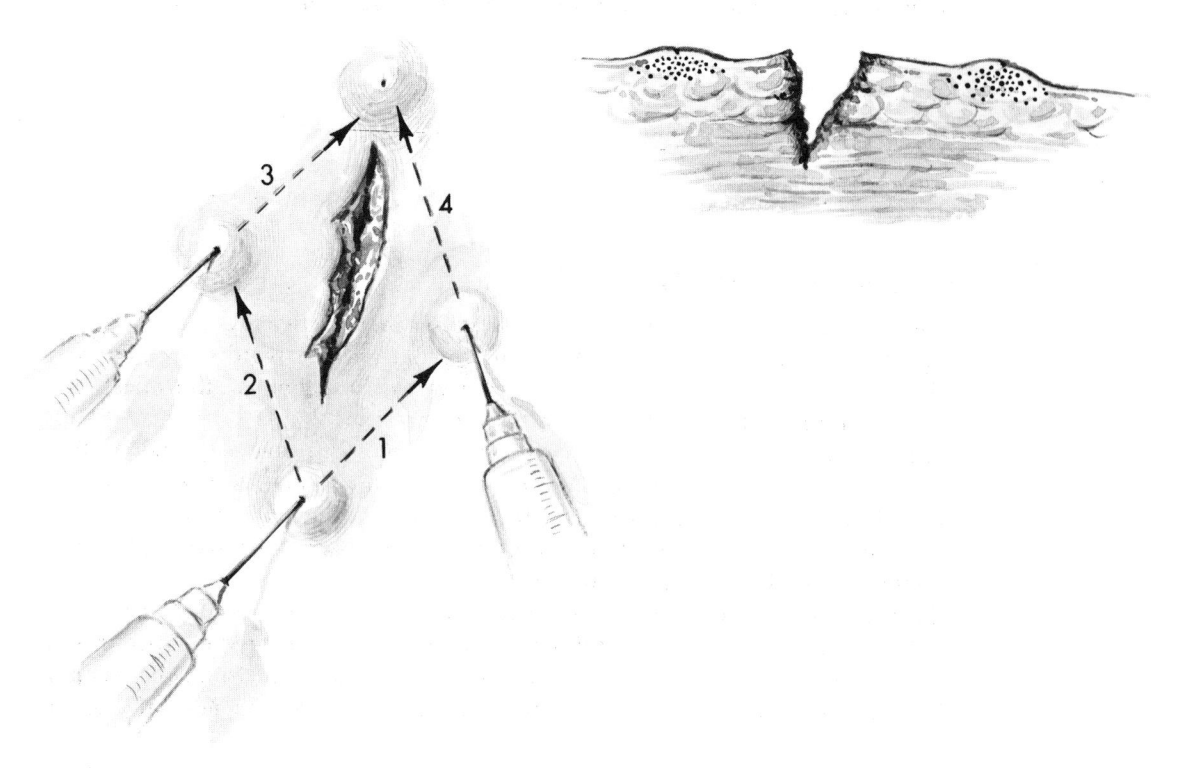

5. Inject 0.2 to 0.3 cc of anesthetic agent until the skin blanches and a small raised area appears which resembles an orange peel. This raised area is the wheal and should measure approximately 1 cm in diameter.
6. During this portion of the procedure, the patient may experience a rather intense burning sensation at the injection site. Advance preparation of the patient and calm reassurance by the physician may allay undue fear, apprehension, and pain.
7. After developing the appropriate wheals, replace the 25-gauge needle with the 22-gauge 1½-inch needle.
8. Introduce this syringe-needle assembly into one wheal and penetrate to the subcutaneous tissue at a 45-degree angle. Aspirate in two planes, and, if no blood is recovered, inject a small amount of solution (0.5 cc).
9. Continue to introduce the needle in the direction of an adjacent wheal, alternately aspirating and injecting the solution along this line until the next wheal is reached. As the injection continues, palpate the skin overlying the tip of the needle to identify the solution in the subcutaneous tissue and be sure the lesion is completely surrounded.
10. To minimize patient discomfort, introduce the larger needle through the skin only at the site of the skin wheal.
11. Upon completion of the ring injection, redirect the needle to the tissues deep to the lesion and deposit some anesthetic agent after aspiration.

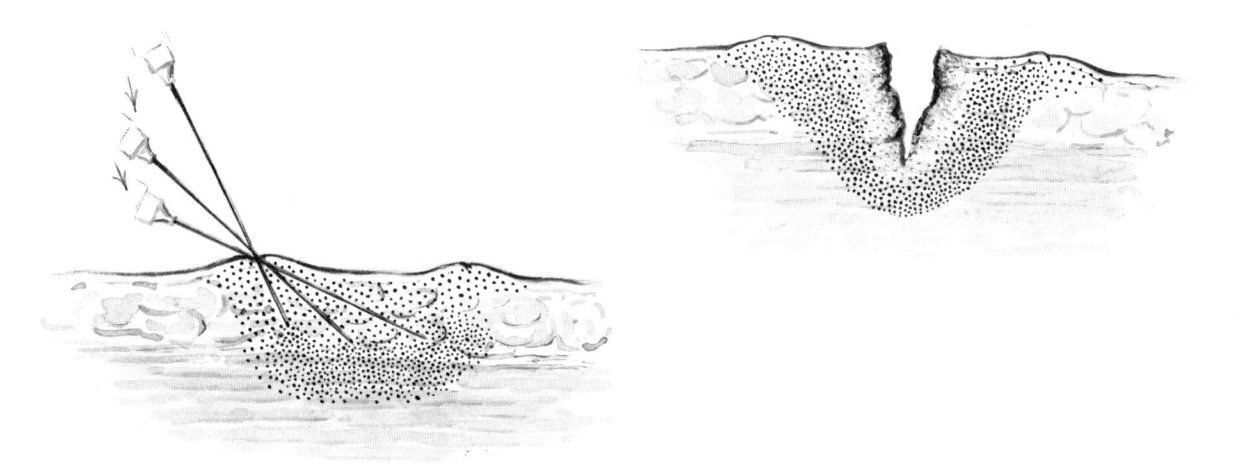

12. When the field block is completed, test the skin within the area for pin prick sensation using the point of the needle. Before proceeding, wait until the pin prick is no longer detected by the patient, usually in 3 to 5 minutes.

NOTE: If a large area must be blocked, keep in mind the total dose of anesthetic agent used, to minimize untoward reactions. For this type of block, a dilute solution (0.25%) is all that is required. The effect of the agent may be prolonged by the addition of epinephrine 1:100,000. In vascular areas, such as the scalp, the use of anesthetic agent with epinephrine will produce local vasoconstriction and thus lessen bleeding from the operative site. Avoid placing the anesthetic agent too close to the edges of the laceration or incision site to minimize tissue swelling.

41 SUPRAORBITAL NERVE BLOCK

INDICATION
Anesthesia of the upper eyelid and the medial aspect of the frontal area.

EQUIPMENT
1. Local set (see page 181)
2. 1% anesthetic agent

ANATOMICAL CONSIDERATIONS
1. The supraorbital nerve lies in a groove easily palpated on the superior rim of the orbit approximately 2.5 cm from the midline of the face.

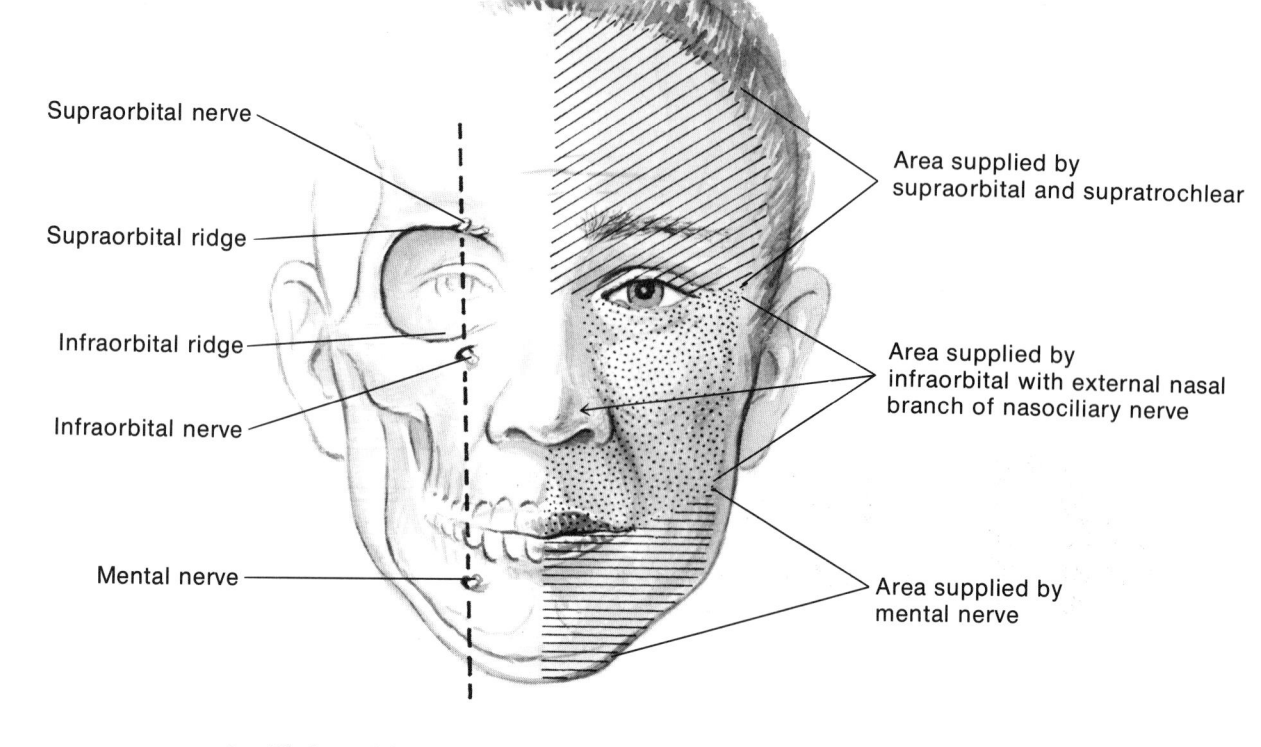

Labels on diagram:
- Supraorbital nerve
- Supraorbital ridge
- Infraorbital ridge
- Infraorbital nerve
- Mental nerve
- Area supplied by supraorbital and supratrochlear
- Area supplied by infraorbital with external nasal branch of nasociliary nerve
- Area supplied by mental nerve

2. If the midline of the frontal area is to be anesthetized, the supratrochlear nerve must also be blocked. This nerve lies just medial to the supraorbital nerve.

PROCEDURE

1. Prep the skin about the eyebrow and upper eyelid with povidone-iodine.
2. Palpate the supraorbital ridge and identify the notch in which the supraorbital nerve courses. This notch is located approximately 2.5 cm on either side of the midline.

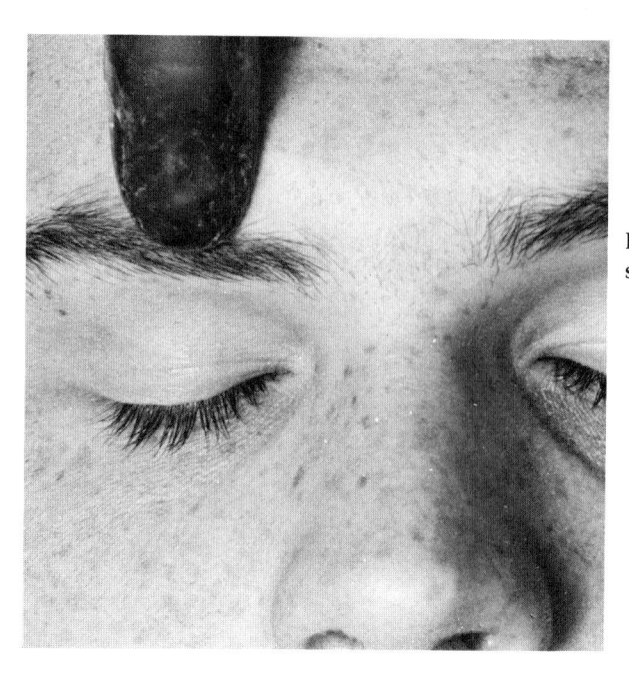

Finger palpation of supraorbital notch

3. Draw 5 cc of anesthetic agent into the syringe.
4. Attach the 25-gauge needle to the syringe, introduce it into the skin directly over the supraorbital ridge, and advance it to the frontal bone. If the nerve is touched by the needle, the patient may note a paresthesia of the frontal area.
5. Aspirate in two planes.

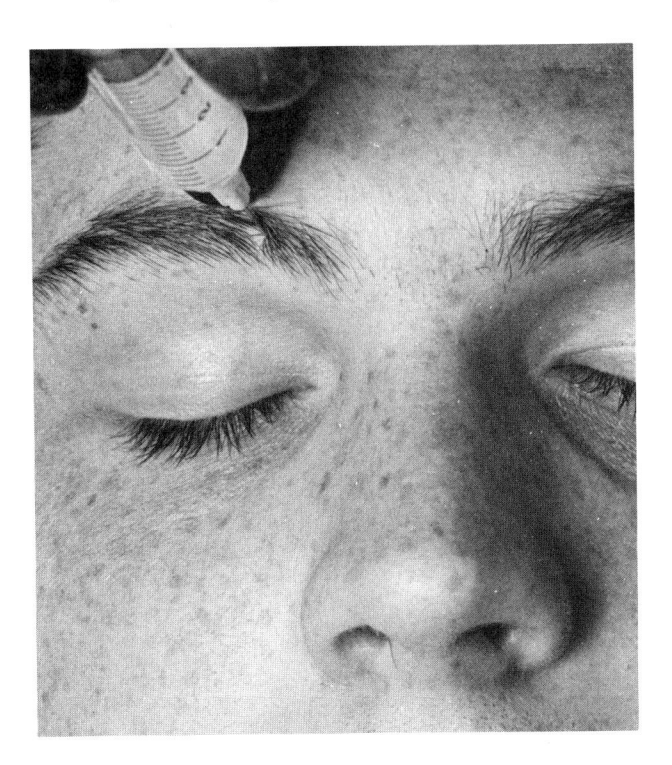

6. If no blood is recovered, inject 2 to 3 cc of anesthetic agent. This should effectively block the nerve.
7. Redirect the needle medially and inject 2 to 3 cc of anesthetic agent along the medial half of the supraorbital ridge to block the supratrochlear nerve.

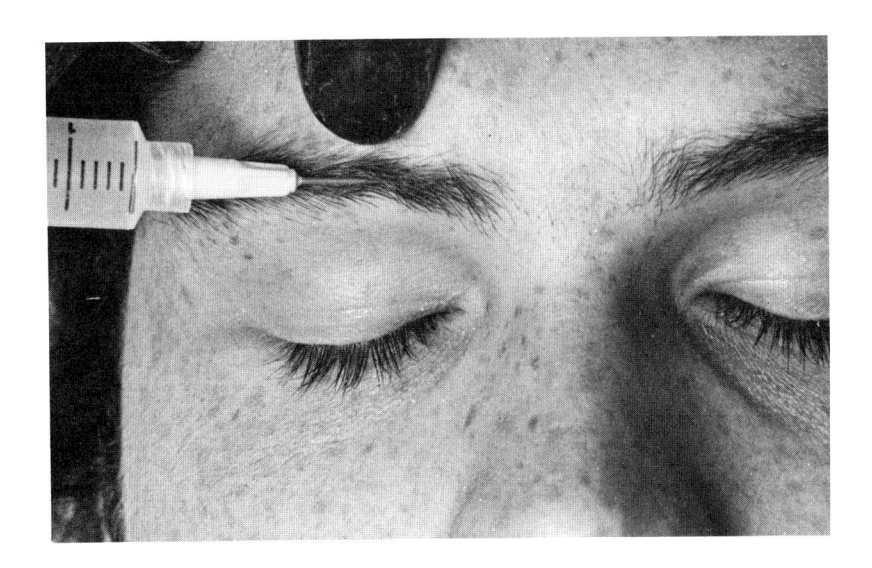

42 INFRAORBITAL NERVE BLOCK

INDICATION
Anesthesia of the lower eyelid, infraorbital region, and upper lip.

EQUIPMENT
1. Local set (see page 181)
2. 1% anesthetic agent

ANATOMICAL CONSIDERATIONS
1. The infraorbital nerve emerges from the infraorbital foramen and branches to supply the skin of the lower lid, infraorbital area, upper lip, and nose (with the terminal branches of the nasociliary nerve.

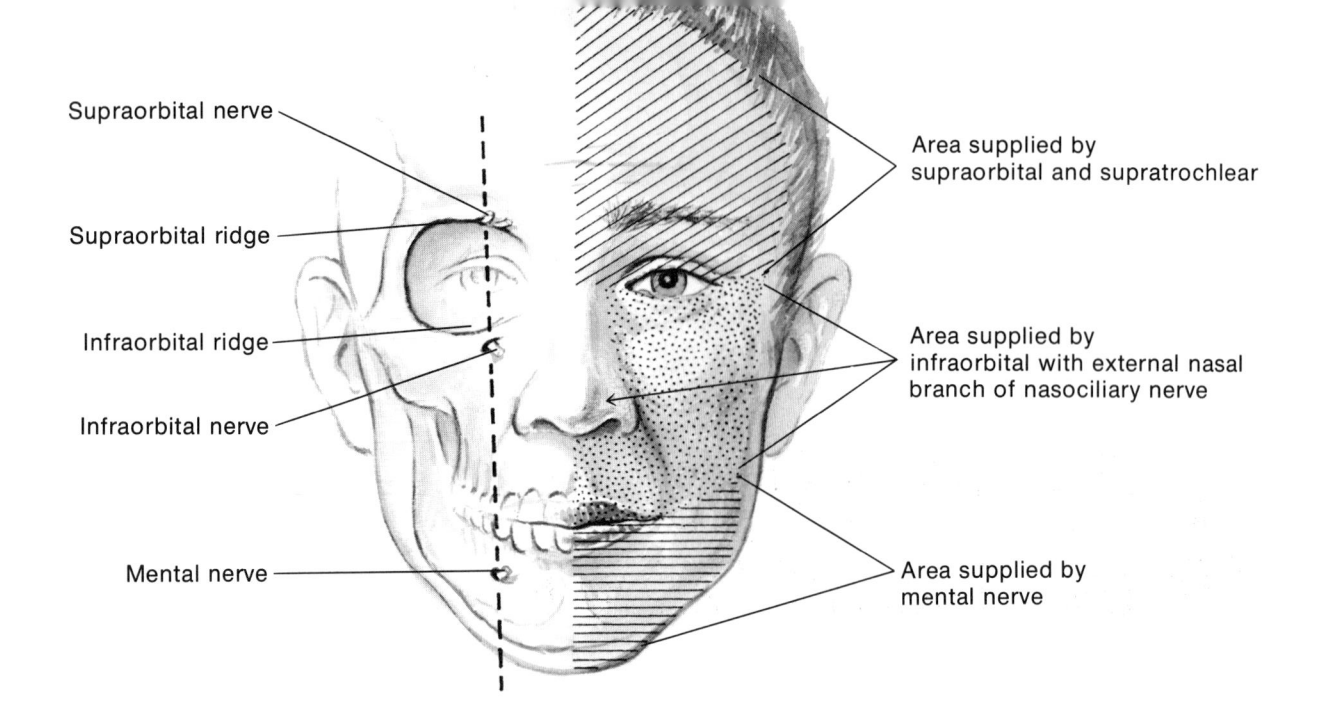

Supraorbital nerve
Supraorbital ridge
Infraorbital ridge
Infraorbital nerve
Mental nerve

Area supplied by supraorbital and supratrochlear

Area supplied by infraorbital with external nasal branch of nasociliary nerve

Area supplied by mental nerve

2. The infraorbital foramen is located just below the infraorbital ridge approximately 2.5 cm lateral to the midline of the face. It is felt as a small depression in this area.
3. The infraorbital canal courses upward and backward at an angle of 45 degrees and laterally 25 degrees.

PROCEDURE

1. Prep the skin of the cheek with povidone-iodine.
2. With the index finger of the left hand, identify the infraorbital foramen.

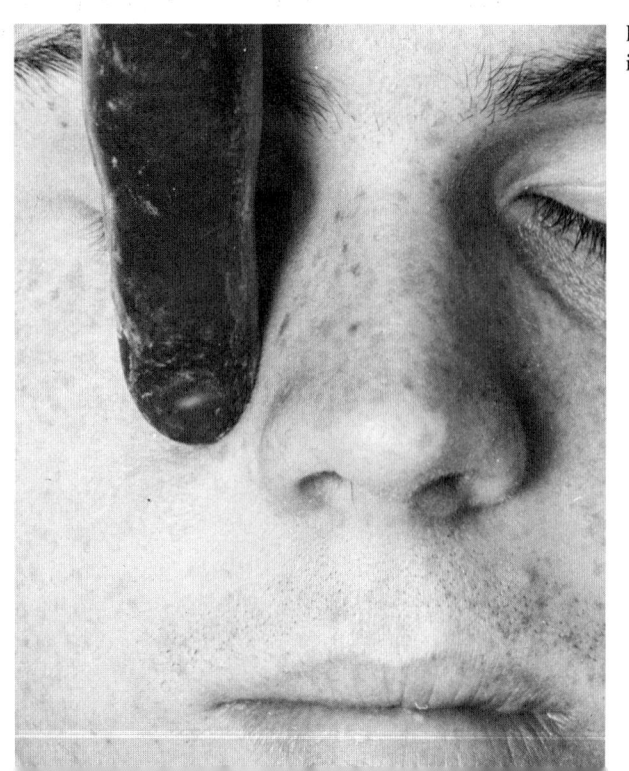

Finger palpation of infraorbital foramen

3. Attach the 25-gauge needle to the syringe and introduce this through the skin into the infraorbital foramen. (The needle should be inserted at an angle of 45 degrees to the skin and 25 degrees medial to an imaginary perpendicular line joining the supraorbital notch and the infraorbital and mental foramina.) When the nerve is touched, a paresthesia will be elicited along the distribution of the nerve. While some prefer to raise a skin wheal prior to probing the foramen, the author has found that this may subsequently hinder locating the foramen.

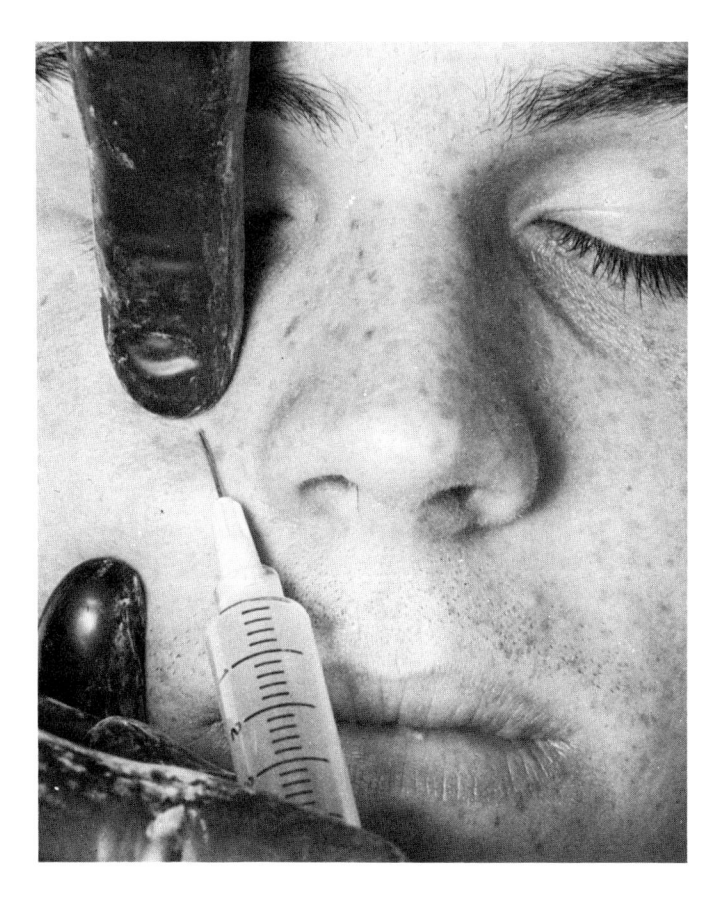

4. When the foramen is entered, inject 1 to 2 cc of anesthetic agent into the canal. Do not advance the needle into the foramen more than ¼ inch to avoid damage to the contents of the orbit.

NOTE: For anesthesia of the skin of the nose, the external nasal branches of the nasociliary nerve must be blocked. This can be done by swabbing the mucosa of the nose using cotton-tipped applicators dipped in 4% cocaine or 2% pontocaine.

43 MENTAL NERVE BLOCK

INDICATION
Anesthesia of the skin and mucous membranes of the area of the mandible and lower anterior teeth.

EQUIPMENT
1. Local set (see page 181)
2. 1% anesthetic agent

ANATOMICAL CONSIDERATIONS
1. The mental nerve emerges from the mental foramen and branches to supply the skin of the lower lip and jaw.
2. The mental foramen is located approximately 2.5 cm lateral to the midline of the face. It can be located easily by drawing an imaginary vertical line between the lower bicuspid teeth, perpendicular to the inferior margin of the mandible. The midpoint between the upper and lower borders of the mandible is identified and an imaginary line drawn through this point, perpendicular to the vertical line. The mental foramen is located at the point of intersection of these two lines.

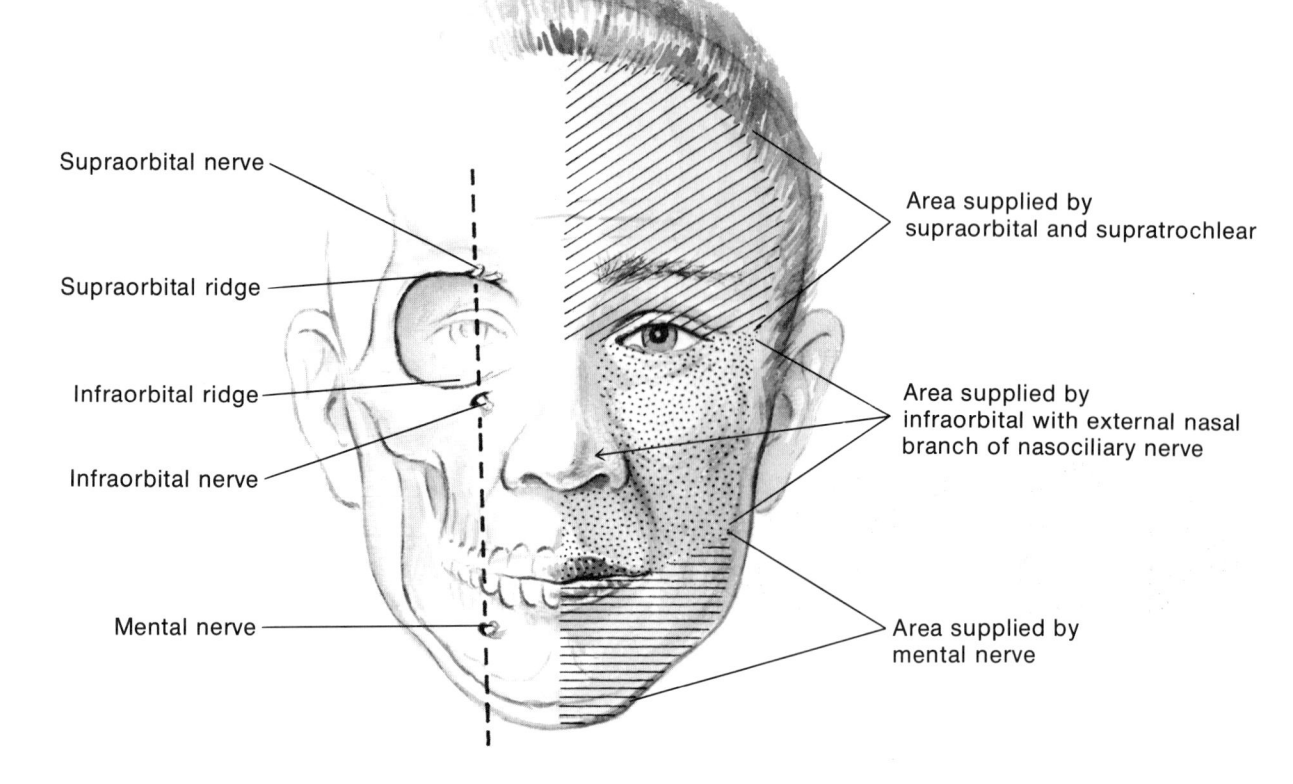

Labels on diagram:
- Supraorbital nerve
- Supraorbital ridge
- Infraorbital ridge
- Infraorbital nerve
- Mental nerve
- Area supplied by supraorbital and supratrochlear
- Area supplied by infraorbital with external nasal branch of nasociliary nerve
- Area supplied by mental nerve

3. The mental foramen should be cannulated at an angle of 45 degrees to the skin.
4. For anesthesia near the midline of the chin or lower lip, bilateral mental nerve block is necessary because of overlapping innervation.

PROCEDURE

1. Prep the skin of the lower cheek and jaw with povidone-iodine.
2. Identify the mental foramen with the left index finger.

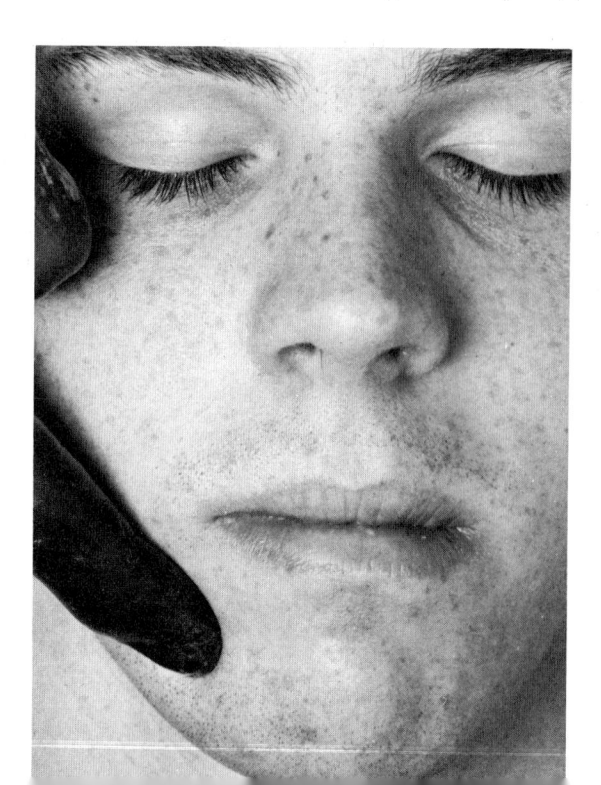

3. Using a 25-gauge needle, penetrate the skin of the lower jaw at a 45-degree angle downward and parallel to the horizontal ramus of the mandible and enter the mental foramen. Use of this small-bore needle can be painless and obviates the need for a skin wheal which may obscure identification of the mental foramen.

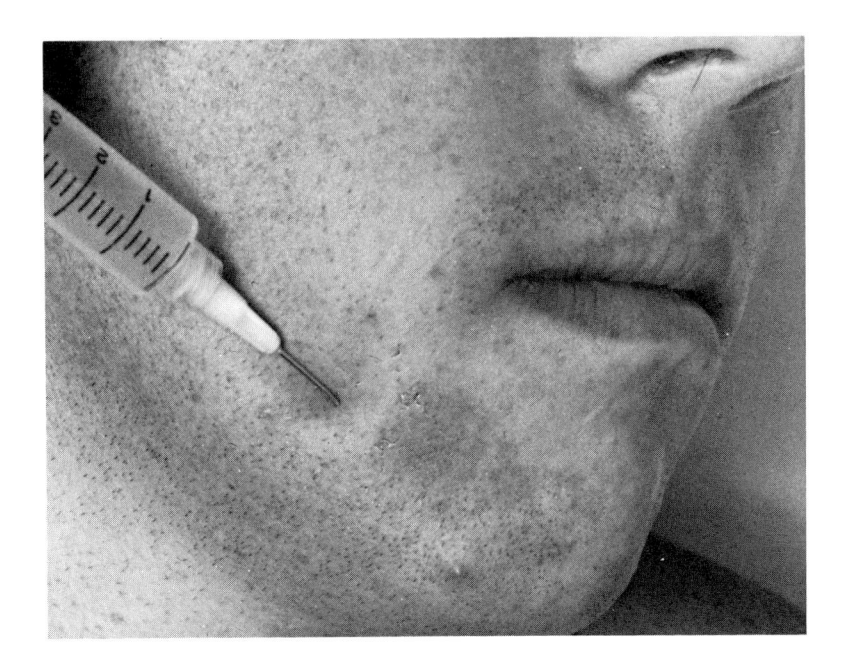

4. A paresthesia may be elicited in the distribution of the mental nerves.
5. Inject 2 cc of 1% anesthetic agent.
6. Repeat the procedure on the opposite side if anesthesia is required close to the midline.

44 INTERCOSTAL NERVE BLOCK

INDICATIONS
1. Fractures of the chest wall, ribs, or costal cartilages.
2. Severe contusion of the chest wall.

EQUIPMENT
1. Local set (see page 181)
2. 1% anesthetic agent

ANATOMICAL CONSIDERATIONS
1. The intercostal nerve lies deep to the interior margin of each rib, in company with the intercostal artery and vein (intercostal neurovascular bundle).

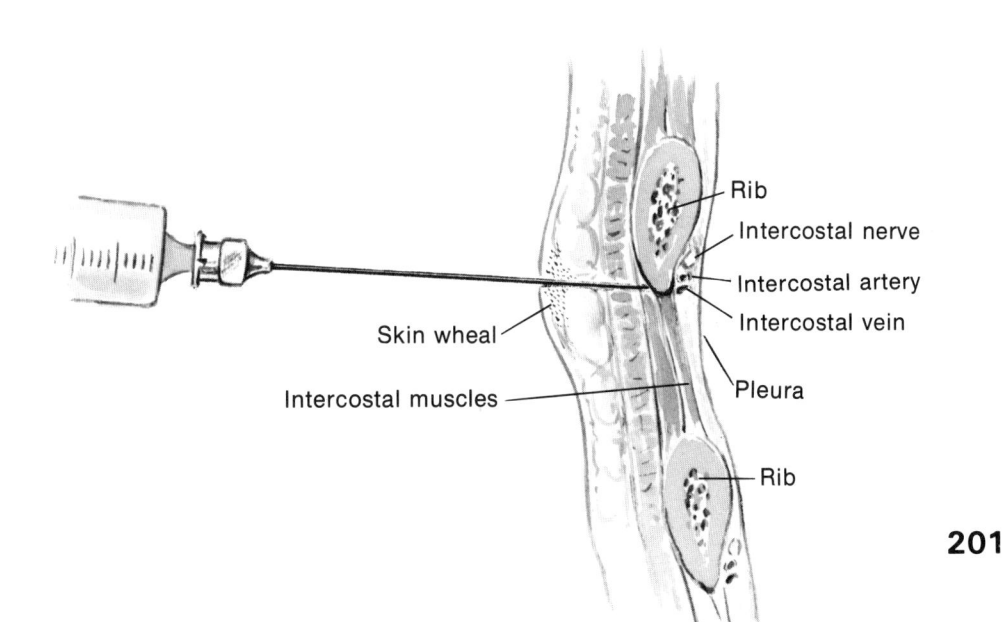

2. The nerve should be blocked between the site of fracture or injury and the root of the nerve.
3. The block should be injected in the axillary line or near the posterior angle of the rib where the least amount of overlying muscle is encountered.

PROCEDURE

1. Infiltrate the intercostal nerve serving each fractured rib, along with the nerve serving the rib immediately above and below the level of fracture. When several intercostal nerves are to be blocked, keep in mind the total amount of anesthetic agent delivered to the patient.
2. Identify the level of rib fracture by clinical examination and x-ray studies.
3. Palpate the rib to identify the nerve(s) to be blocked.
4. Raise a skin wheal over each rib which corresponds to the intercostal nerve to be blocked, using a small amount of anesthetic agent and a 25-gauge needle.
5. Attach a 21-gauge or 22-gauge needle to the syringe and introduce it through the skin wheal until the surface of the rib is encountered.

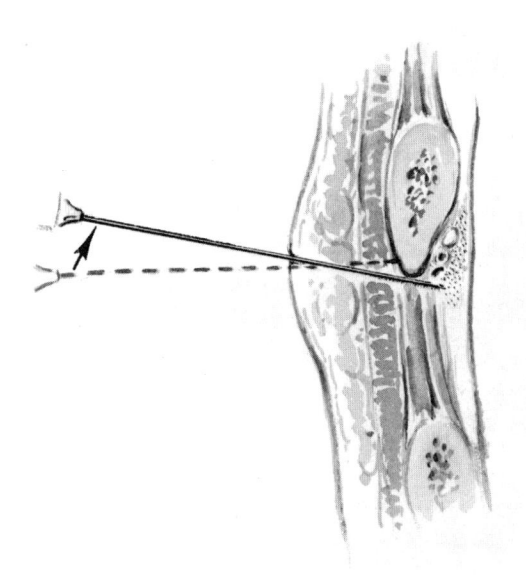

6. By gentle and careful manipulation alternately withdrawing the needle slightly and reinserting it in a more caudal direction, locate the lower margin of the rib. Then carefully introduce the needle 2 to 3 mm deeper to reach the depth of the intercostal nerve.
7. Aspirate in two planes (180 degrees) to be certain the needle is not in a vessel. Slowly inject 2 to 3 cc of anesthetic agent.
8. Repeat the procedure as indicated, to include one rib above and one below the level(s) of fracture.
9. Following the procedure, take an x-ray film of the chest to be certain a pneumothorax was not accidentally produced.

45 MEDIAN NERVE BLOCK

INDICATIONS
1. Repair of lacerations in parts of the hand in the distribution of the median nerve.
2. Minor surgical procedures involving the palm of the hand.

EQUIPMENT
1. Local set (see page 181)
2. 1% anesthetic agent

ANATOMICAL CONSIDERATIONS
1. The median nerve supplies sensation to the volar aspect of the thumb and of the index and middle fingers and the lateral one half of the ring finger.

Sensory distribution of median nerve

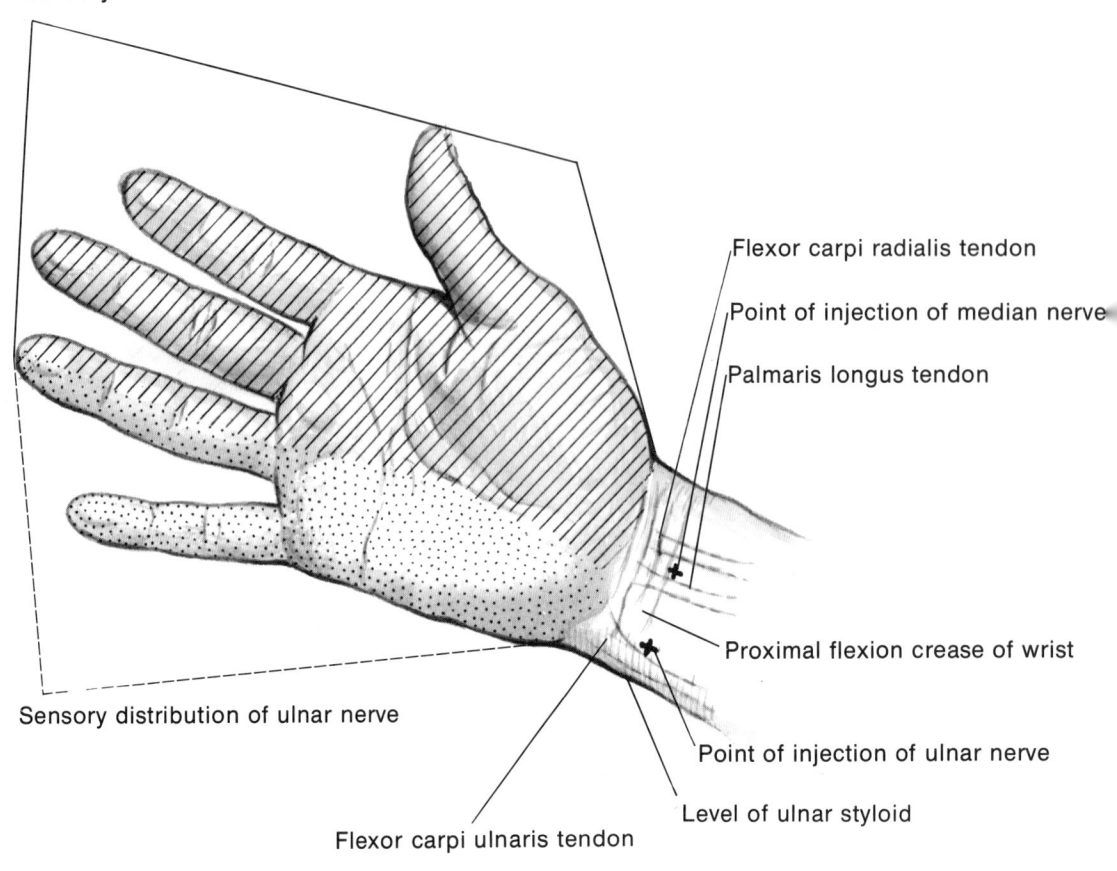

Flexor carpi radialis tendon
Point of injection of median nerve
Palmaris longus tendon
Proximal flexion crease of wrist
Point of injection of ulnar nerve
Level of ulnar styloid
Flexor carpi ulnaris tendon
Sensory distribution of ulnar nerve

2. The median nerve is usually blocked at the wrist.
3. The nerve at this level lies deep to the transverse carpal ligament in a position lateral to the palmaris longus tendon and medial to the flexor carpi radialis.
4. The palmaris longus tendon is easily identified by having the patient oppose the thumb and small finger with the wrist held in 20 to 30 degrees of flexion. It follows a longitudinal course in the midline of the volar aspect of the wrist.

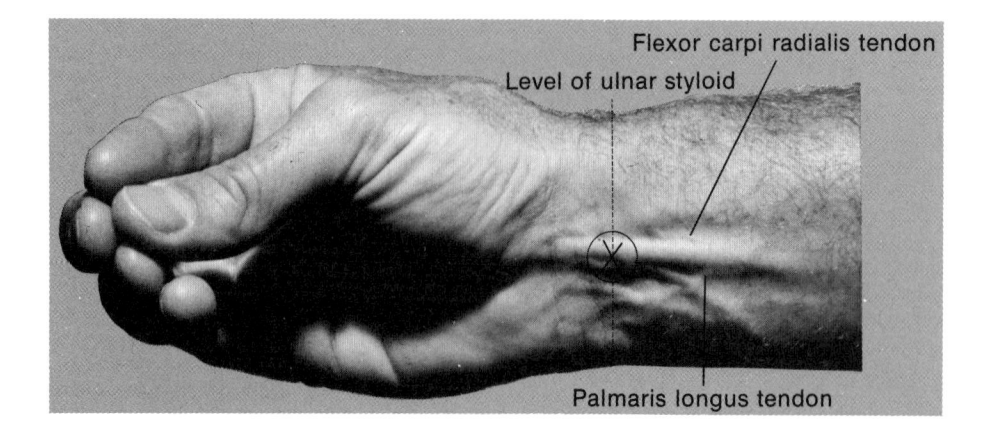

Flexor carpi radialis tendon
Level of ulnar styloid
Palmaris longus tendon

5. The flexor carpi radialis runs parallel and just lateral to the palmaris longus.
6. A narrow groove can be palpated between these two tendons. The nerve lies deep in this groove, beneath the transverse carpal ligament.
7. The injection should be made at the level of the proximal flexion crease of the wrist which is approximately at the level of the ulnar styloid.

NOTE: The radial and ulnar nerves may also be blocked at the same time, depending upon the innervation of the operative site.

PROCEDURE

1. Ask the patient to oppose the thumb and small finger and identify the groove between the palmaris longus and flexor carpi radialis tendons.
2. Draw an imaginary line transversely on the volar aspect of the wrist at the level of the ulnar styloid.
3. Prep the wrist with povidone-iodine.
4. Raise a skin wheal using the 25-gauge needle in the palmaris-radialis groove.
5. Introduce the 22-gauge needle through the skin wheal perpendicularly and penetrate the deep fascia.

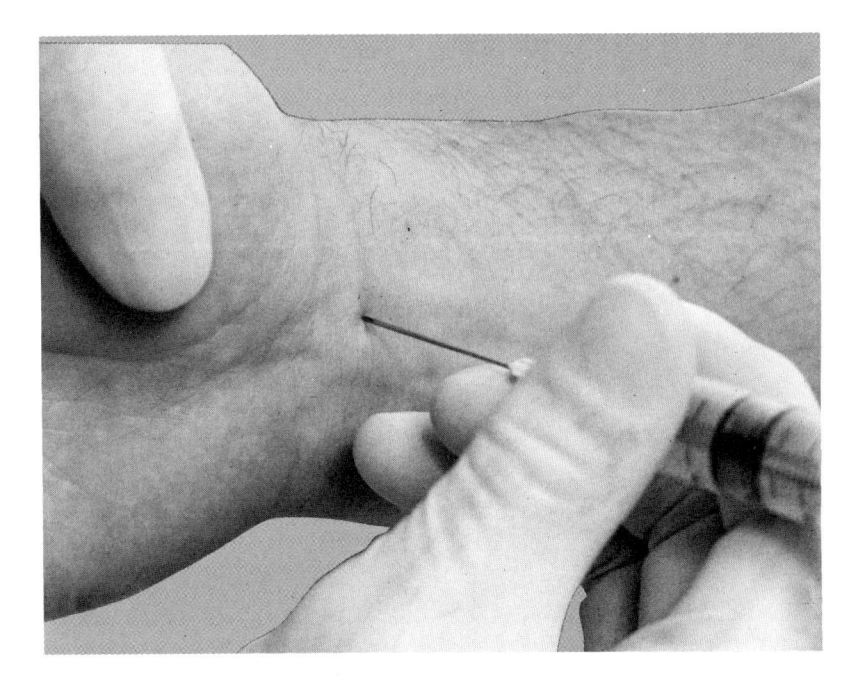

6. Inject 3 to 4 cc of 1% anesthetic agent after aspirating in two planes.
7. Withdraw the needle slightly and redirect it to a point deep to the flexor carpi radialis tendon and inject 2 to 3 cc of anesthetic agent at this point.
8. Gently massage the area to hasten diffusion of the anesthetic solution in the tissues.

46 RADIAL NERVE BLOCK

INDICATIONS
1. Repair of lacerations of the hand in the distribution of the radial nerve.
2. Minor surgical procedures involving the radial aspect of the dorsum of the hand.

EQUIPMENT
1. Local set (see page 181)
2. 1% anesthetic agent

ANATOMICAL CONSIDERATIONS
1. The radial nerve supplies sensation to the dorsum of the thumb and of the index and middle fingers and the lateral one half of the ring finger.

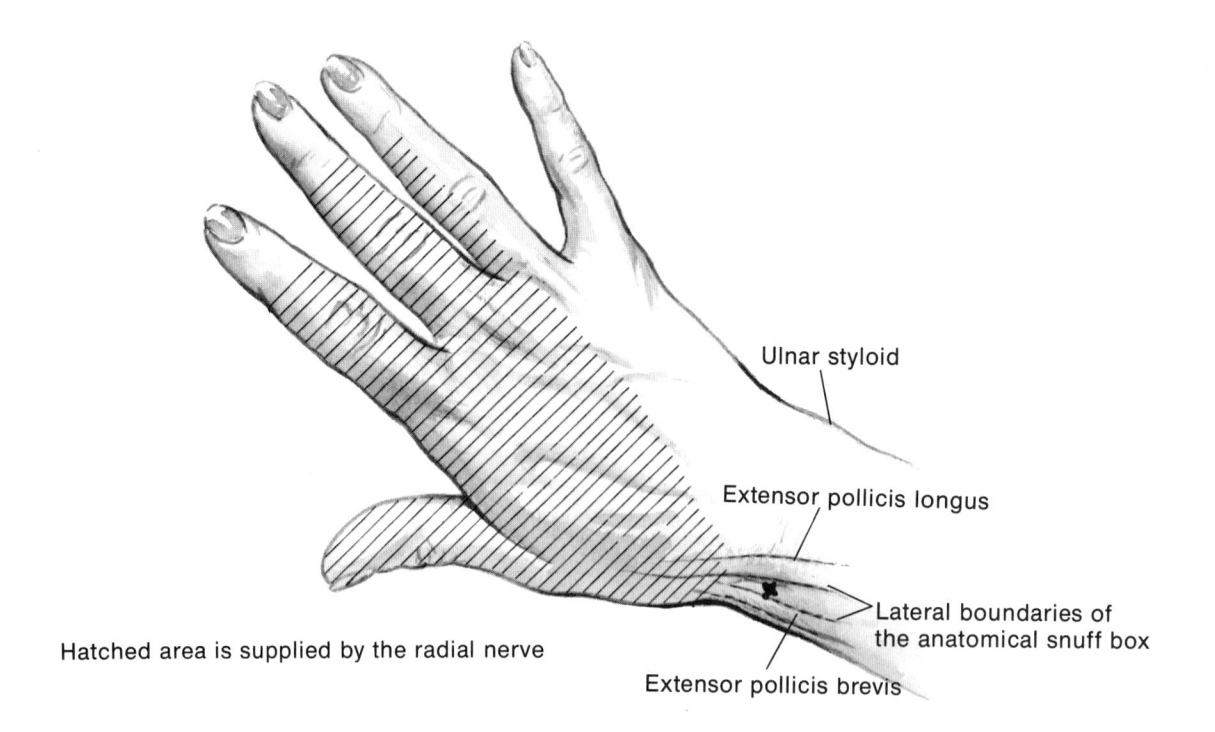

Hatched area is supplied by the radial nerve

Ulnar styloid
Extensor pollicis longus
Lateral boundaries of the anatomical snuff box
Extensor pollicis brevis

2. Just above the wrist, the radial nerve divides into lateral and medial branches.
3. The branches lie in proximity to the anatomical snuffbox.
4. The anatomical snuffbox is identified on the dorsolateral aspect of the wrist between the extensor pollicis longus and brevis tendons. These tendons are more easily seen and palpated by abduction and extension of the thumb.

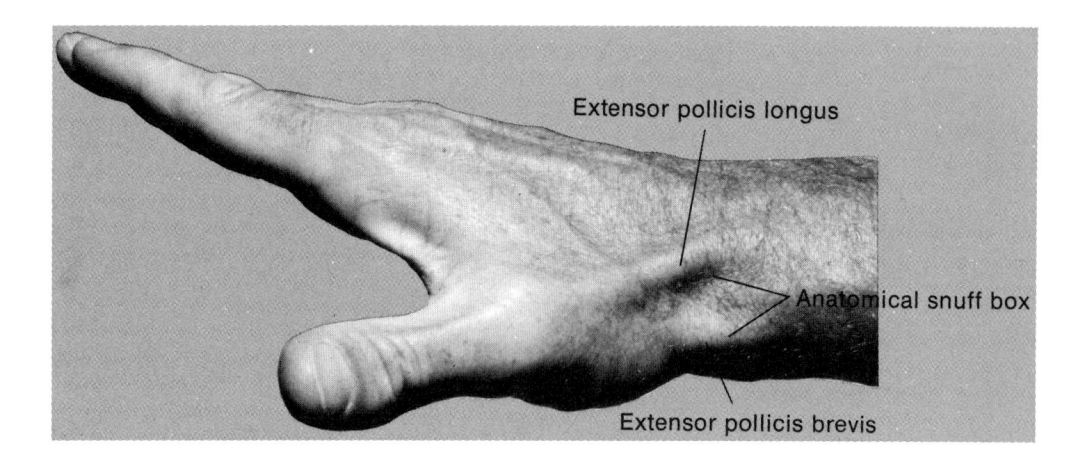

Extensor pollicis longus
Anatomical snuff box
Extensor pollicis brevis

PROCEDURE

1. Prep the hand with povidone-iodine.
2. Ask the patient to abduct and extend the thumb. Palpate the extensor tendons of the thumb forming the "snuffbox."
3. Raise a skin wheal using the 25-gauge needle at the base of the triangle just medial to the extensor pollicis brevis tendon.
4. Using the 22-gauge needle, infiltrate in a perpendicular line through the skin wheal to a depth of 1 to 2 cm with 2 cc of 1% lidocaine. This will effectively

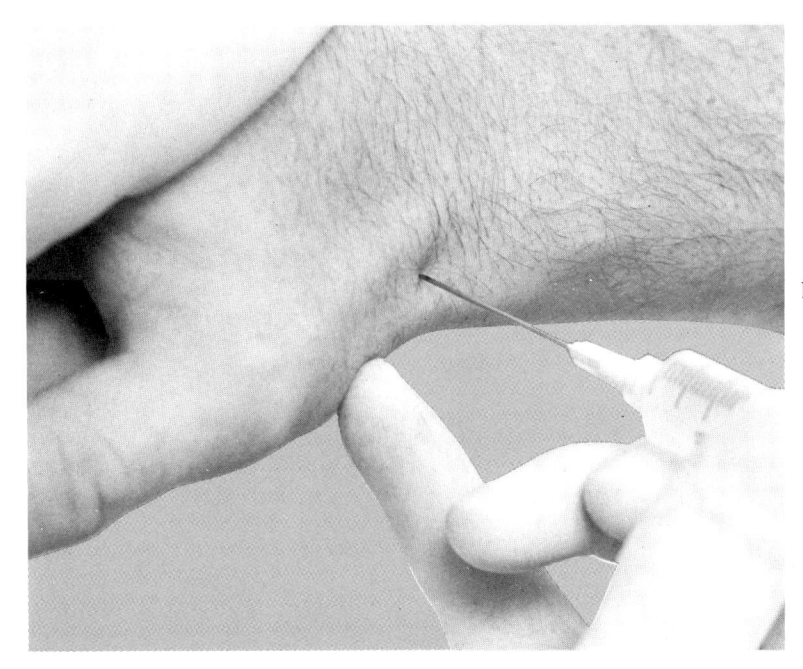

Lateral branch

block the lateral branch.
5. To block the medial branch, infiltrate along the lateral aspect of the extensor pollicis longus tendon.

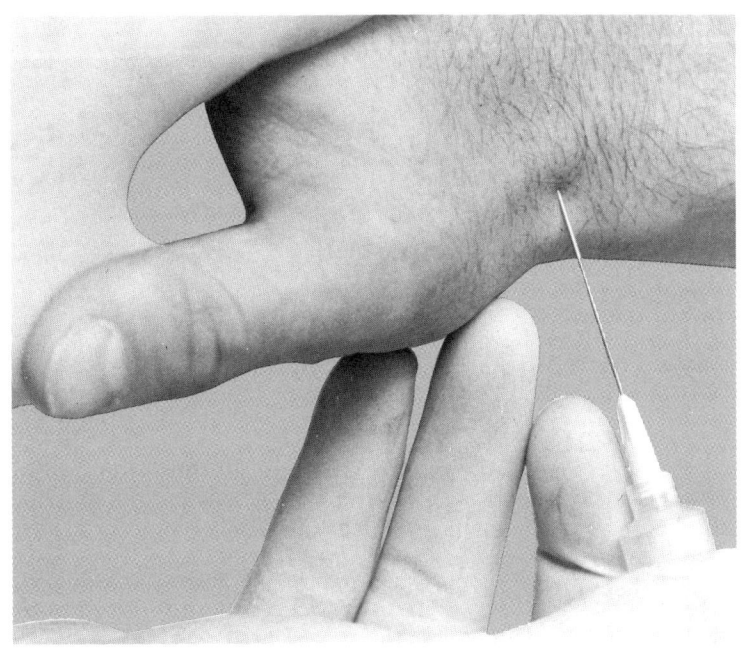

Medial branch

BIBLIOGRAPHY

Burton, R. L. and Kamell, W. M. Hand surgery: Distal conduction anesthesia. Contemp. Surg. 6:46, 1975.

47 ULNAR NERVE BLOCK

INDICATIONS
1. Repair of lacerations of the hand in the distribution of the ulnar nerve.
2. Minor surgical procedures involving the small finger.

EQUIPMENT
1. Local set (see page 181)
2. 1% anesthetic agent

ANATOMICAL CONSIDERATIONS
1. The ulnar nerve supplies motor sensation to the intrinsic muscles of the hand and sensation to the little finger and medial one half of the ring finger, both dorsal and volar aspects.

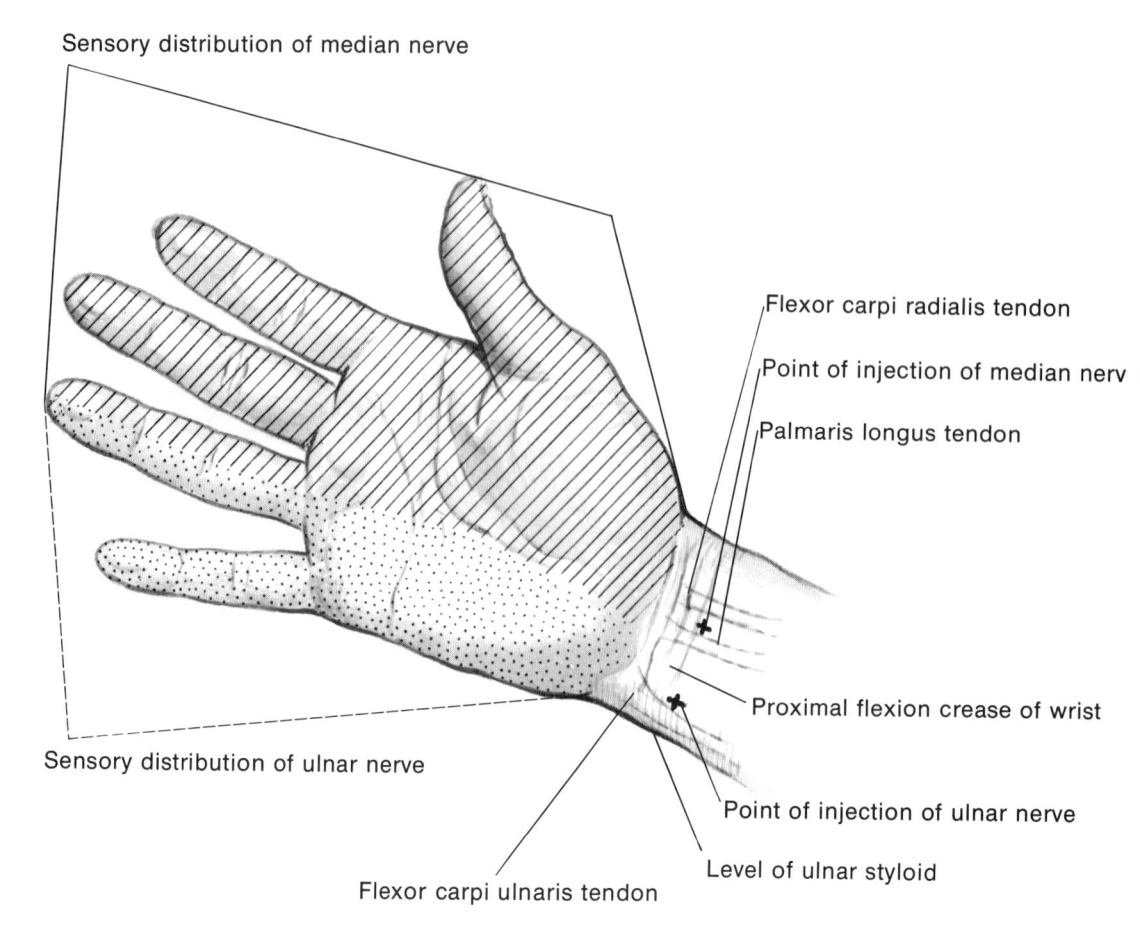

Sensory distribution of median nerve

Flexor carpi radialis tendon
Point of injection of median nerv
Palmaris longus tendon

Proximal flexion crease of wrist

Sensory distribution of ulnar nerve

Point of injection of ulnar nerve
Level of ulnar styloid
Flexor carpi ulnaris tendon

2. At the proximal flexion crease of the wrist (usually at the level of the ulnar styloid) the ulnar nerve is located just lateral and deep to the flexor carpi ulnaris tendon.
3. The flexor carpi ulnaris tendon may be found on the medial aspect of the wrist, just lateral to the ulnar styloid.
4. If the wrist is dorsiflexed approximately 45 degrees, a longitudinal groove is found on the medial aspect of the wrist. The nerve lies deep in this groove.

PROCEDURE

1. Prep the wrist with povidone-iodine and place in palm up position.
2. Palpate the flexor carpi ulnaris tendon at the proximal flexion crease of the wrist at a level just lateral to the ulnar styloid.

Level of ulnar styloid

Flexor carpi ulnaris tendon

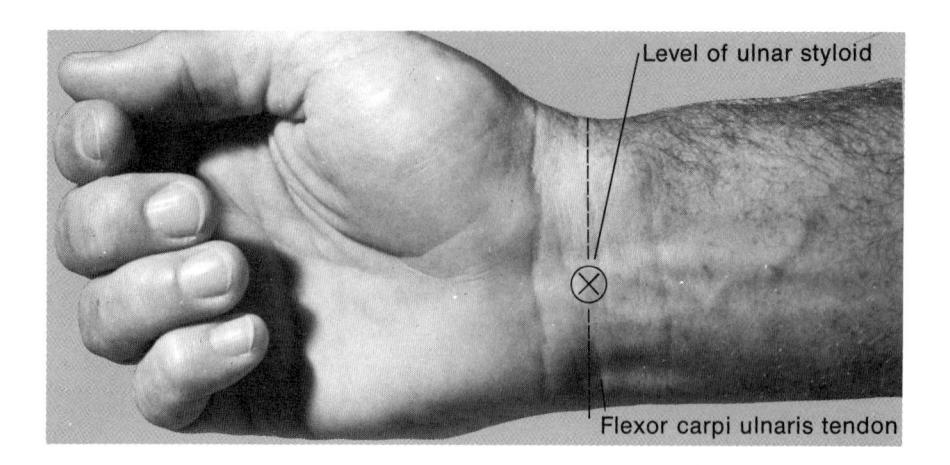

3. Raise a skin wheal with the 25-gauge needle just lateral to the flexor carpi ulnaris tendon in the longitudinal groove.
4. Introduce the 22-gauge needle perpendicularly through the skin wheal beneath the deep fascia.
5. A paresthesia may be elicited along the distribution of the ulnar nerve. Inject 3 to 4 cc of anesthetic agent at this point.

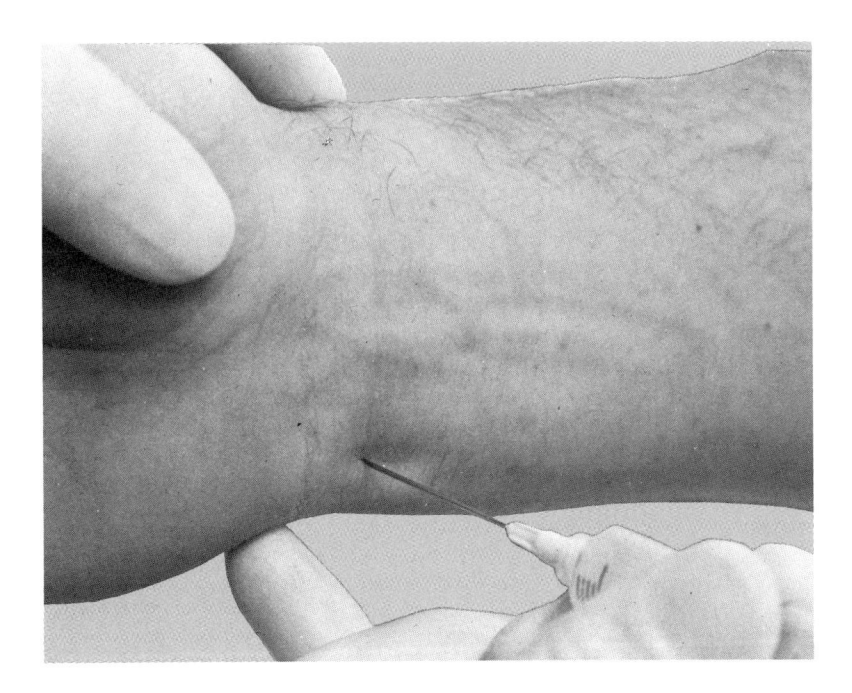

6. Massage the site gently to diffuse the anesthetic solution.

48 DIGITAL NERVE BLOCK

The digital nerve(s) may be blocked at one of two levels, depending on the needs of the patient. If anesthesia of one or more entire fingers (toes) is indicated, the appropriate digital nerves may be blocked at the level of the midlength of the metacarpal (metatarsal) bones. If anesthesia of the distal three-fourths of a finger (toe) is required, the digital nerves may be blocked at the proximal end of the finger (toe).

INDICATIONS

1. Anesthesia of the fingers or toes.
2. Repair of lacerations of the fingers or toes.
3. Minor surgical procedures involving the fingers or toes.

EQUIPMENT

1. Local set (see page 181)
2. 0.5 or 1% anesthetic agent

ANATOMICAL CONSIDERATIONS

1. The digital nerves which supply the fingers and toes are located in the interspaces between the metacarpal (metatarsal) bones. Each digital nerve bifurcates near the metacarpophalangeal (metatarsophalangeal) joint to supply sensation to opposing sides of adjacent digits. For example, the digital nerve in the third metacarpal (metatarsal) space supplies sensory innervation to the medial aspect of the middle finger (toe) and the lateral aspect of the third finger (toe). This must be kept in mind when selecting the nerve(s) to be blocked at the base of each finger (toe).

2. There are four digital nerves supplying each digit, each of which is located in a quadrant of the finger (toe). Thus, there are two volar and two dorsal digital nerves supplying each finger (toe).
3. The digital nerves should be approached from the dorsal aspect of the hand (foot) and fingers (toes) rather than from the volar side, because of the greater elasticity of the dorsal skin and less dense subcutaneous tissue. The injection can be done with a minimum of discomfort to the patient using this approach. The ideal level for digital nerve block at the metacarpal (metatarsal) area is the midpoint of the length of the metacarpal (metatarsal) and, at the digital area, the proximal end of the proximal phalanx.

PROCEDURE

DIGITAL NERVE BLOCK AT THE METACARPAL (METATARSAL) LEVEL

1. Prep the dorsum of the hand (foot) with povidone-iodine.
2. Select the appropriate nerves to be blocked.
3. Raise a skin wheal at the midpoint of each metacarpal (metatarsal) **interspace** selected using a 25-gauge needle.

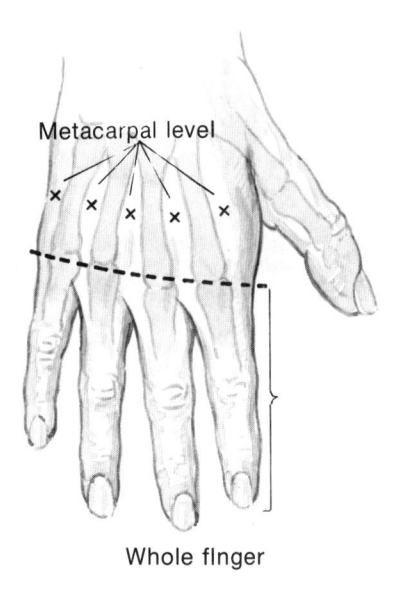

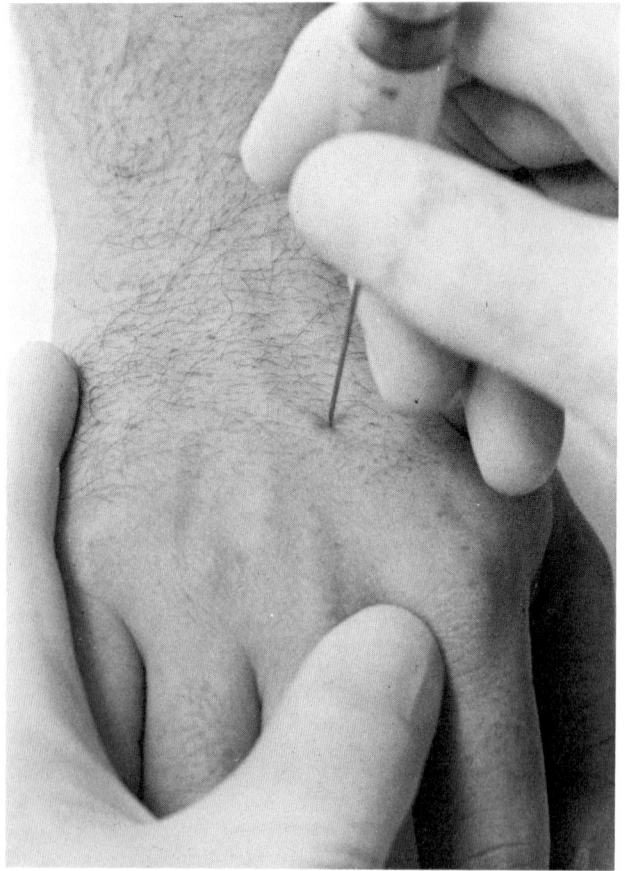

4. Change to the 22-gauge needle and introduce this through the skin wheal perpendicular to the skin. The entire depth of the interspace should be flooded with the anesthetic agent; 3 to 4 cc may be used in each space. Before each injection, aspirate in two planes to avoid intravascular deposition of the anesthetic agent. Carry the injection as close to the palmar (plantar) aspect of the hand (foot) as possible.

DIGITAL NERVE BLOCK AT THE DIGITAL LEVEL

1. Prep the finger (toe) to the metacarpophalangeal (metatarsophalangeal) joint with povidone-iodine.
2. Raise a skin wheal on the dorsomedial and dorsolateral aspects of each finger (toe) as close as possible to the base of the finger (toe) using the 25-gauge needle.
3. Change to the 22-gauge needle and introduce this through the wheal at a 45-degree angle, to the depth of the periosteum of the proximal phalanx. Withdraw 1 to 2 mm, aspirate in two planes, and inject 1 to 2 cc of solution to block the digital nerve.

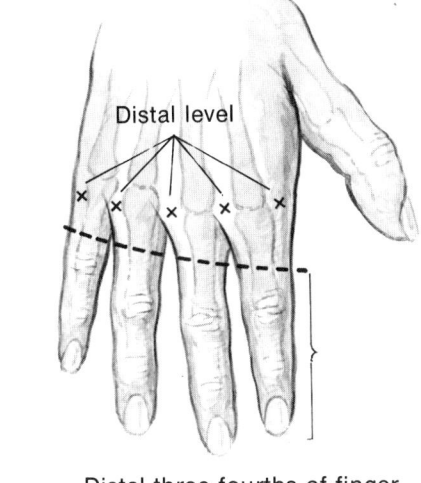

Distal level

Distal three-fourths of finger

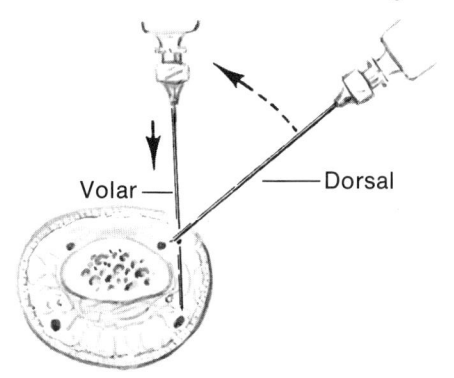

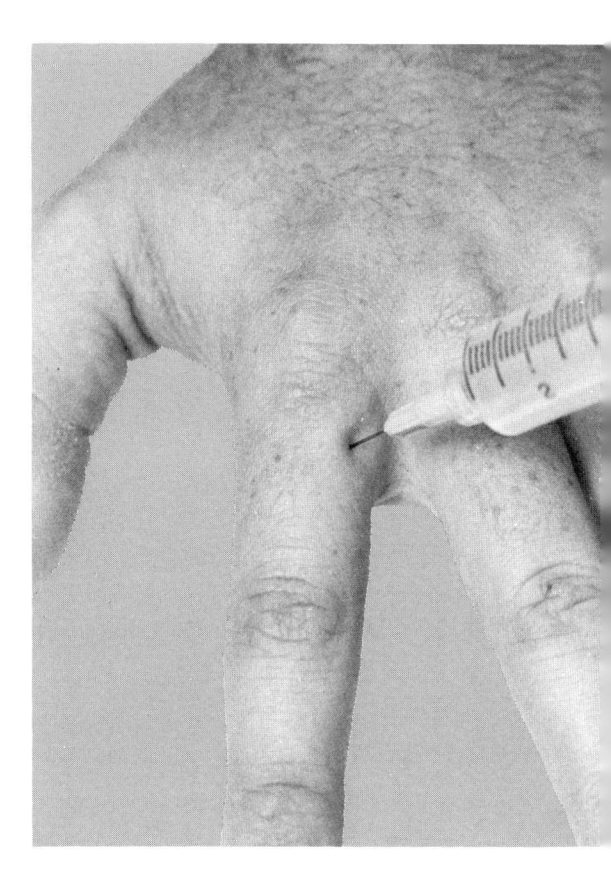

Volar — Dorsal

4. With the needle still in the dorsal quadrant, bring it to the perpendicular position and introduce it deeper into the volar quadrant; aspirate in two planes and inject 1 to 2 cc of solution to block the volar digital nerve.

217

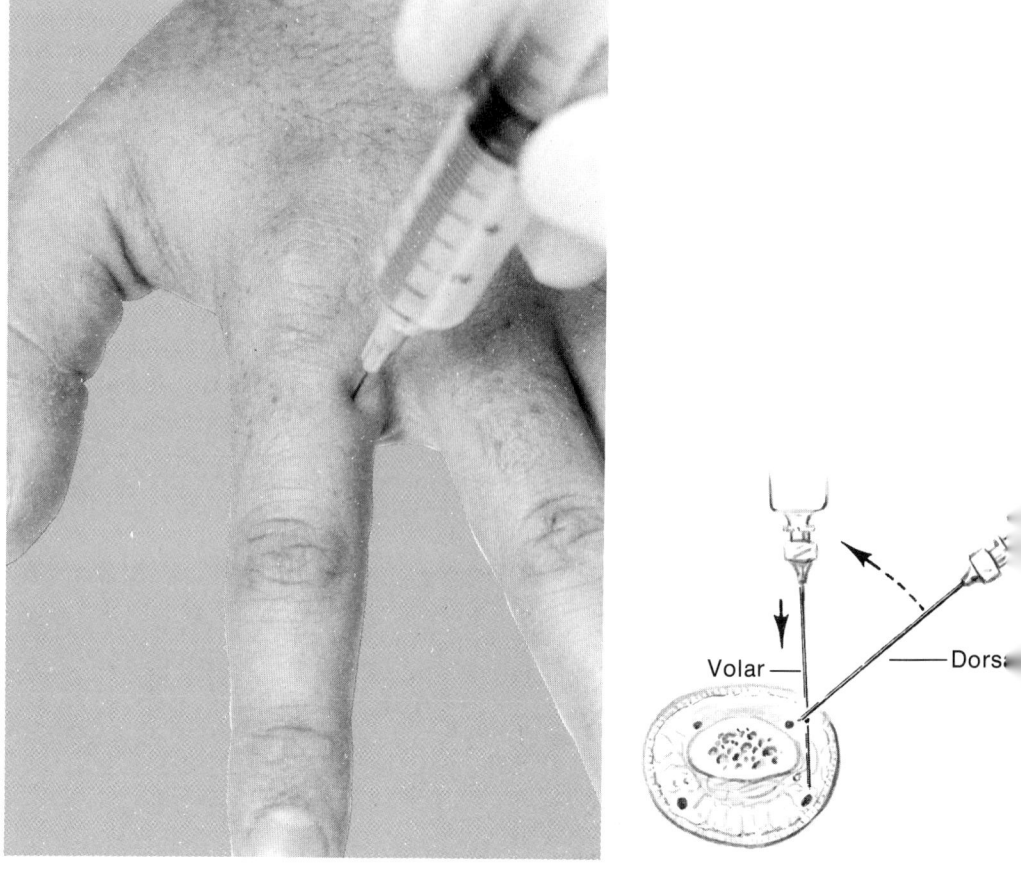

5. Repeat the procedure on the other side of the finger (toe).

NOTE: A vasoconstrictor agent (epinephrine) should not be used in conjunction with any procedure involving the hands, feet, or digits. The digital arteries are end arteries and have few, if any, collateral anastomoses. Thus, constriction of these vessels may cause severe degrees of impairment of blood supply which could cause gangrene of the involved digits. The digital nerve may also be blocked by injection into the appropriate interdigital web space(s).

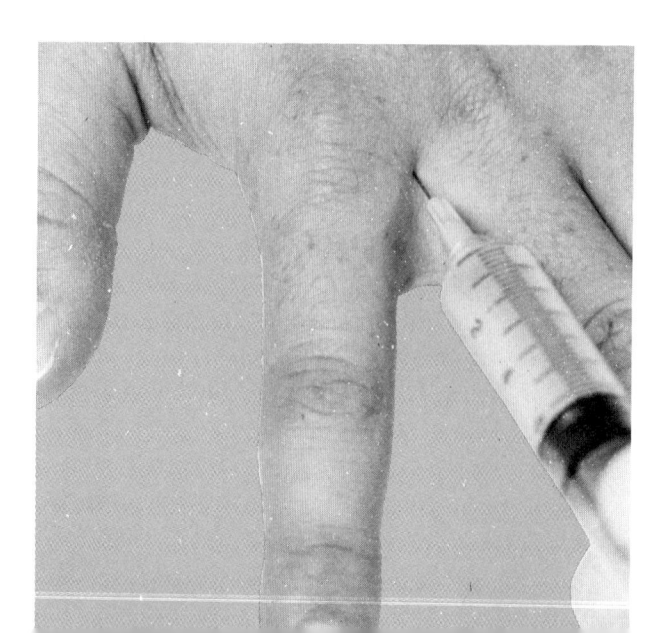

218

49 LUMBAR PUNCTURE

INDICATIONS
1. To obtain cerebrospinal fluid for diagnostic purposes.
2. To measure cerebrospinal fluid pressure.
3. To give medication intrathecally.

EQUIPMENT
1. 25-gauge needle for skin wheal
2. 22-gauge 1½-inch needle for deeper infiltration
3. 21-gauge 3½-inch spinal needle with obturator (25 gauge for pediatric patients)
4. 10 cc syringe for skin anesthesia
5. Four sterile towels
6. Sample bottles, sterile
7. 0.5% lidocaine solution for the anesthesia
8. 3-way stopcock
9. Manometer

ANATOMICAL CONSIDERATIONS
1. The spinal cord usually terminates at the level of the second lumbar vertebra. Therefore, the subarachnoid space must be entered below the level of the second lumbar vertebra to avoid injury to the cord.
2. The preferred site for lumbar puncture is the interspace between the spinous processes of the third and fourth (L3 to L4) or fourth and fifth vertebrae (L4 to L5).
3. The fourth lumbar vertebra is at the level of the iliac crest.
4. The subarachnoid space is entered by a midline or a midlateral approach in the interspinous space.

PROCEDURE

MIDLINE APPROACH

1. Place the patient in the full lateral position, with the back at the edge of the table. To assure the spine is not twisted, check to see that the shoulders are at the level of the iliac crest.
2. The patient is held by an assistant with the head in flexion and the knees drawn up in acute flexion. This position enhances flexion of the vertebral column and widens the interspaces between the posterior spinous processes.
3. Prep the skin of the back with povidone-iodine and drape.
4. Palpate the interspace between the spinous processes of L4 and L5.
5. Raise a skin wheal in the midline of the interspinous space with a 25-gauge needle; then, using the 22-gauge needle, infiltrate into the deeper tissues directing the needle cephalad at a 45-degree angle.

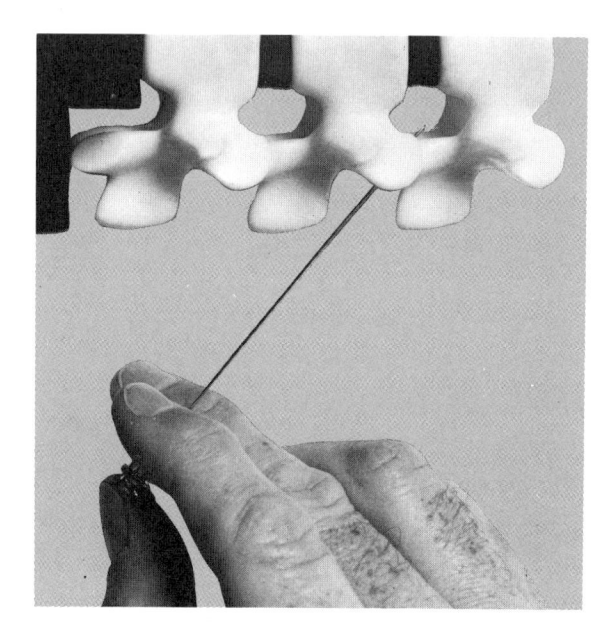

6. Introduce the 21-gauge spinal needle with obturator into the wheal and advance it cephalad at approximately 45 degrees until the dura is entered. If bone is encountered, withdraw the needle slightly, change the angle, and reinsert.
7. As the dura is reached, a sense of resistance is encountered which passes when the needle penetrates the dura. Then advance the needle another 4 to 5 mm to the subarachnoid space.
8. Withdraw the obturator. Cerebrospinal fluid will drop from the needle. If none is obtained, replace the obturator, rotate the needle 90 to 180 degrees, and aspirate gently.
9. When spinal fluid is obtained, attach the 3-way stopcock and manometer and measure the spinal fluid pressure. After obtaining the baseline pressure, ask the patient to strain slightly (Valsalva's maneuver). With this maneuver, the spinal fluid pressure will normally rise unless there is a block in the spinal canal. In adults or children who are unable to cooperate, apply finger

pressure to both internal jugular veins. Obstruction of these veins will also be reflected by a rise in cerebrospinal fluid pressure unless there is a block in the spinal canal. This is called Queckenstedt's test.
10. Collect 1 to 2 ml aliquots of spinal fluid in sterile tubes for cell study, analysis, and culture.
11. After collecting adequate samples, inject medication as indicated. Inject the fluid slowly in order to minimize discomfort to the patient.
12. When the procedure is completed, withdraw the needle and place a dry sterile dressing over the puncture site.
13. The patient should be instructed to remain recumbent for 6 to 12 hours.

LATERAL APPROACH

This may be used when the midline approach is not successful.
1. Position the patient as described above.
2. Identify the interspace chosen for puncture (L3 to L4 or L4 to L5).
3. With the thumb of the left hand in the center of the interspinous space, select a point 2 cm lateral to this midline point. It is technically easier if the lateral point is <u>below</u> the left thumb.

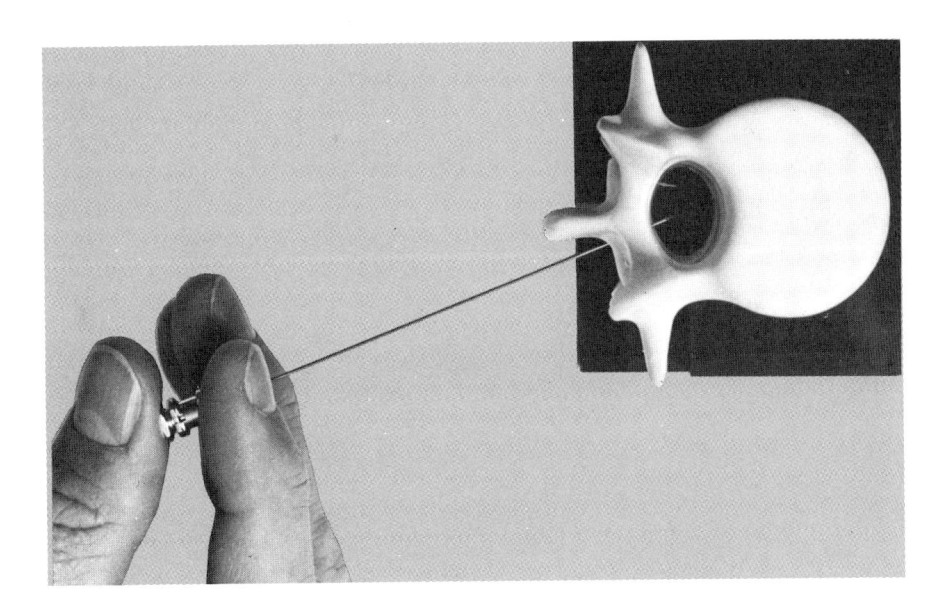

4. Raise a skin wheal at this lateral point using the 25-gauge needle.
5. Change to the 22-gauge needle and infiltrate the deeper tissues toward the midline and cephalad.
6. Introduce the 21-gauge spinal needle with obturator through the wheal, advancing it toward the midline at an angle of 25 degrees and cephalad 45 degrees. If bone is encountered, withdraw the needle a few millimeters, alter the angle slightly, and reinsert.
7. Continue to advance the needle slowly until the dura is penetrated and the subarachnoid space entered.
8. Withdraw the obturator and the cerebrospinal fluid will drop from the needle. If none is obtained, rotate the needle 90 to 180 degrees and aspirate gently.

When spinal fluid is obtained, <u>follow steps 9 through 13 described above</u>.

50 REMOVAL OF FOREIGN BODIES IN EAR AND NOSE

A variety of foreign bodies may be introduced into the nasal passage or external auditory meatus. While many of these, such as insects, may enter the passage accidentally, most foreign bodies are introduced by the patient. The majority of cases occur in children and the mentally retarded.

The presence of the foreign body may produce inflammation, especially when the object has been present for a long period of time. In right-handed children, the foreign body is usually inserted into the right nostril or external auditory meatus. Unilateral obstruction of either passage should cause one to suspect the presence of a foreign body.

Diagnosis is based on careful examination of the patient. In the case of a small child, it may be necessary to restrain the patient to complete an adequate examination.

In a cooperative patient, the foreign object may be removed without anesthesia; however, in apprehensive patients and particularly in pediatric patients, local or general anesthesia may be necessary.

Caution and skill are the keys to safe removal of such foreign bodies.

REMOVAL OF FOREIGN BODY IN THE NOSE

A foreign body retained in the nose is seen more commonly in children than adults. Although most objects enter through the anterior nares, some may enter the nose via the posterior choanae during the act of vomiting.

Unilateral purulent drainage from the nose, especially in a child, should cause one to suspect the presence of a foreign body.

EQUIPMENT

1. Head mirror and light source
2. Nasal speculum
3. Alligator forceps

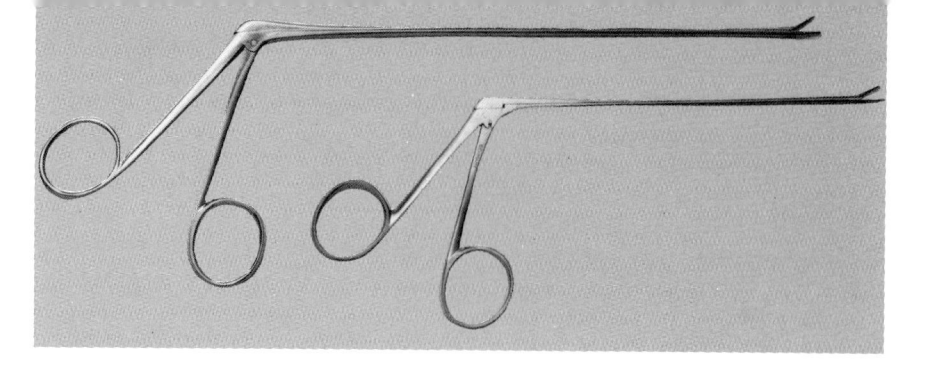

4. Suction tip
5. Right-angled blunt hook

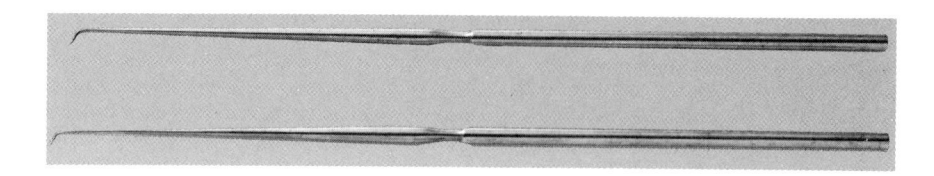

6. Tongue retractor
7. Papoose Board

ANATOMICAL CONSIDERATION

The foreign body may be located anywhere in the nasal passage, but most often is trapped in the inferior meatus, located beneath the inferior turbinate.

PROCEDURE

1. If the patient is an uncooperative child, he should be restrained on a Papoose Board or with sheets to prevent injury.
2. Carefully inspect the nasal passage.
3. The foreign body may be covered by purulent secretions. If so, suction these secretions to expose the retained object.
4. Grasp the foreign body with a suitable forceps and carefully extract it.
5. If the object has a perforation (e.g., a bead), an angled blunt hook may be used to extract it.
6. Avoid pushing the object posteriorly into the pharynx. If this occurs, it will usually be swallowed harmlessly. However, in a small child, the object could be aspirated into the trachea. To avoid this, place the child in a slight Trendelenburg's position and have an assistant be prepared to grasp the object if it falls into the oropharynx. This is best done by having the assistant place a tongue retractor in the mouth so that the pharynx is clearly visualized.

REMOVAL OF FOREIGN BODY IN THE EAR

Foreign bodies which may be retained in the ear include insects, toys, beads, vegetable matter, to name but a few.

The following general principles of management should be observed.

1. Insects should be killed by instilling a small amount of ether or alcohol into the external auditory canal.
2. A foreign body near the external auditory meatus or one which is loose and does not completely occlude the canal may be removed by irrigation.
3. A small, smooth object, such as a bead, may be difficult to remove with forceps; in this case, a right-angled blunt hook may be the instrument of choice.
4. The object should not be pushed deeper into the canal since the tympanic membrane may be damaged.
5. A foreign body present for a long period of time may be covered with cerumen.

EQUIPMENT

A number of instruments should be available to remove the foreign object. The indications for each will depend on the type and location of the retained object.
1. Otoscope
2. Ear syringe
3. Irrigation fluid (water or saline)
4. Alligator forceps
5. Right-angled blunt hook

ANATOMICAL CONSIDERATIONS

1. The external auditory canal in adults is a fibrocartilaginous osseous tunnel 2.5 to 3.5 cm long which courses anteriorly and inferiorly, in a somewhat circuitous fashion. For this reason, if the canal is to be adequately examined, the external ear must be gently pulled posteriorly and superiorly.
2. In a child, the canal is much more horizontal with the tympanic membrane placed at the level of the external meatus. Thus, the external ear is pulled posteriorly and downward for visualization of the canal.
3. The canal narrows at the junction of the external (cartilaginous) and internal (osseous) segments. This area is the isthmus. Objects impacted deep to the isthmus are best treated by an otolaryngologist.
4. Many foreign objects will be found near the external meatus. The objects must not be pushed deeper into the canal with the otoscope.
5. At times, objects impacted deep in the auditory canal may not be removed without damage to the tympanic membrane. In such patients, a postauricular incision may be needed; thus, the services of an otolaryngologist may be called for.

PROCEDURE

1. To avoid injury, keep the patient perfectly still during the examination and extraction process. If the patient is unable to cooperate, do not attempt the extraction procedure in the emergency department. In this case, schedule the procedure under general anesthesia in the operating room.
2. Locate the foreign object by careful examination of the external auditory canal with the otoscope.

REMOVAL BY IRRIGATION

1. If the object is near the external meatus, and does not fully occlude the canal, or if it is small, irrigate the canal with water or alcohol.

NOTE: Water should not be used if the foreign object is vegetable matter which is hydroscopic.

2. Irrigate, place the tip of the ear syringe in the meatus, and aim the stream of fluid toward the open (nonoccluded) portion of the canal. In this way, the fluid will fill the canal behind the foreign body and force it out. Do not occlude the canal with the syringe tip.
3. Do not be too forceful in introducing the irrigating fluid.
4. When the object is evacuated, re-examine the canal to be sure it is clear and there is no damage to the lining.
5. Instill antibiotic medication if necessary.

REMOVAL BY INSTRUMENTATION

1. If the object is large or completely occludes the canal, a number of instruments may be used to remove it.
2. If the object has a perforation, such as a bead, use a right-angled blunt hook. If the material is cerumen or vegetative, imbed the hook in the material and remove it in this manner.
3. If the object is large, use smooth forceps to grasp and remove it.

NOTE: Forceps should probably not be used for removing a round, smooth object because it may be forced deeper into the canal.

4. After removal, inspect the canal for any damage.
5. Instill antibiotic medication if needed.

BIBLIOGRAPHY

Ballantyne, J. and Groves, J. Diseases of the Ear, Nose & Throat, ed. 3, Vol. 2. Philadelphia: J. B. Lippincott Co., 1971.

Serio, J. C. The Practice of Emergency Nursing. In J. H. Cosgriff, Jr. and D. L. Anderson, eds. Philadelphia: J. B. Lippincott Co., 1975.

———. Personal communication.

Wilson, T. G. Diseases of the Ear, Nose & Throat In Children. London: William Heinemann Ltd., 1955.

51 ANTERIOR NASAL PACKING

INDICATIONS
1. Bleeding from the anterior nares uncontrolled by external pressure or cautery.
2. For use in conjunction with posterior packing.

EQUIPMENT
1. Nasal speculum
2. Bayonet forceps
3. Cotton balls
4. Suction tip
5. Head mirror and light source
6. Scissors
7. Twelve 4 × 4-inch gauze bandages
8. Kidney basin and tissues
9. Six packs of ½ × 72-inch sterile Vaseline gauze
10. 4% cocaine (no more than 5 cc)
11. Adrenalin 1:1000

ANATOMICAL CONSIDERATIONS
1. Anterior nasal bleeding may arise from the most forward portion of the septum (Kiesselbach's area) which is often arrested by firmly pinching the nostrils between the thumb and index fingers for 5 to 10 minutes.

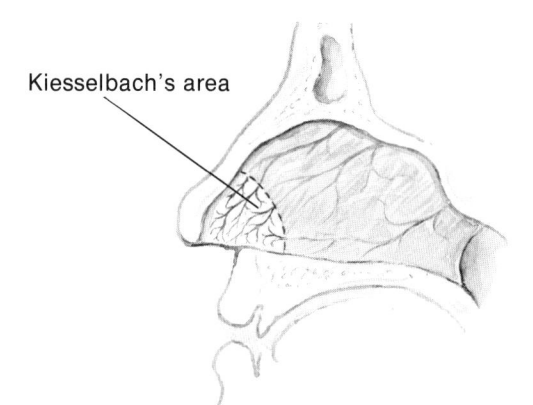

Kiesselbach's area

2. Bleeding may also arise from the anterior superior area of the nasal cavity, from branches of the anterior ethmoidal artery.
3. Bleeding may originate from one or both nostrils.

PROCEDURE

1. Seat the patient in a chair with the head held in slight extension and placed in a head rest.
2. Have a good light source. Use a head mirror or a head light for illumination.
3. Allow the patient to hold the kidney basin and tissues and advise him to expectorate when necessary. He should not swallow the blood since it may lead to nausea and emesis.
4. Spread the nares gently with a nasal speculum and try to identify the bleeding source. It is only necessary to pack the side which is bleeding.
5. Moisten a cotton ball with a small amount of cocaine solution and apply it to the nasal mucous membrane. This has both anesthetic and vasoconstrictive properties.
6. Remove the cotton ball.
7. Place the ½-inch Vaseline gauze in the affected side with bayonet forceps, in a layered fashion. The gauze should be placed in the nose as far as the posterior tips of the turbinates. Layer the gauze until the nasal passage is completely filled.

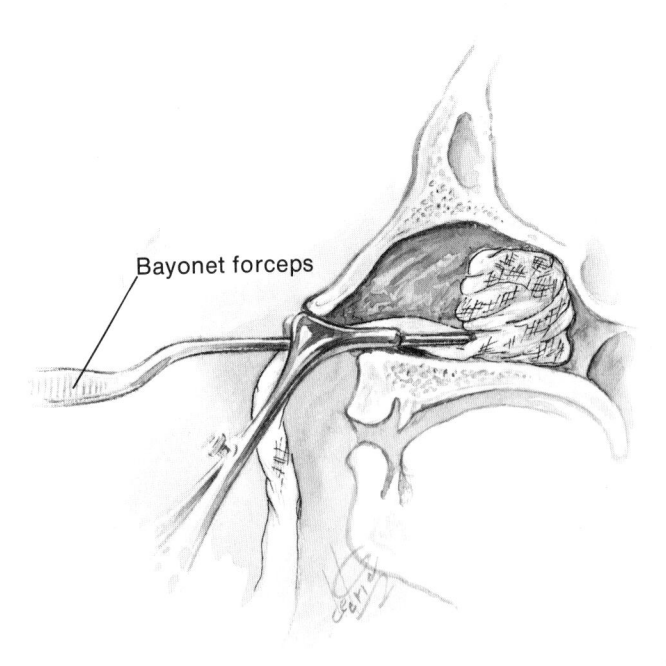

8. Also pack the superior recess of the nasal cavity and anterior to the middle and superior turbinates.
9. When the packing is completed, observe the patient for at least 15 to 20 minutes to be certain bleeding is controlled. If it is not, the pack must be removed and replaced after placing a posterior pack.

52 POSTERIOR NASAL PACKING

INDICATIONS

1. Severe bleeding from the posterior nares.
2. Bleeding uncontrolled by anterior packing.

EQUIPMENT

1. Nasal speculum
2. Bayonet forceps
3. Sponge forceps
4. Cotton balls
5. Two medicine glasses
6. Two 8-inch Kelly curved hemostats
7. Suction tip
8. Head mirror
9. Scissors
10. Twelve 4 × 4-inch gauze pads
11. Kidney basin and tissues
12. Two 10 to 12 Fr. straight (Robinson) urethral catheters
13. ½-inch sterile vaseline gauze
14. Umbilical tape
15. 4% cocaine
16. Adrenalin 1:1000
17. 4% lidocaine spray

ANATOMICAL CONSIDERATIONS

1. Severe epistaxis may originate from the anterior or posterior portion of the nares.

2. The posterior pack must be secured in position above the soft palate, completely occluding both nasal passages.
3. An anterior pack must be inserted with a posterior pack.

PROCEDURE

1. This procedure sometimes requires general anesthesia especially in a child; however, in adults, with gentle care, it can be completed using a topical anesthetic and sedation such as diazepam.
2. Prepare the pack by rolling a 4 × 4-inch gauze pad and cutting it to the size of the nasopharynx. Bind the gauze roll with three separate pieces of umbilical tape, leaving the ends at least 8 to 10 inches long.

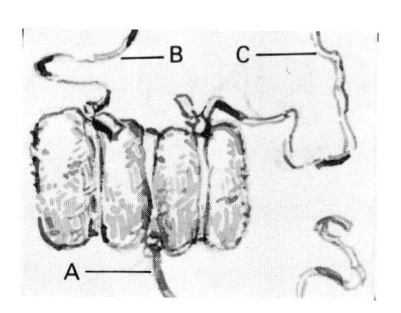

3. Spray each nasal cavity with 4% lidocaine spray for topical anesthesia.
4. Insert a gauze pad or cotton moistened with 4% cocaine into each nasal cavity. This has both anesthetic and vasoconstrictive properties.
5. Lubricate the rubber catheters and insert into each nasal passage until they are seen in the pharynx.
6. Grasp the catheters with bayonet forceps or sponge forceps and deliver them through the mouth.

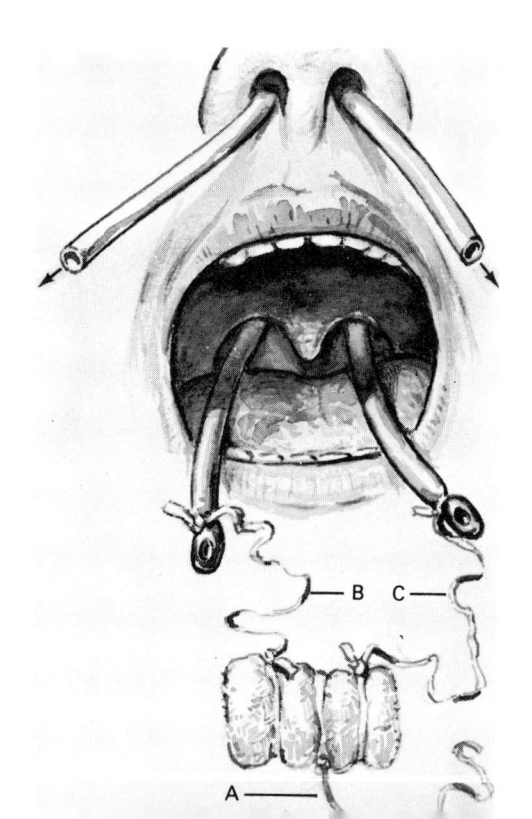

7. Tie two of the three free ends of the tape on the gauze roll to the rubber catheters.

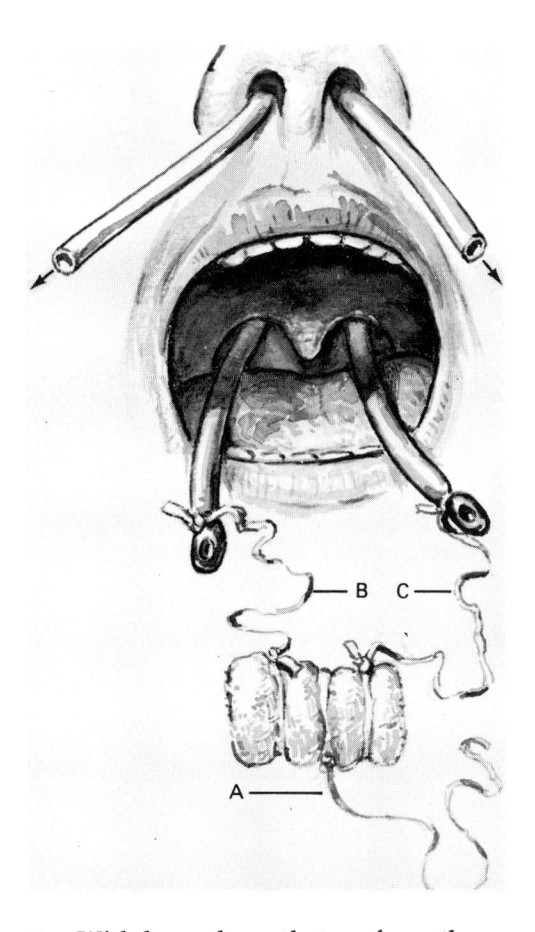

8. Withdraw the catheters from the nares, drawing the pack into the mouth.
9. Then place the pack in position in the nasopharynx. This can be done by grasping it with a long curved hemostat and placing it above the soft palate, using gentle traction on the tapes exiting from the nares.

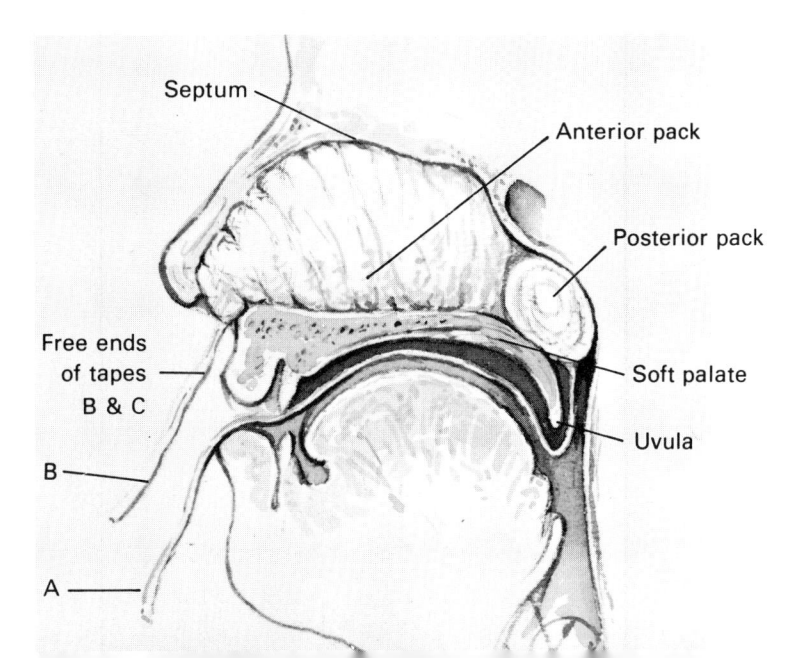

10. Tie the two nasal tapes at the columella, over a dental roll.
11. Tape the third tape to the cheek. This is used to facilitate removal of the pack.

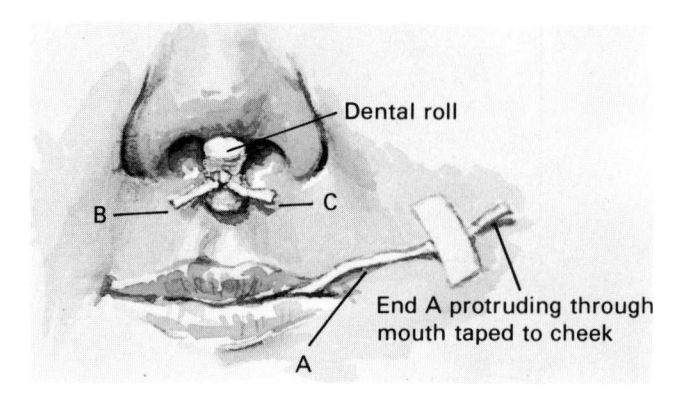

12. Then pack the anterior nares firmly with Vaseline gauze. The ½-inch Vaseline gauze is usually packaged in 72-inch lengths and is put into place in each nostril in layered fashion.

53 INDIRECT (MIRROR) LARYNGOSCOPY

Indirect laryngoscopy is an important diagnostic maneuver used to examine and evaluate suspected lesions of the epiglottis, glottis, and vocal cords. With experience and care it can be performed with a minimum of discomfort to the patient and may provide significant information. In most patients, it is done without anesthesia, but, when necessary, a topical anesthetic agent may be used.

INDICATIONS

1. Unexplained hoarseness for two weeks or more.
2. Suspected tumor of the epiglottis or vocal cords.
3. Suspected foreign body retained in the hypopharynx.

EQUIPMENT

1. Laryngeal mirror (several sizes should be available)
2. Light source—an uncovered bulb preferably of the clear type
3. Head mirror (or a head light)
4. Warm water (to heat the mirror)
5. 4 × 4-inch gauze pads
6. Tongue blade
7. Topical anesthetic agent (1% tetracaine or lidocaine viscous) (optional)
8. Examining chair

ANATOMICAL CONSIDERATIONS

1. The mucous membrane of the soft palate and oropharynx is sensitive to touch (the gag reflex). This reflex varies in intensity from one individual to another.
2. The patient must be comfortably seated with the head fixed in position. Ideally, the patient should be sitting erect, with his spine against the back of

the chair and his head and shoulders thrust forward approximately 10 to 12 inches from the back of the chair. Extension of the neck may limit examination.
3. Recall that the anatomical landmarks are visualized in the mirror in the reverse of their actual anteroposterior position; the left and right sides are not altered.

PROCEDURE

1. Reassure the patient and place him erect in a straight-backed chair. The head rest is usually not required for this examination.
2. If the patient has a particularly active gag reflex, give him 5 cc of lidocaine viscous. Have the patient slosh the liquid about in his mouth and swallow it. Omit this step if the patient can tolerate the procedure without anesthesia.
3. Have a bare light bulb source at the right side of the patient's head and adjust your head mirror to reflect the light at a focal length of 14 to 18 inches.
4. With a tongue blade, retract the cheeks carefully and examine the entire mouth, the gums, and the tonsils.
5. Heat the laryngeal mirror in the warm water bath to prevent fogging by the patient's breath. Shake the mirror to remove the excess water. Do not rub the mirror.
6. Ask the patient to stick out his tongue and fold the gauze pad over the end of it, covering both top and bottom. Gently but firmly hold the tongue with slight tension in the protruded position. Avoid any pressure on the undersurface of the tongue against the lower incisor teeth. Ask the patient to breathe quietly.
7. While directing the reflected light from the head mirror into the oral cavity, and with gentle traction on the tongue, carefully introduce the mirror into the mouth with the lens facing the upper surface of the tongue.

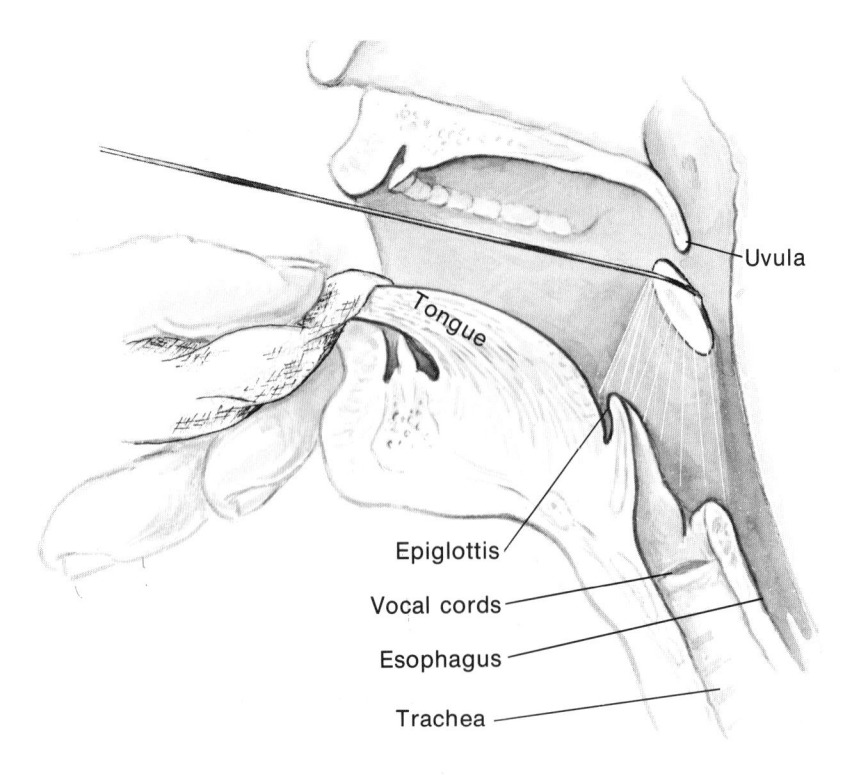

8. First examine the base of the tongue and the superior surface of the epiglottis.
9. Insert the mirror deeper into the mouth toward the posterior wall of the pharynx and by rotating the mirror from side to side, examine the pyriform sinuses and the lateral walls of the pharynx.
10. With the mirror in the midline of the pharynx, the vocal cords should be visible, below the epiglottis. Remember the actual anatomy will be reversed in the laryngeal mirror. Examine the cords and observe the movement of each with respiratory activity. Also examine the structures about the cords including the arytenoids, commissures, and the aryepiglottic folds. Ask the patient to take a deep breath and note movement of each vocal cord. The cords should separate during inspiration.

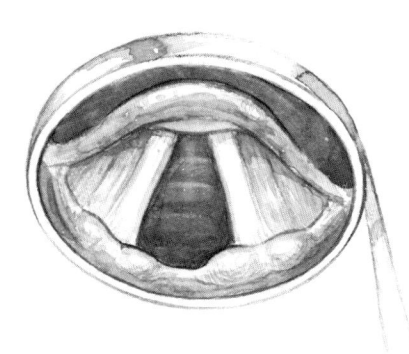

Cords abducted

11. Ask the patient to say "E-e-e-e-e" and observe whether the vocal cords properly oppose (adduct). Failure of the cords to adduct, indicates recurrent laryngeal nerve palsy.

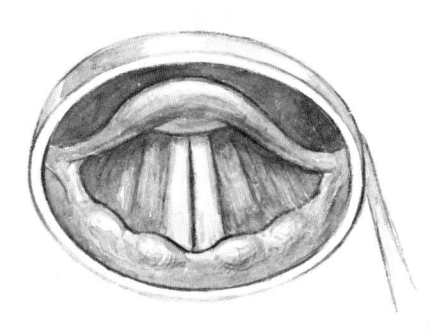

Cords adducted

12. Look carefully for any lesions or retained foreign bodies in the area examined.
13. As the vocal cords open (abduct), the upper portion of the trachea may be visualized.
14. If any lesions are identified, direct laryngoscopy is required for further evaluation.
NOTE: If topical anesthesia is used, the patient should be advised not to take food or drink for 3 to 4 hours.

54 PERICARDIOCENTESIS

INDICATIONS
1. Drainage of hemopericardium.
2. Relief of cardiac tamponade.

EQUIPMENT
1. Local set
2. 18- or 19-gauge 4-inch spinal needle, short bevel, with obturator
3. 30 cc syringe
4. 0.5% lidocaine

ANATOMICAL CONSIDERATIONS
1. The approach of choice is through the left costoxiphoid angle. This approach is least likely to cause vascular injury to the coronary vessels.

Xiphoid process
Costal margin

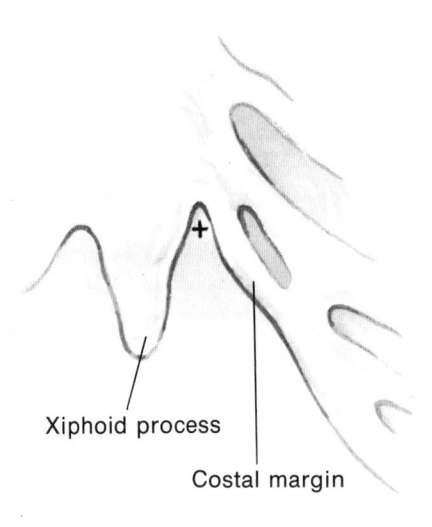

2. A secondary approach is via the fourth or fifth left intercostal space. This method could possibly penetrate the internal mammary vessels or the coronary vessels.

PROCEDURE

1. Prep the skin about the xiphoid process with povidone-iodine.
2. Raise a skin wheal using a small amount of 0.5% lidocaine at a point approximately 2.0 cm below the costal margin, to the left of the xiphoid process.
3. Introduce the 4-inch needle with obturator upward toward the pericardial cavity at an angle of approximately 45 degrees to the skin. The needle should pass anterior to the liver, through or above the diaphragm, and be aimed toward the left midclavicular line.

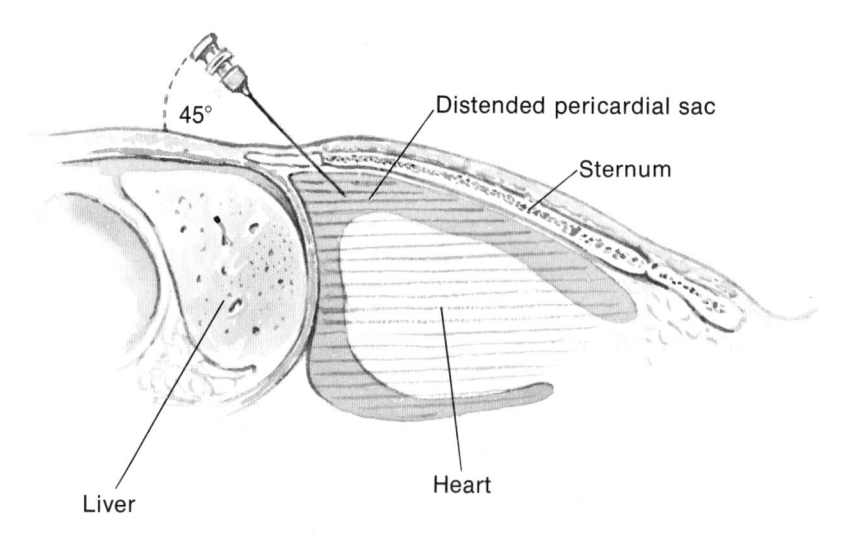

4. As the pericardial sac is encountered, a sense of resistance is noted and then relieved.
5. Upon entering the pericardial cavity, remove the obturator, attach the syringe, and aspirate.
6. If blood is not recovered, withdraw and reinsert the needle.
7. Aspirate as much blood as possible. Free blood from the pericardial cavity usually will not clot, whereas blood from the cardiac chamber will clot.
8. If the needle abuts against the wall of the ventricle, the thrust of the ventricle can be felt. In this case, withdraw the needle slightly until the cardiac movement is no longer felt.

NOTE:
1. Remarkable clinical improvement is noted with removal of as little as 20 to 30 cc of blood.
2. As a variation of the method described above, thread a small plastic catheter through the needle and leave the catheter in position in the pericardial sac. With the tube in place, you can observe for continuous bleeding.
3. If more than 200 cc of blood is recovered or if tamponade recurs, urgent thoracotomy is indicated.
4. Using an alligator clip, attach an anterior chest electrocardiographic lead to the needle. In this way changes in the EKG are shown which may indicate penetration of the myocardium. These changes include an increase in QRS voltage, alteration of the ST segments, or occurrence of ectopic beats. If any of these occur, withdraw the needle a few mm until the EKG changes are no longer seen.

BIBLIOGRAPHY

Bains, M. S. and Beattie, E. J., Jr. Cardiac tamponade. Hosp. Med. 12:47, 10, 1976.
Simpson, J. S. Thoracic injuries in Care of the Injured Child. Baltimore: Williams & Wilkins, 1975, p. 139.

55 NEEDLE DRAINAGE OF THE PLEURAL CAVITY

This procedure is a life-saving temporary measure only. Closed chest drainage by tube thoracostomy and underwater drainage should be accomplished as soon as possible. Anesthesia is rarely required.

INDICATIONS
1. Tension pneumothorax.
2. Need for emergency evacuation of air from the pleural cavity when adequate instruments are not available.
3. Massive pneumothorax with mediastinal shift.

EQUIPMENT
1. 13- to 14-gauge needle
2. Prep

ANATOMICAL CONSIDERATIONS
1. Drainage is preferably initiated through an upper intercostal space.

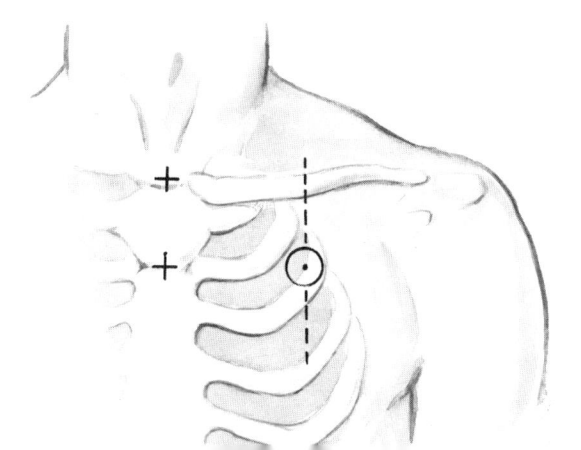

2. The intercostal neurovascular bundle runs in a groove of each rib at its inferior margin.
3. Place the needle close to the upper margin of the third rib in the midclavicular line.
4. Identify by palpation the sternomanubrial junction (angle of Lewis) at the junction of the upper and middle thirds of the breastbone. By moving the fingers laterally, the second intercostal space is palpated. The index finger is on the angle of Lewis, the middle finger in the second intercostal space.

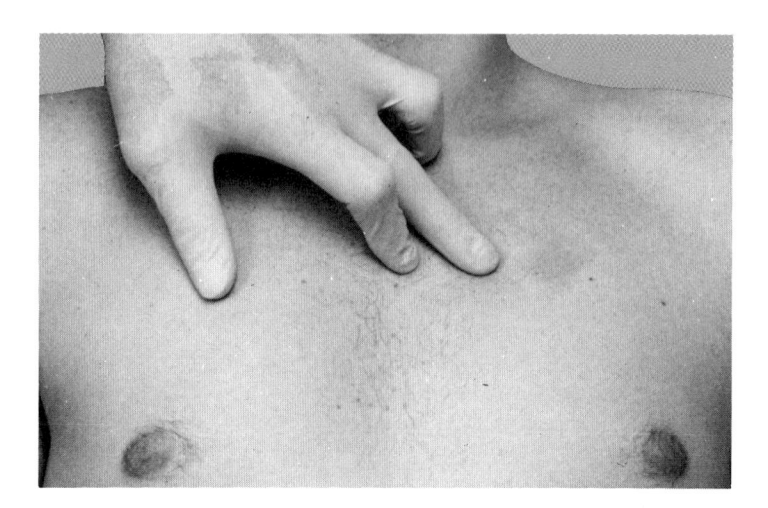

5. The internal mammary vessels course vertically close to the lateral borders of the sternum and should be avoided.

PROCEDURE

1. These patients are often in extremis and time may not permit use of local anesthesia.
2. Prep the upper chest wall anteriorly.
3. Locate the sternomanubrial junction and the second intercostal space.
4. Palpate the upper edge of the third rib in the midclavicular line. This is the point of entry.
5. Firmly insert the needle into the pleural space in an upward direction.

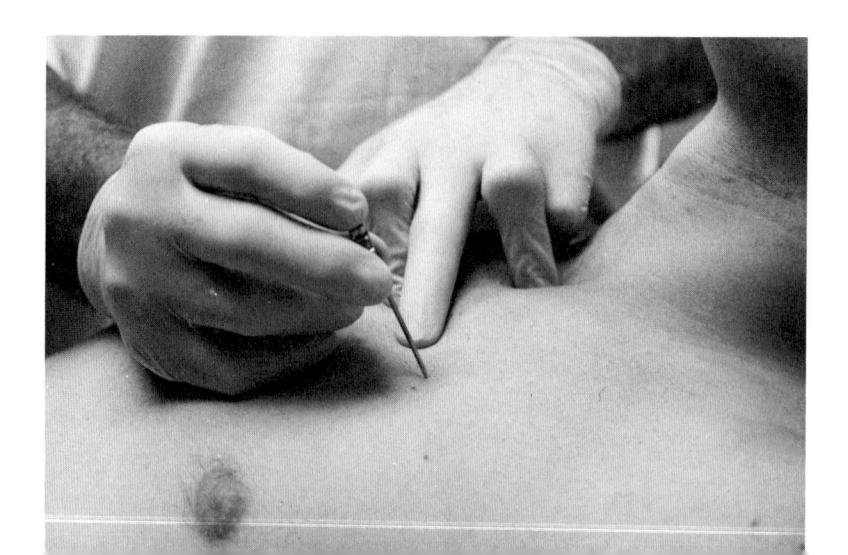

6. When the needle is in the pleural cavity, a sudden release of air will occur through the needle and the patient's condition will improve immediately.

NOTE:
1. As soon as possible, closed chest drainage with underwater seal should be initiated.
2. A variation of the method described above is to utilize a one-way valve device attached to the needle (see below).
3. Use a sterile finger cot or cut a finger from a sterile surgical glove and cut the closed end off.

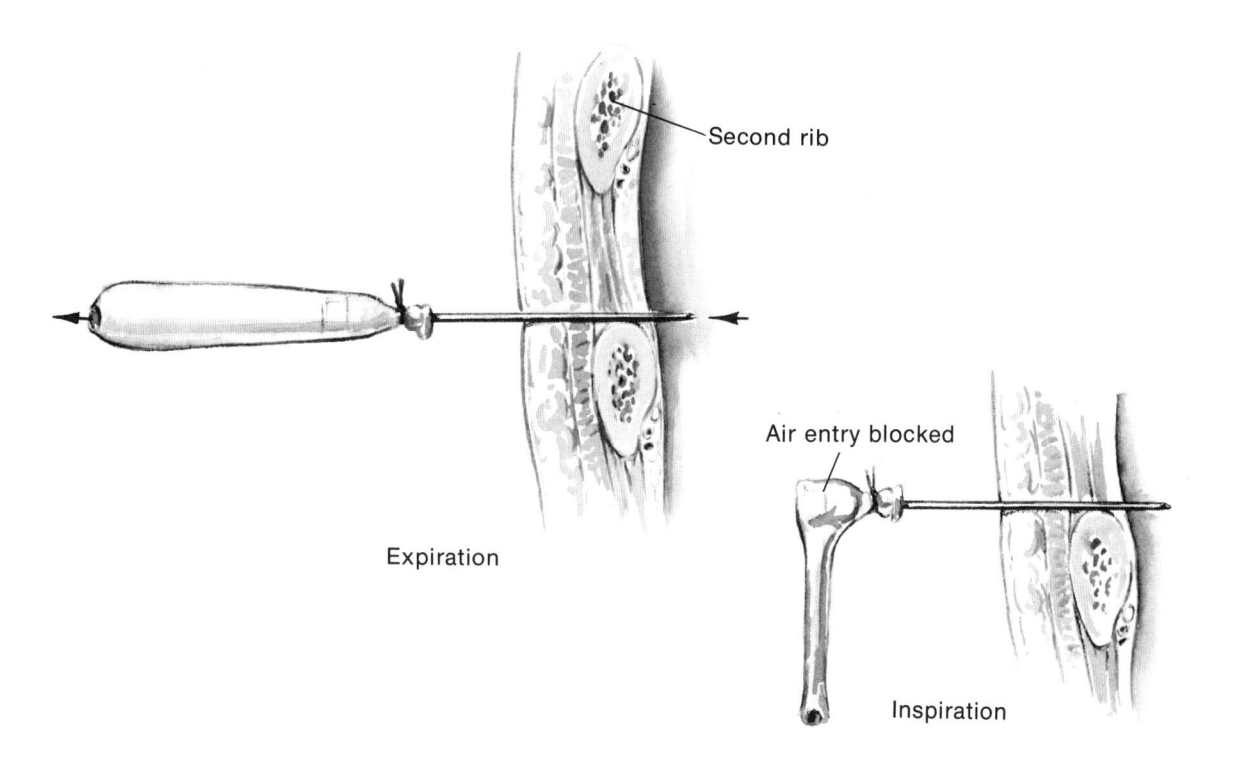

Second rib

Expiration

Air entry blocked

Inspiration

4. Tie one open end to the hub of the needle.
5. With expiration air will pass outward through the needle-valve assembly.
6. With inspiration, the rubber valve will collapse against the hub of the needle and prevent entry of air into the pleural space.

56 THORACENTESIS

INDICATIONS

1. Accumulation of fluid in the pleural cavity (pleural effusion) with impairment of respiration.
2. Accumulation of blood in the pleural cavity (hemothorax) with impairment of respiration.
3. Removal of fluid for diagnostic purposes.

EQUIPMENT

1. Local set
2. 50 cc syringe
3. 15- or 16-gauge 2-inch needle, short bevel
4. 3-way stopcock
5. Connecting tubing
6. Medicine glass
7. Twelve 4 × 4-inch gauze pads
8. Towels
9. Povidone-iodine
10. Calibrated metal pitcher
11. Large curved hemostat
12. Collection bottles for special studies (chemistry, bacteriology, pathology)
13. Collecting basin

ANATOMICAL CONSIDERATIONS

1. The site for thoracentesis should be determined by careful study of posteroanterior and lateral x-ray films of the chest combined with thorough physical examination to determine the extent and the location of the fluid. The fluid

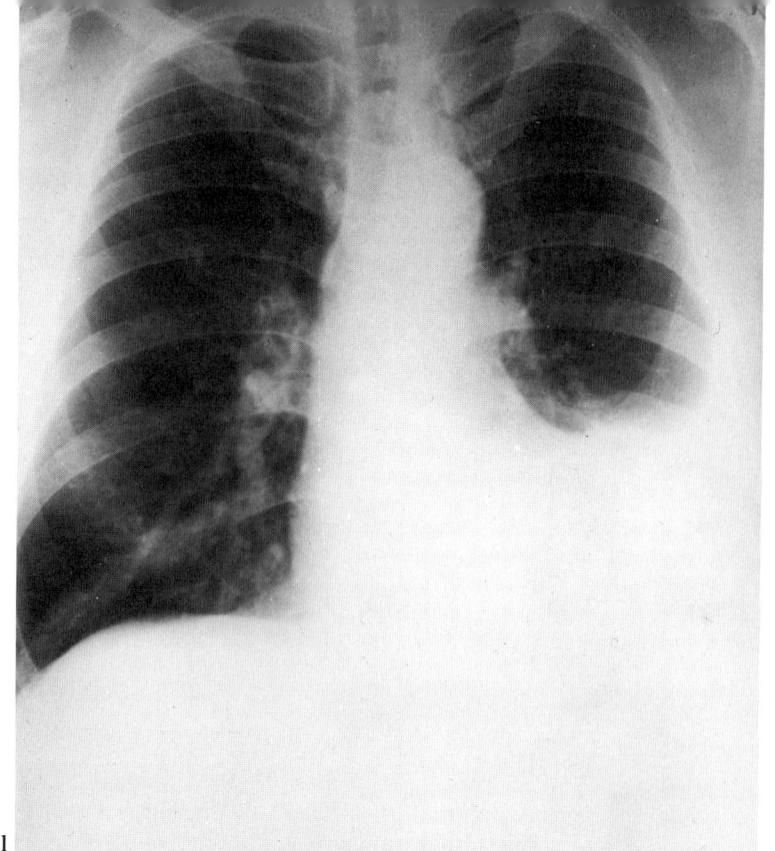

Fluid level

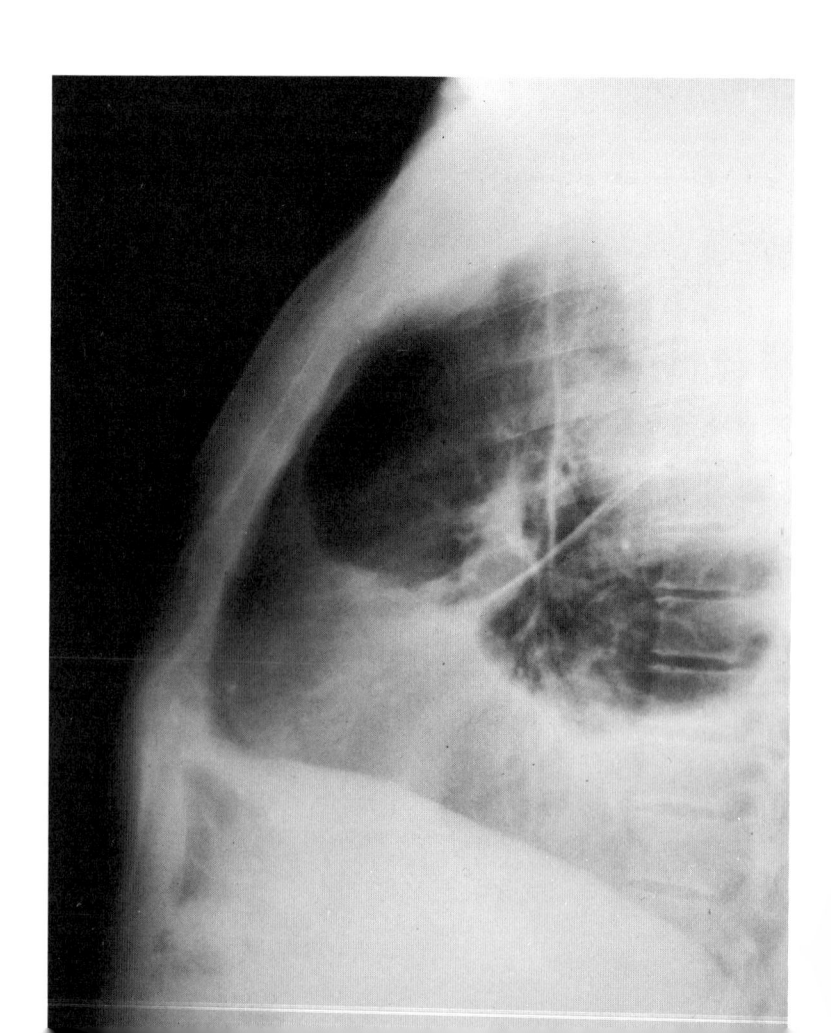

may at times be located in one specific area of the pleural cavity.
2. The base of the pleural space is usually located at the level of the ninth intercostal space in the posterior axillary line. This is variable however and may be ascertained by careful study of the x-ray film of the chest.
3. To avoid injury to the intercostal vessels, puncture of the pleural space should be done in the intercostal space just above the superior border of the rib.
4. To allow the fluid to gravitate to the lowermost portion of the pleural space, the patient should be placed in a comfortable sitting position.
5. The needle is introduced into the fluid collection only deep enough to easily withdraw the fluid.
6. As fluid is removed, the lung re-expands into the area. Care must be taken not to puncture the lung and cause an air leak.

PROCEDURE

1. Place the patient in a comfortable sitting position.
2. Examine the patient by percussion and auscultation to determine the location and level of the fluid.
3. Confirm this by careful study of posteroanterior and lateral x-ray films of the chest, and palpation of the ribs. Count the ribs in the back, from the twelfth upward.
4. Select the site for thoracentesis. It should be done in the lower portion of the fluid collection, near the superior surface of the diaphragm.
5. Prep the skin of the chest wall with povidone-iodine.
6. Drape the area with sterile towels.
7. Raise a skin wheal with 0.5% lidocaine using a 5 or 10 cc syringe and a 25-gauge needle.
8. Change to the 22-gauge 1½-inch needle and introduce this through the wheal into the lowermost portion of the intercostal space. If the rib is encountered, "walk" the needle upward until the superior margin of the rib is identified.
9. Introduce the needle deeper into the intercostal space, aspirate in two planes, and infiltrate with the anesthetic agent through the full thickness of the intercostal muscle layers.
10. Warn the patient that as the needle nears the pleura, he may experience a sudden "twinge" of sharp pain. Infiltrate at this level after aspirating in two planes.
11. Introduce the needle through the parietal pleura and aspirate. If the fluid collection has been entered, a small amount should be recovered. If no fluid is recovered, redirect the needle in a downward or upward direction.
12. If fluid is recovered, the site of the collection is thus identified. Withdraw the needle completely.
13. Attach the 3-way stopcock and the 15- or 16-gauge short bevel needle to the 50 cc syringe and introduce this needle into the pleural collection through the skin wheal. First contact the rib and "walk" the needle into the interspace above it.

Skin wheal and local infiltration

Rib

Intercostal bundle (nerve, artery, vein)

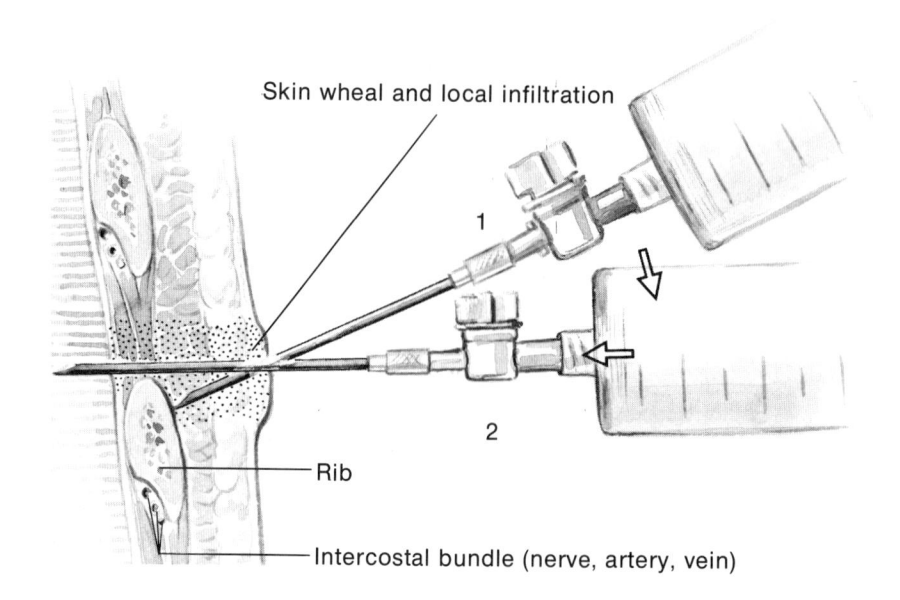

14. Once fluid is recovered, place the curved hemostat on the needle at skin level to prevent further penetration.
15. Attach the connecting tubing to the sidearm of the stopcock and place the free end into the collecting basin.

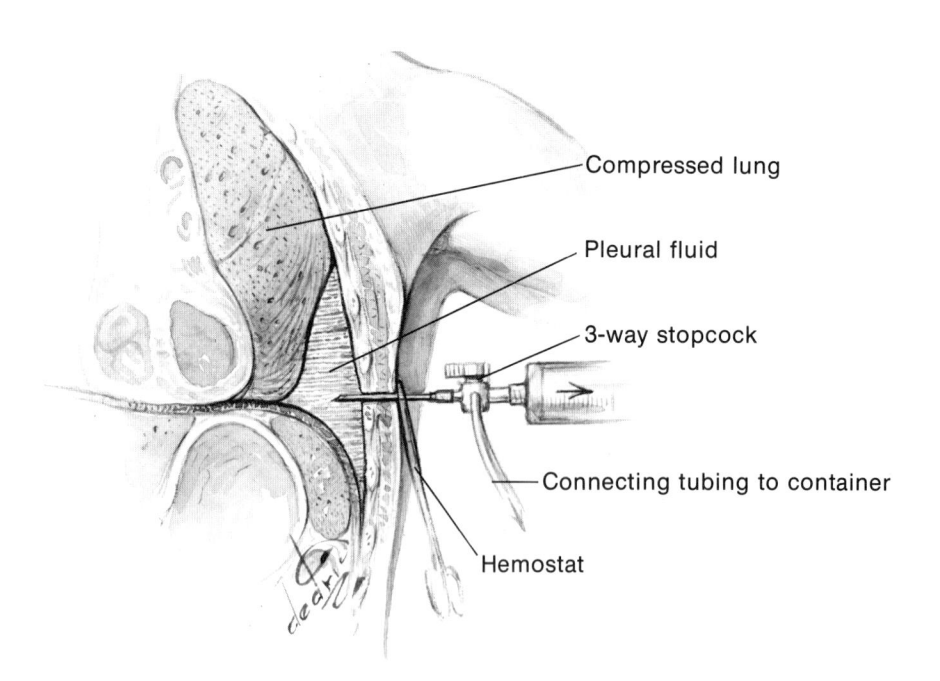

Compressed lung

Pleural fluid

3-way stopcock

Connecting tubing to container

Hemostat

16. Alternately aspirate the fluid into the syringe and rotate the stopcock to empty it into the collecting basin.
17. Place samples of the fluid in appropriate receptacles for study. These include chemistry, bacteriology and histopathologic study as indicated.
18. Repeat the aspiration and evacuation process until no more fluid is recovered. Measure and record the total amount removed.

19. At this point, remove the needle and syringe assembly and place a dry sterile dressing over the site.
20. Repeat the posteroanterior and lateral chest x-ray studies to evaluate the amount of clearing and check for pneumothorax.

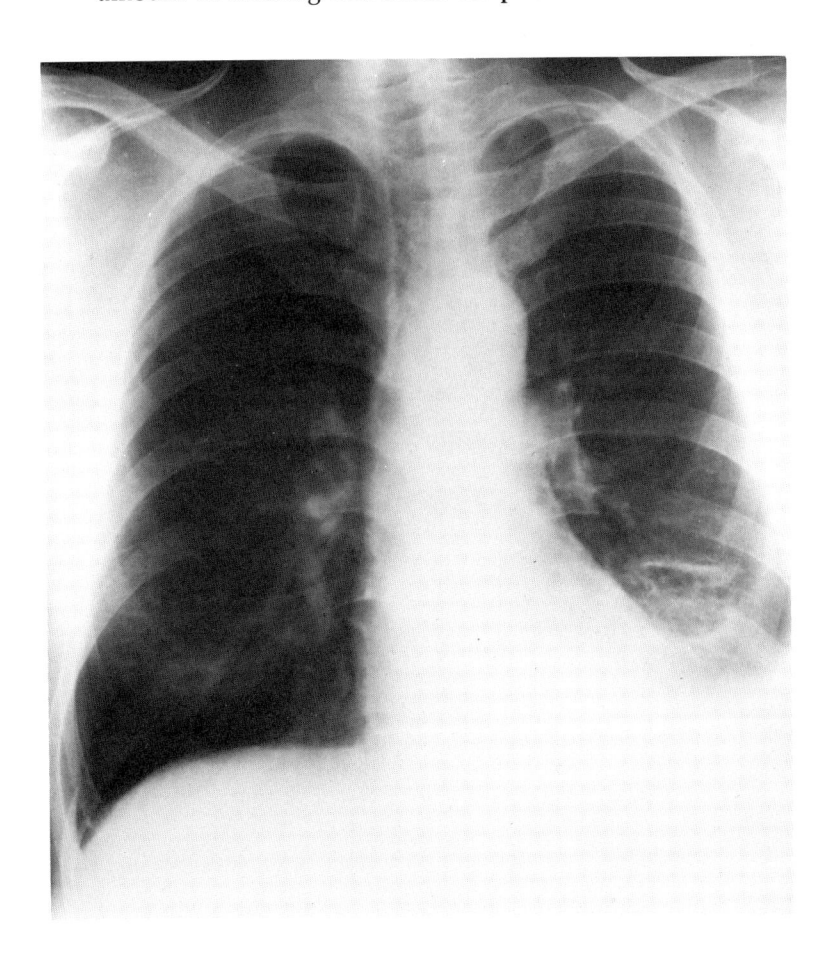

NOTE: The operator must be familiar with the use of the 3-way stopcock. Caution must be used to insure that no communication is inadvertently established between the pleural space and the atmosphere, allowing for pneumothorax to develop.

57 CLOSED THORACOSTOMY

INDICATIONS

1. Pneumothorax of sufficient degree to warrant closed chest drainage.
2. Hemothorax.
3. Drainage of the pleural cavity may be indicated to evacuate air and/or fluid.

EQUIPMENT

1. 10 cc syringe
2. 25-gauge ⅝-inch needle
3. 22-gauge 1½-inch needle
4. Four towels
5. #3 scalpel handle with #15 blade
6. Twelve 4 × 4-inch gauze sponges
7. 24 Fr. Foley catheter with 5 cc bag (smaller catheter for children); 24 Fr. straight catheter with additional holes cut in the tip
8. Large curved hemostat
9. Chest trocar

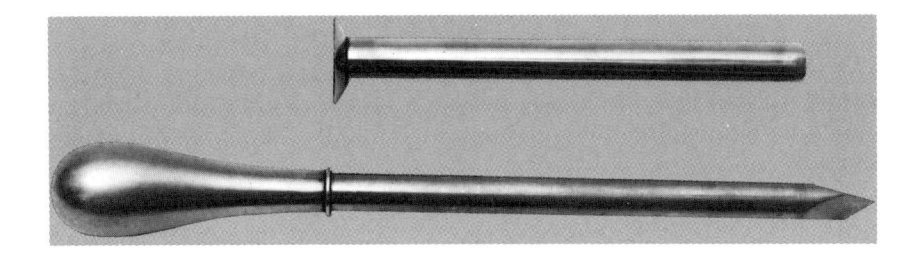

251

10. Needle holder
11. Suture scissors
12. 3-0 silk suture on cutting needle
13. Chest bottle with sterile fluid (disposable equipment is available)
14. Connecting tubing

EVACUATION OF PNEUMOTHORAX
ANATOMICAL CONSIDERATIONS

1. Since air rises, the site of drainage is an upper anterior intercostal space. Usually the first or second interspace is used.
2. The point of insertion of the catheter is in the midclavicular line, thus avoiding the internal mammary vessels.

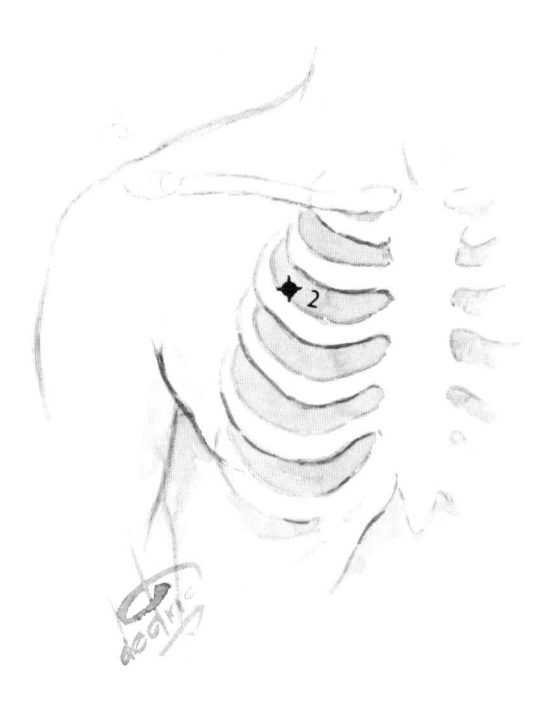

3. Pleural adhesions identified on x-ray examination of the chest should be avoided.
4. Penetration of the interspace should be done at the upper border of the ribs to lessen the possibility of damage to the intercostal vessels.
5. In female patients, the catheter may be inserted in the third or fourth intercostal space in the axillary line to avoid unsightly scarring of the anterior chest wall.

PROCEDURE

1. Shave the skin about the site. Place the patient in a semirecumbent position so the air rises to the apex of the pleural space.

2. Prep the skin of the chest wall with povidone-iodine.
3. Identify the second intercostal space with the middle finger while palpating the sternomanubrial angle (angle of Lewis) with the index finger.

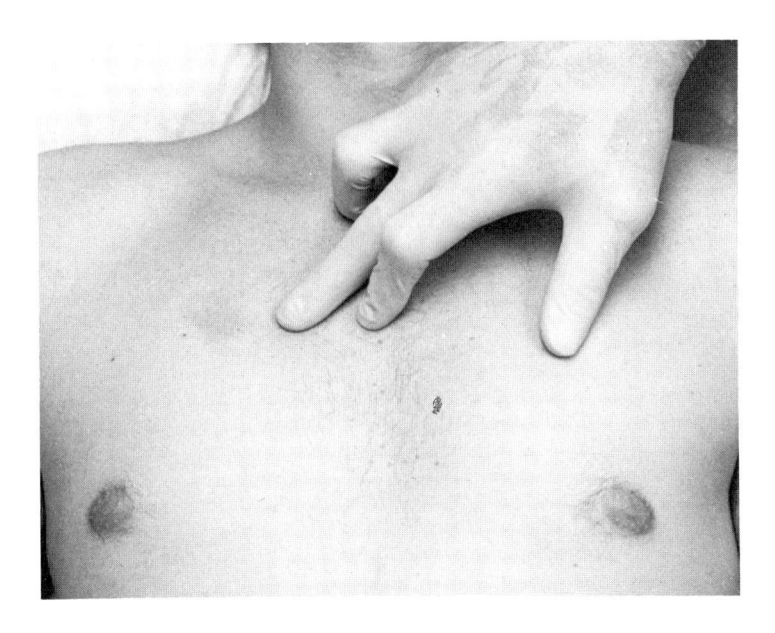

4. Raise a skin wheal above the superior border of the first or second rib in the midclavicular line using the 25-gauge needle.
5. Infiltrate the deeper layers of the interspace to the pleura using the longer 22-gauge needle.
6. Make a small (1/4 to 1/2-inch) nick in the skin wheal and deepen this into the intercostal muscles. Avoid the lower border of the rib.
7. Gently but firmly force the curved hemostat through the skin incision into the pleural space, spread it, and withdraw it.

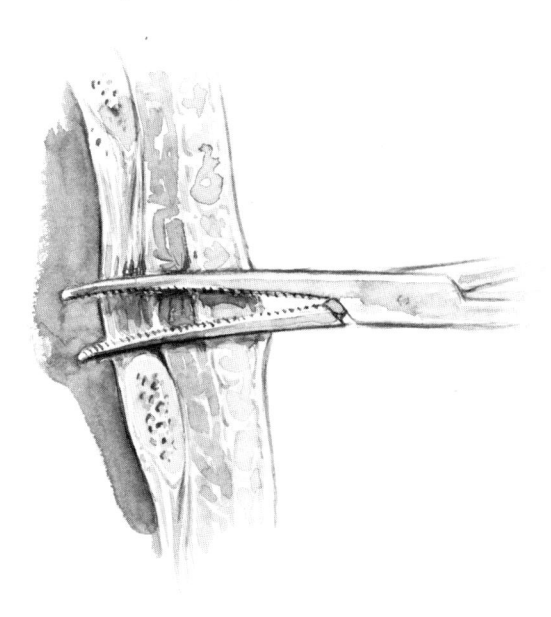

8. Grasp the tip of the Foley catheter (beyond the bag) in the hemostat and pass this into the pleural cavity in an upward direction.

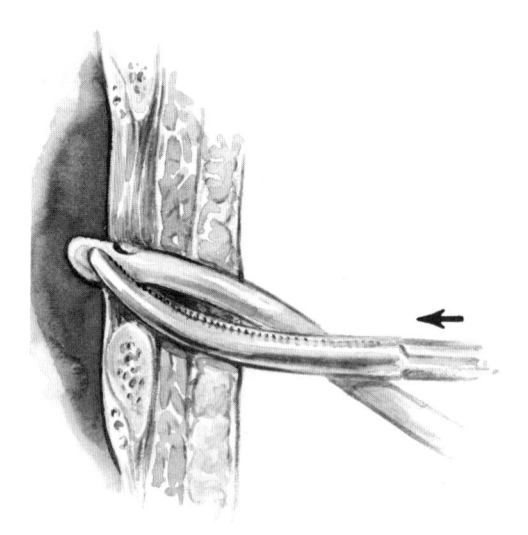

9. Remove the hemostat. Air will escape from the pleural cavity.
10. Inflate the balloon on the catheter with 5 cc of sterile saline and withdraw the catheter until the balloon is cinched against the parietal pleura. A sense of resistance will be felt.
11. Place a silk suture through the skin margins and leave long to wrap around the catheter as it exits from the skin. This is used to close the skin when the catheter is removed. Apply a sterile dressing to the area.

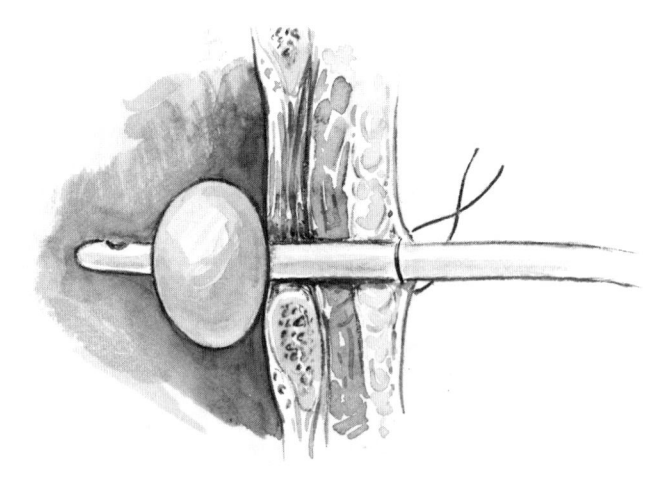

12. Attach the catheter to an underwater seal drainage bottle that is partially filled with water. The end of the drainage tube should extend 1 cm below the level of the water. Thus if the intrapleural pressure rises above 1 cm, air will be evacuated from the pleural cavity into the bottle. A simple device (Heimlich valve) can be attached to the end of the thoracostomy tube and

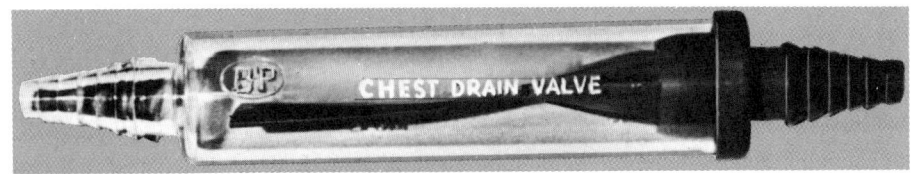

Heimlich valve

allow evacuation of air, without connection to an underwater seal. This permits the patient to be ambulatory.
13. In many instances, the intrapleural air will be completely evacuated by having the patient cough several times.
14. Follow-up upright chest x-ray examination should be done to ascertain whether the lung has completely re-expanded.

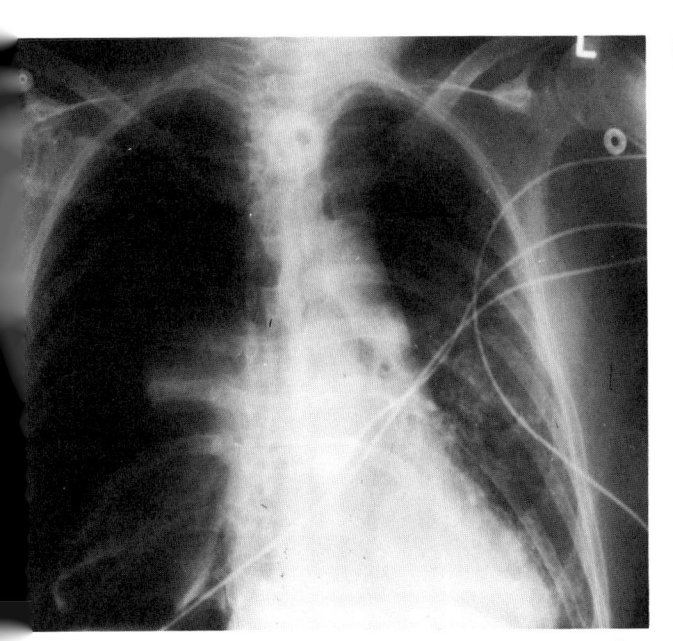

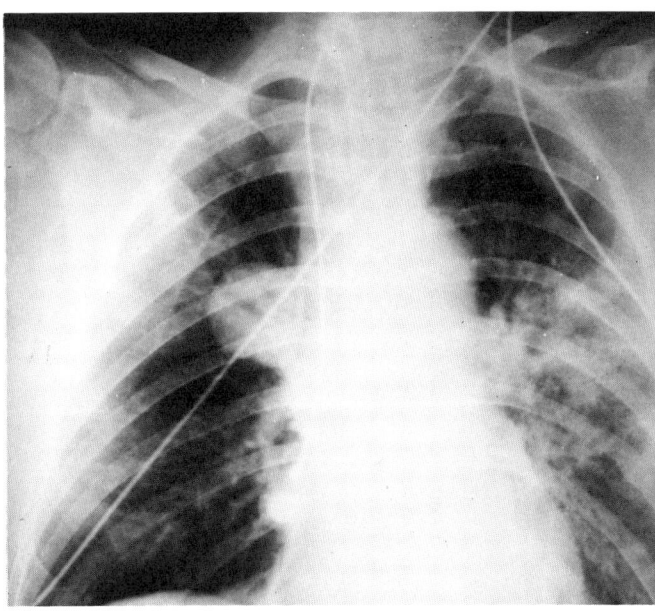

(Left) Massive right pneumothorax with mediastinal shift to left. Lung fully collapsed. (Right) Postoperative. Mediastinum in midline; right lung reexpanded.

15. The leak in the lung will be sealed as the lung re-expands and the visceral and parietal pleura contract. If the leak in the lung is sufficiently large, sealing will not be complete and there may be no significant decrease in the amount of pneumothorax. A vacuum pump may be attached to the drainage bottle and 15 to 20 cm of negative pressure applied to evacuate the pneumothorax.

EVACUATION OF HEMOTHORAX
ANATOMICAL CONSIDERATIONS
1. Fluid within the chest cavity, unless loculated, will gravitate to the lowest portion of the pleural space.

2. To evacuate fluid collection, the drainage tube should be placed in a lower posterior intercostal space. Usually the ninth intercostal space is chosen, in the posterior axillary line.

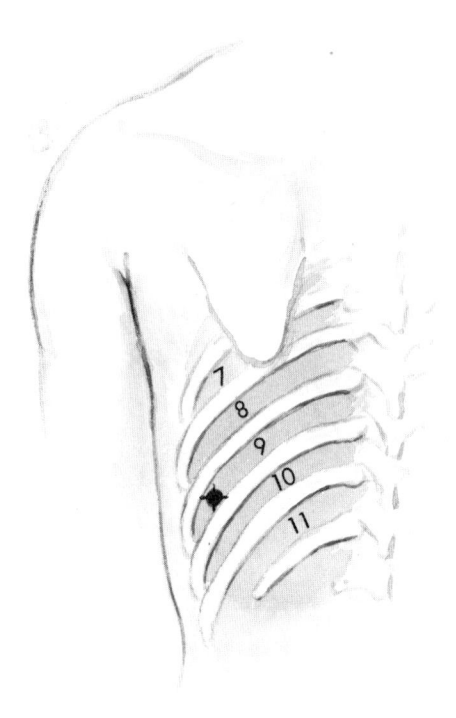

3. Catheter placement in the interspace should be done as described in drainage of a pneumothorax.
4. Location of the fluid can be identified by upright chest x-ray examination.

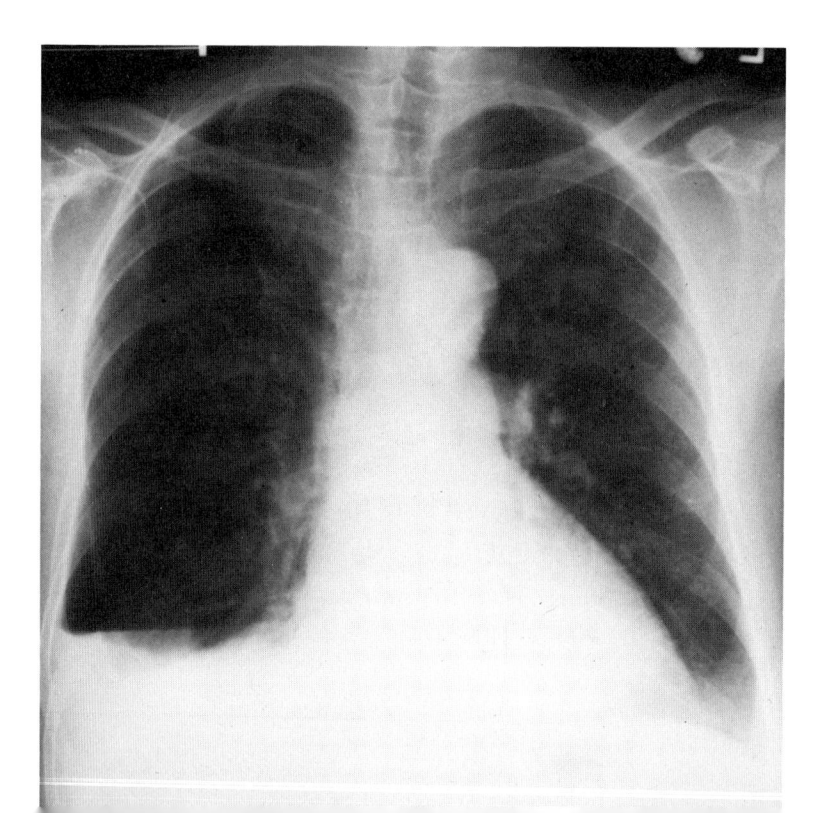

PROCEDURE

1. Identify the ninth intercostal space in the posterior axillary line by first finding the twelfth rib posteriorly and counting upward.
2. Place the patient in the sitting position, if possible.
3. Prep the skin of the lateral and posterior chest with povidone-iodine.
4. Raise a skin wheal in the ninth interspace and inject the anesthetic agent deeper into the intercostal muscles to the pleura.
5. Aspirate the pleural cavity. If blood is obtained, introduce a 24 Fr. Foley catheter as described for evacuation of pneumothorax and attach the catheter to an underwater seal.
6. If no blood or fluid is aspirated, repeat the procedure at the next higher interspace until the lower level of fluid is found, then introduce the catheter and attach to a drainage bottle.
7. A silk suture should be placed through the wound margins, left long, and wrapped about the catheter as it exits from the skin. Apply a sterile dressing to the area.
8. A follow-up chest x-ray examination should be done.

ALTERNATE PROCEDURE FOR THORACOSTOMY (TROCAR)

1. Before starting the procedure, determine that the entire length of the straight catherer passes through the trocar. Do not use a Foley catheter, because it will not pass through the trocar.
2. Select the site for thoracostomy, positioning the patient as necessary for evacuation of pneumothorax or fluid.
3. Prep the chest wall at the site with povidone-iodine and drape.
4. Raise a skin wheal and infiltrate the deeper tissues to the pleura.
5. Make a ½ to ¾-inch incision in the skin and subcutaneous tissue.
6. Holding the trocar in the hand with the handle of the obturator against the heel of the hand, firmly thrust the trocar through the intercostal space at the upper margin of the rib and into the pleural cavity.

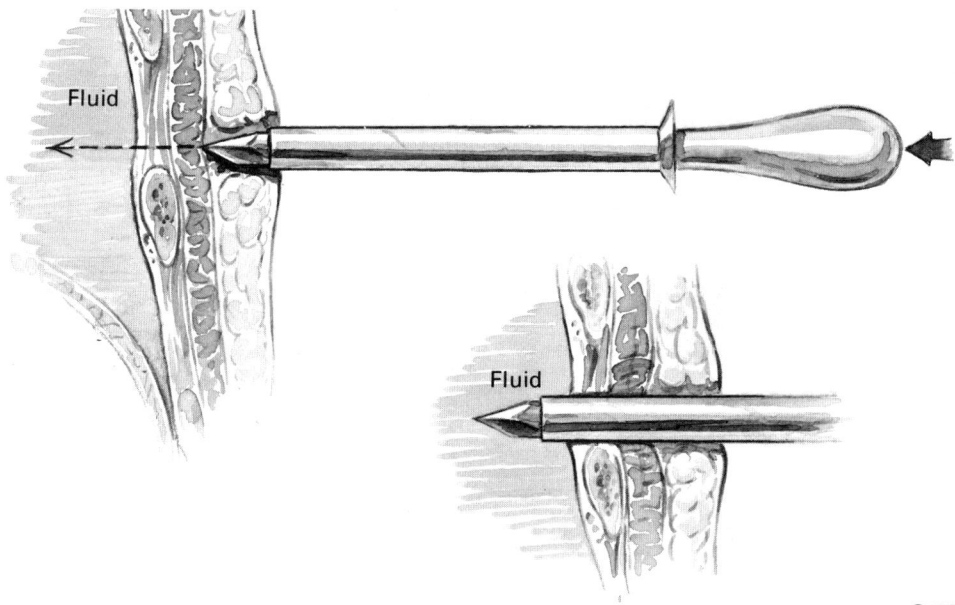

7. Withdraw the obturator and insert the straight catheter through the trocar barrel into the pleural space.

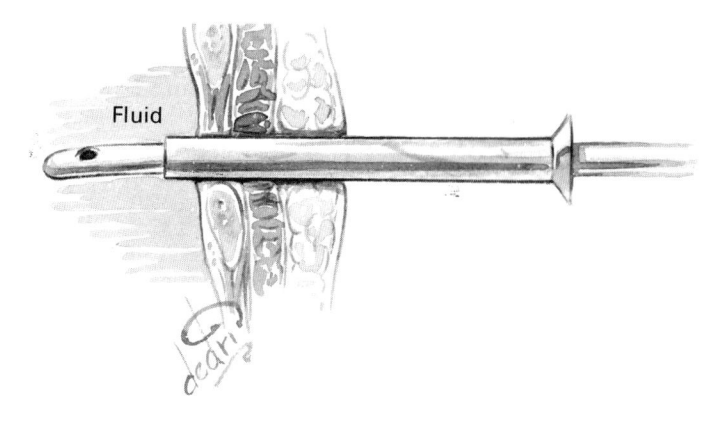

Fluid

8. Hold the protruding portion of the catheter in one hand to maintain it in position, and, with the other, remove the trocar barrel. Place a suture through the wound margins and about the catheter to prevent accidental removal.
9. Apply a sterile dressing over the wound.

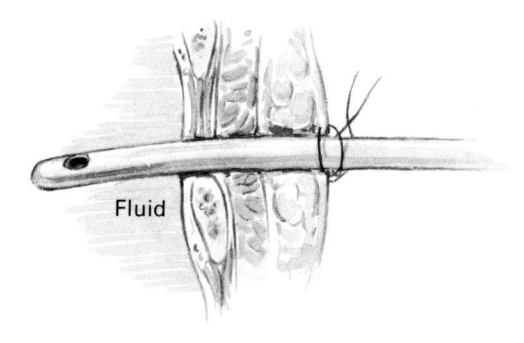

Fluid

10. Attach the free end of the catheter to an underwater seal as previously described.
11. Obtain a follow-up upright chest x-ray film.

58 PERITONEAL FLANK TAP

This procedure is similar to the four-quadrant tap. Some favor this approach.

INDICATIONS
1. Blunt abdominal trauma with suspicion of intraperitoneal injury.
2. Suspected intraperitoneal bleeding.
3. Unconscious patient with possible intraperitoneal injury.

EQUIPMENT
1. Three 10 cc syringes
2. Two 19-gauge 3½ to 4-inch spinal needles with obturator
3. Local set
4. Sample tubes

ANATOMICAL CONSIDERATION
Flank tap should be done in the lateral aspect of the anterior abdominal wall in the anterior axillary line midway between the costal margin and the iliac crest.

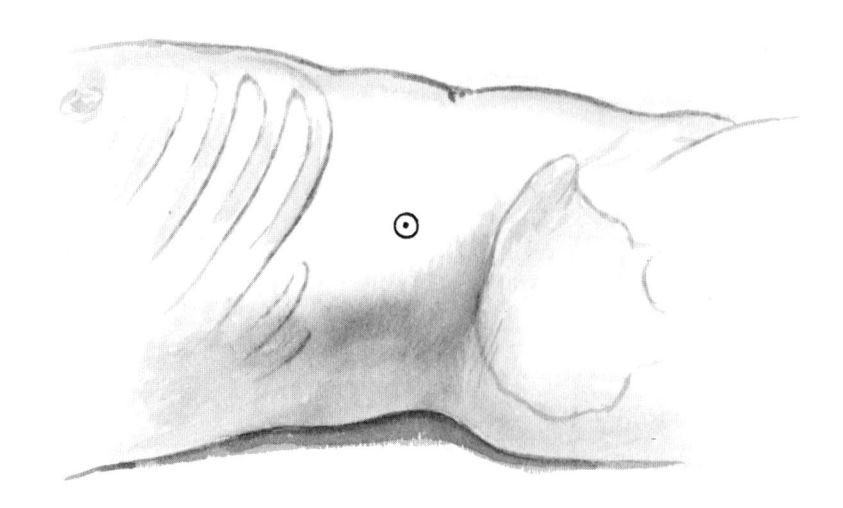

PROCEDURE

1. Select the site for the tap, prep an area 8 to 10 inches square about the site with povidone-iodine and drape.
2. Raise a skin wheal in each flank.
3. Infiltrate the deeper tissues of the abdominal wall to the peritoneum along the intended line of insertion of the spinal needle.
4. Insert the spinal needle with obturator into the skin wheal and advance it toward the peritoneal cavity.
5. As the peritoneum is encountered, note a feeling of slight resistance. Advance the needle slowly through the peritoneum.
6. Once the peritoneal cavity is entered, remove the obturator and attach a clean 10 cc syringe.
7. Aspirate gently in two planes (aspirate, then rotate the needle 180 degrees and aspirate again).
8. If nonclotting blood or bloody fluid is obtained, the tap is positive and the procedure may be discontinued. If no fluid is obtained, repeat the procedure on the opposite flank.
9. Analyze the fluid as outlined in "Four-quadrant Tap".

BIBLIOGRAPHY

Baker, R. J. Newer techniques in evaluation of injured patients. Surg. Clin. N. Am. 55:31, 1975.

59 PERITONEAL FOUR-QUADRANT TAP

INDICATIONS
1. Blunt abdominal trauma with suspicion of intraperitoneal injury.
2. Suspected intraperitoneal bleeding.
3. Unconscious patient with suspected intraperitoneal bleeding.

EQUIPMENT
1. Five 10 cc syringes
2. Four 19-gauge 3½ to 4-inch spinal needles with obturator
3. 25-gauge needle
4. 22-gauge 1½-inch needle
5. Sample tubes
6. 0.5% lidocaine

ANATOMICAL CONSIDERATIONS
1. Peritoneal tap should be done in the anterior abdominal wall lateral to the rectus sheath.
2. Penetration of the rectus sheath may damage the epigastric vessels resulting in a false positive tap and/or hematoma formation.
3. It is imperative to avoid any operative scar where intraperitoneal adhesions may be encountered.

PROCEDURE
1. Prep the entire abdominal wall with povidone-iodine.
2. Raise a skin wheal with 0.5% lidocaine in each quadrant of the abdomen, lateral to the rectus sheath.

3. Make deeper infiltration into the subcutaneous and muscular layers at each wheal site.
4. Insert a spinal needle with obturator into the skin wheal in one quadrant and pass it into the deeper tissues of the abdominal wall. The point of entry is approximately the center of each quadrant. As the peritoneum is penetrated resistance is encountered momentarily and is relieved.

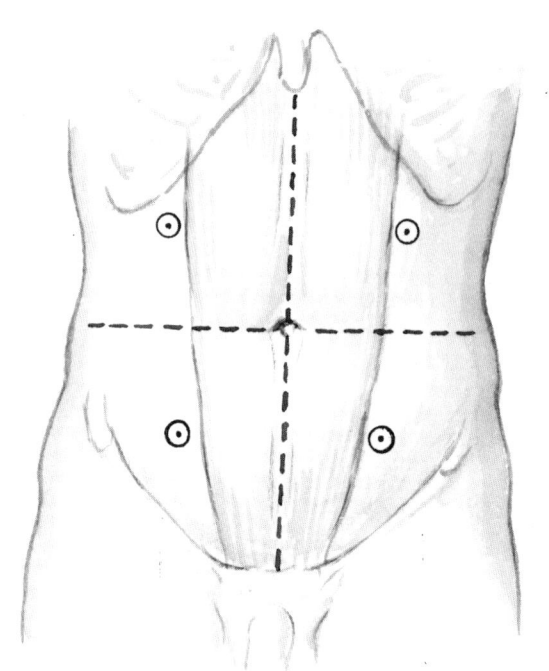

5. Once the needle is in the peritoneal cavity, remove the obturator, attach a 10 cc syringe and gently aspirate. If blood or bloody fluid is recovered, the tap is positive.
6. Place a small amount of aspirate in a clear tube and observe whether it clots. Typically intraperitoneal blood will not clot. Blood recovered by accidental puncture of a mesenteric or abdominal wall vessel will clot.
7. Examine any fluid recovered microscopically after appropriate staining. If a sufficient amount is obtained, amylase or other biochemical tests may be carried out.
8. Inadvertent puncture of the intestine is usually of no consequence.
   If no intraperitoneal fluid is recovered, repeat the procedure in another quadrant, using a fresh needle and syringe.
9. Failure to recover any fluid is considered a negative tap and has no significance.
10. When nonclotting blood or bloody fluid is recovered, the tap is considered positive. Experience has shown a positive tap to be accurate in the diagnosis of intra-abdominal injury in 80 percent of patients.

NOTE: Indications for exploratory laparotomy in a patient with a positive peritoneal tap should include complete clinical assessment of the abdomen.

BIBLIOGRAPHY

Draponas, T. and McDonald, J. Peritoneal tap in abdominal trauma. Surgery 50:742, 1961.

Olsen, W. R. and Haldreth, D. H. Abdominal paracentesis and peritoneal lavage in blunt abdominal trauma. J. Trauma 11:824, 1971.

60 PERITONEAL LAVAGE

INDICATIONS
1. Blunt abdominal trauma and suspected intraperitoneal injury.
2. Unexplained shock in a patient with multiple organ system injury.
3. Unconscious patient with possible intraperitoneal injury.
4. Suspected intraperitoneal injury with a negative four-quadrant or flank tap.

CONTRAINDICATIONS
1. Multiple abdominal scars.
2. Pregnancy.

EQUIPMENT
1. Local set with prep
2. #3 scalpel handle with #11 or #15 blade
3. Standard peritoneal dialysis catheter with stylet and connector (Stylocath-Abbott)
4. 1,000 cc normal saline or Ringer's lactate (for adults)
5. Normal saline or Ringer's lactate (for children 10 to 20 cc/kg of body weight)
6. One strand 4-0 silk suture and swedged needle, needle holder, scissors
7. Intravenous tubing
8. 10 cc syringe
9. 0.5% lidocaine with epinephrine

PROCEDURE

1. The bladder should be emptied by spontaneous micturition or drained by a catheter.
2. Prep the abdomen with povidone-iodine and drape the area with sterile towels.
3. Infiltrate the midline of the lower abdomen about 3 cm below the umbilicus using 0.5% lidocaine with epinephrine.
4. Make a stab wound at the site of the skin wheal.

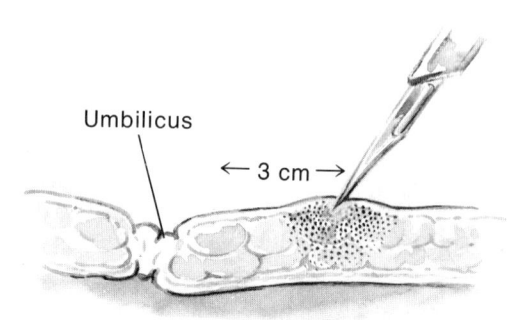

5. Insert the peritoneal dialysis catheter and stylet into the incision and advance with firm pressure in a twisting motion until the peritoneum is entered. There will be a sudden lessening of resistance as the peritoneum is penetrated. Once the peritoneum is entered, withdraw the stylet 1 cm and direct the device at a 45-degree angle toward the lower abdomen.

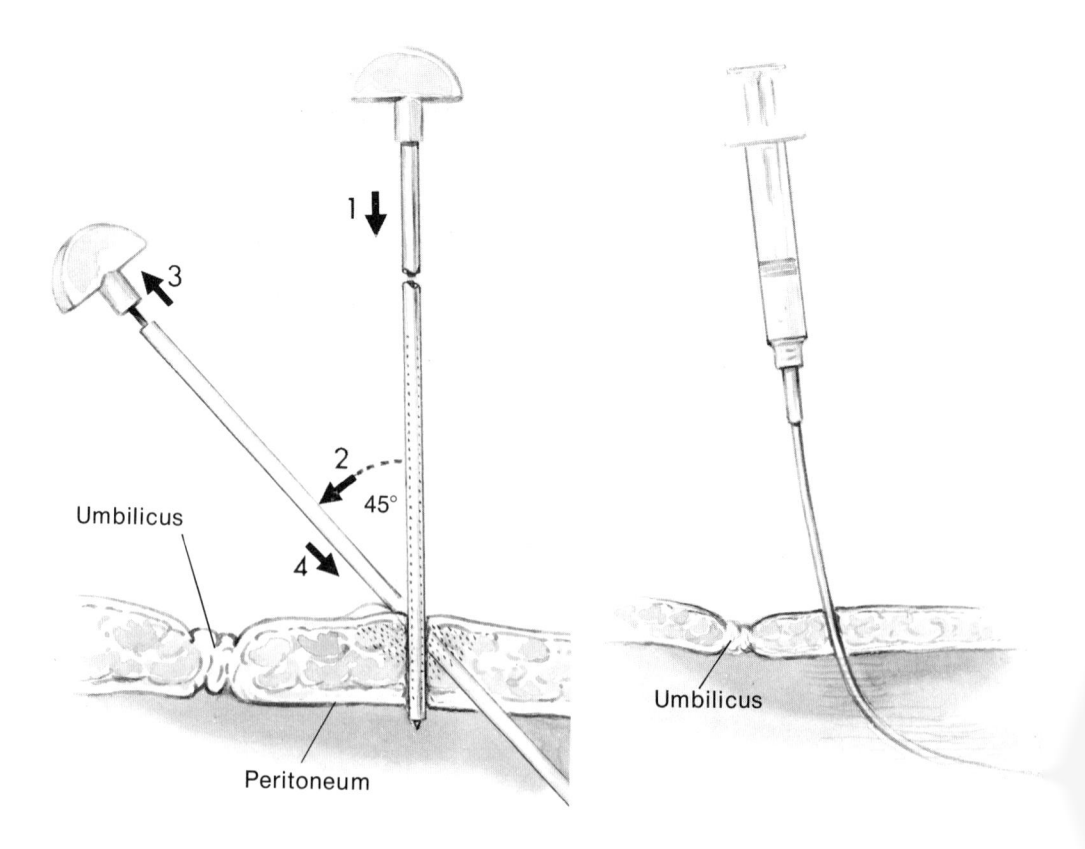

6. Remove the stylet and connect the connector.
7. Attach the 10 cc syringe and aspirate the peritoneal cavity. If nonclotting blood is obtained, the study is positive and there is no indication for lavage.
8. If no blood is aspirated, attach the intravenous tubing to the connector and allow 1,000 cc of normal saline or Ringer's lactate to infuse into the peritoneal cavity. (In children use 10 to 20 cc/kg of body weight.)

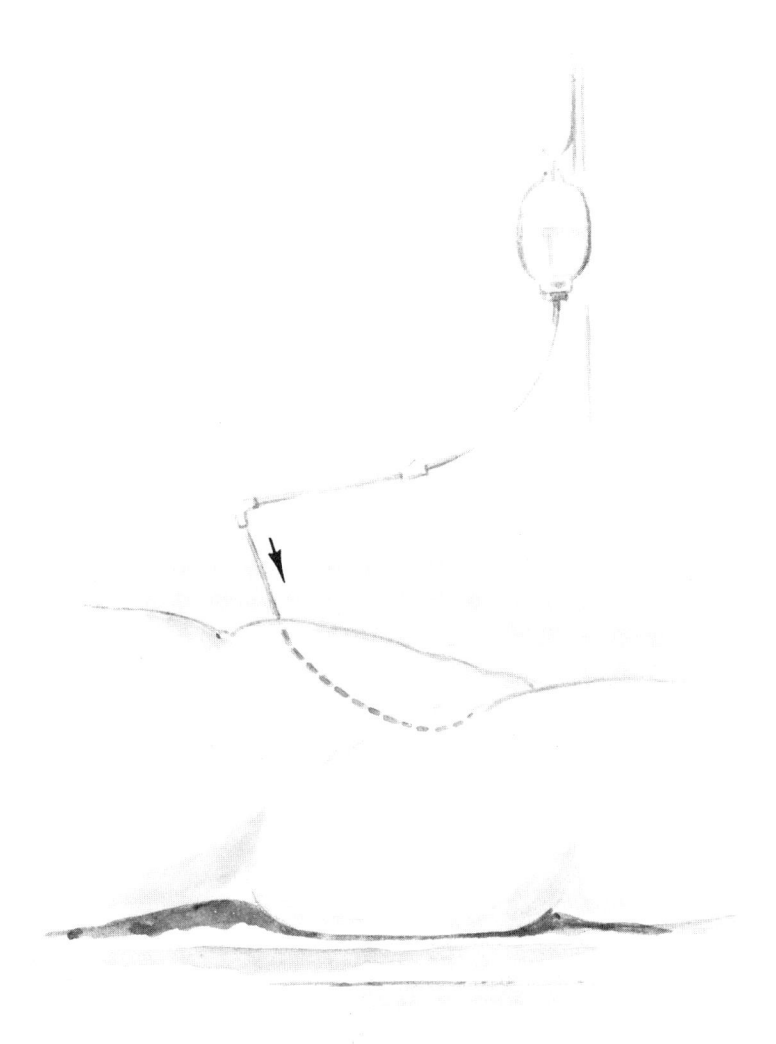

9. When the infusion is complete, turn the patient from side to side to diffuse the fluid.
10. Place the empty IV bottle on the floor and allow the intraperitoneal fluid to be syphoned.

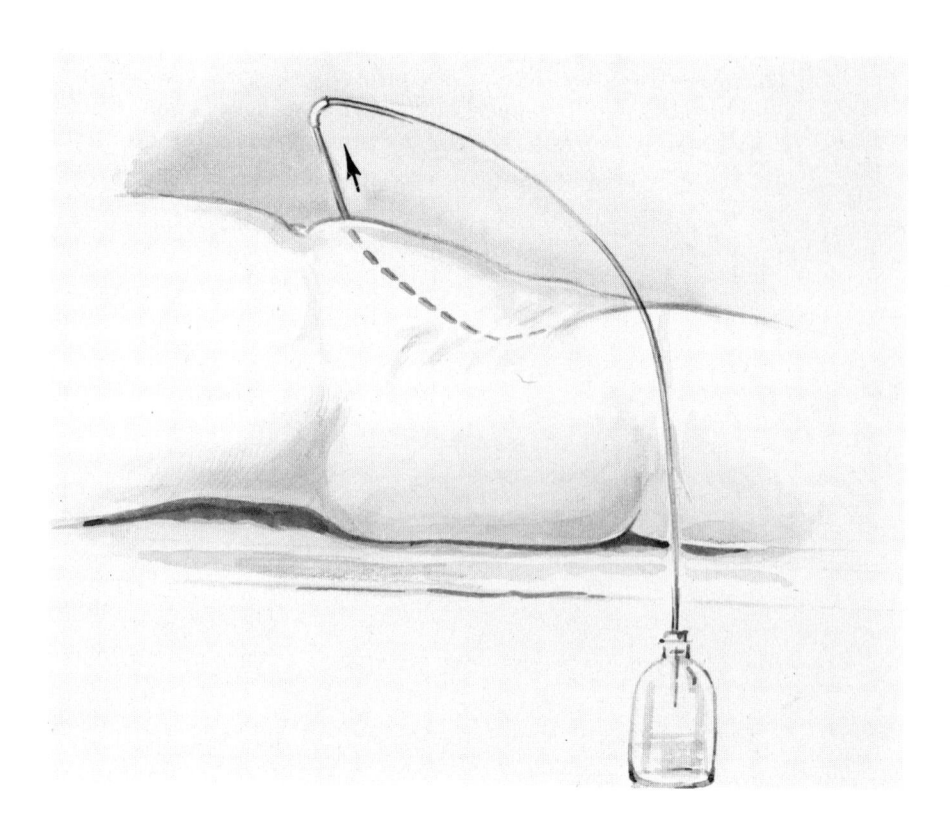

11. Bloody fluid is indicative of a positive lavage.
12. All lavage fluid may not be recovered. When the procedure is completed, close the stab wound with a single silk suture and apply a sterile dressing.
13. Analyze the recovered fluid for red blood cell count, amylase, bile, and culture for bacteria.

BIBLIOGRAPHY

Engrav, L. H., Benjamin, C. J., and Strate, R. G. Diagnostic peritoneal lavage in blunt abdominal trauma. J. Trauma 15:854, 1975.

Kazarian, K. K., Devanesan, J. D., and Mersheimer, W. L. Diagnostic peritoneal lavage. N. Y. State J. Med. 2149, 1975.

Parvin, T. S., Smith, D. E., Asher, W. M., and Virgilio, R. W. Effectiveness of peritoneal lavage in blunt abdominal trauma. Ann Surg. 181:255, 1975.

Perry, J. F., Jr., DeMueles, J. E., and Root, H. D. Diagnostic peritoneal lavage in blunt abdominal trauma. Surg. Gyn. & Obstet. 131:742, 1970.

Root, H. D., Hauser, C. W., McKin, C. R., and Lafare, J. W. Diagnostic peritoneal lavage. Surgery 633, 1965.

61 CUL-DE-SAC ASPIRATION

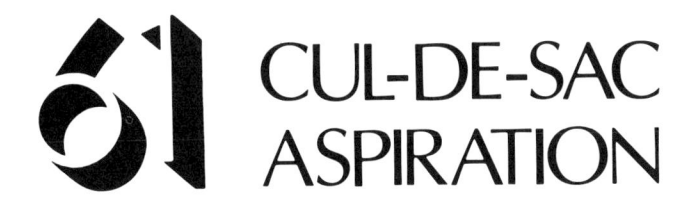

INDICATIONS
1. Suspected ruptured ectopic pregnancy.
2. Suspected intraperitoneal bleeding in a female.
3. Some cases of pelvic inflammatory disease.

EQUIPMENT
1. 5 cc syringe with 25-gauge ⅝-inch needle
2. 10 cc syringe
3. 19-gauge 4-inch spinal needle
4. Vaginal speculum
5. Uterine tenaculum
6. Prep
7. Sponge forceps
8. 1% lidocaine
9. Six 4 × 4-inch gauze pads

ANATOMICAL CONSIDERATIONS
1. The posterior cul-de-sac (pouch of Douglas) is the lowermost extension of the peritoneal cavity in the pelvis. It is located between the posterior wall of the uterus and the anterior wall of the rectum.

Urinary bladder

Posterior lip of cervix

Cul-de-sac

Posterior fornix

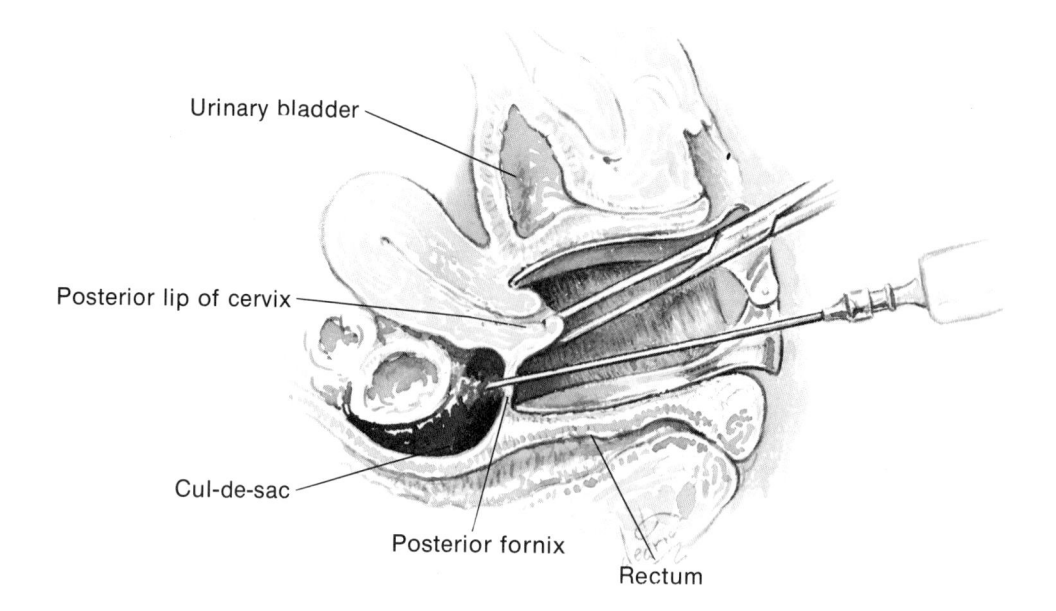

Rectum

2. The inferior border of the cul-de-sac is in close proximity to the superior border of the posterior fornix of the vagina.
3. Free blood within the peritoneal cavity from any source may gravitate to the cul-de-sac but is especially common following an ectopic pregnancy or a ruptured bleeding ovarian cyst.
4. The procedure is contraindicated when adhesions are suspected from prior pelvic injury or endometriosis.

PROCEDURE

1. Place the patient in the lithotomy position.
2. Prep the vagina with povidone-iodine.
3. Insert a lubricated vaginal speculum to obtain exposure of the cervix.
4. Grasp the posterior lip of the cervix with a tenaculum and raise it forward to expose the posterior fornix.
5. Inject 1 to 2 cc of anesthetic agent into the superior wall of the posterior fornix (optional).
6. Insert the 4-inch needle on the 10 cc syringe through the posterior fornix into the cul-de-sac on a plane parallel to the spine. Do not direct the needle posteriorly toward the rectum.
7. If nonclotting blood is obtained, the tap is positive and indicates intraperitoneal bleeding. If pus is recovered, pelvic inflammatory disease is strongly suspected.
8. If no blood is obtained the tap is negative.

NOTE: A negative cul-de-sac aspiration should not in itself be a deterrent to laporatomy but should be considered in conjunction with other clinical findings.

62 STEINMAN PIN INSERTION

INDICATION

Need to initiate and maintain skeletal traction especially in fractures of the long bones of the limbs.

EQUIPMENT

1. Sterile Steinman pins (scored-not scored) and yoke
2. Drill handle, chuck, chuck key
3. #3 scalpel handle with #11 blade
4. 10 cc syringe
5. 25-gauge $5/8$-inch needle
6. 22-gauge $1^{1}/_{2}$-inch needle
7. 0.5% lidocaine
8. Twelve 4 × 4-inch gauze pads
9. Four towels
10. Collodion

ANATOMICAL CONSIDERATIONS

1. The Steinman pin is used for skeletal traction in the upper or lower limbs. In the upper extremity, skeletal traction may be indicated in certain fractures of the humerus. In this instance, the pin is inserted in the olecranon process.
2. In the leg, skeletal traction is used in certain fractures of the femur. The traction pin may be placed through the femoral condyles or the tibial tubercle, depending upon the nature of the fracture. In some patients, the pin may be passed through the calcaneus.
3. The pin should be placed under strict aseptic conditions and be held in position without any slippage.

PROCEDURE

1. Shave the area where the pin is to be inserted.
2. Prep the skin with povidone-iodine.
3. Palpate the level at which the pin is to be placed.
4. Raise a skin wheal using the 25-gauge needle and infiltrate in the deeper tissues to the periosteum.

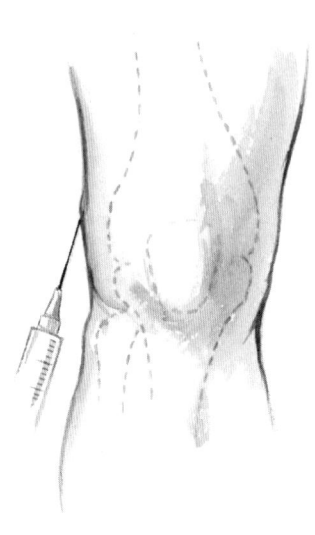

5. Draw the skin upward in the limb so it will be taut at the level of pin insertion.
6. Make a small nick in the skin with the scalpel.
7. Insert the pin through the incision to the periosteum and drill through the bone until the pin points beneath the skin on the opposite side of the extremity.

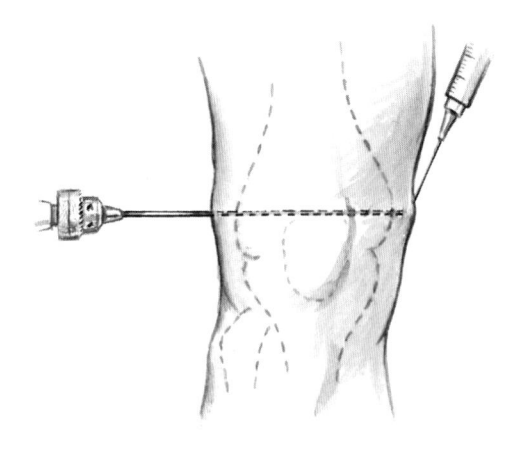

8. Infiltrate this point with local anesthetic.
9. Nick the skin at this point.
10. Drill the pin through the second skin incision.
11. Cut two 2-inch squares from the gauze pad. Moisten these with collodion and place each about the pin where it protrudes from the skin.
12. Attach the yoke firmly to the Steinman pin to prevent slippage.

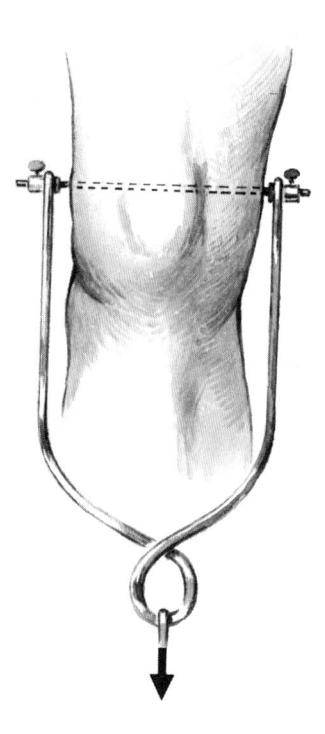

13. Felt pads may be cut to size (1 to 2-inch squares) and placed on the pin between the collodion gauze and the yoke.
14. Attach the yoke to the pulley system.

63 CERVICAL TRACTION

Over the years, a number of devices have been used for skeletal traction in certain injuries of the cervical spine. While these were of great value, their proper application required shaving of portions of the patient's scalp and drilling of the outer table of the cranium.

The Gardner-Wells traction tongs is an instrument of remarkable simplicity and ease of application, consisting of a rigid member shaped to the contour of the calvarium at each end of which is a threaded hole through which spring-loaded, needle-sharp points are placed.

While the entire assembly may be autoclaved, it is not required. The needle-sharp points can be removed and placed in antiseptic solution. These points penetrate the outer table by continuous pressure exerted on a relatively small cross-sectional area and account for the stability of the tongs in the skull. The tongs rarely pull out when applied properly and will tolerate up to 65 pounds of traction.

This device has been left in place for more than eight weeks with no evidence of infection.

INDICATIONS

1. Stabilization of and traction for the cervical spine.
2. Traction for some fractures of the cervical spine.
3. Traction for fracture-dislocation of the cervical spine.

EQUIPMENT

1. Gardner-Wells traction tongs
2. Rope
3. Pulley
4. Weight holder and weights
5. 25-gauge ⅝-inch needle
6. 5 cc syringe
7. 0.5% lidocaine
8. Prep
9. Six 4 × 4-inch gauze pads

ANATOMICAL CONSIDERATIONS

1. The points of the traction tongs are placed in the direction of the pull.

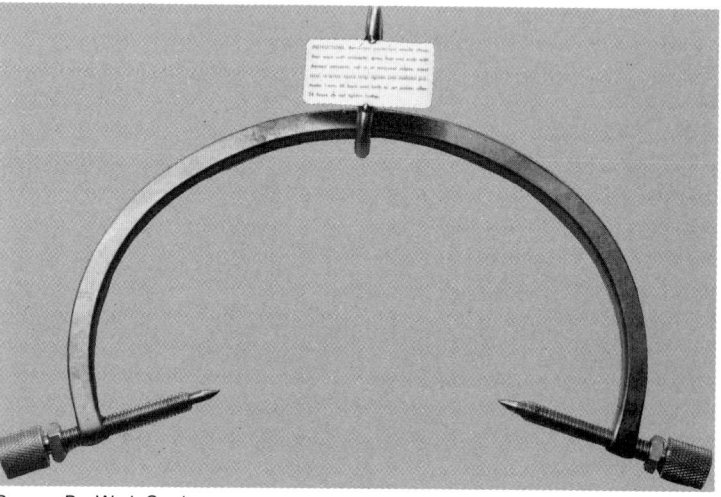

Source: Dr. W. J. Gardner

2. The ridge in the upper portion of the temporal bone is the area to which the tongs should be applied.

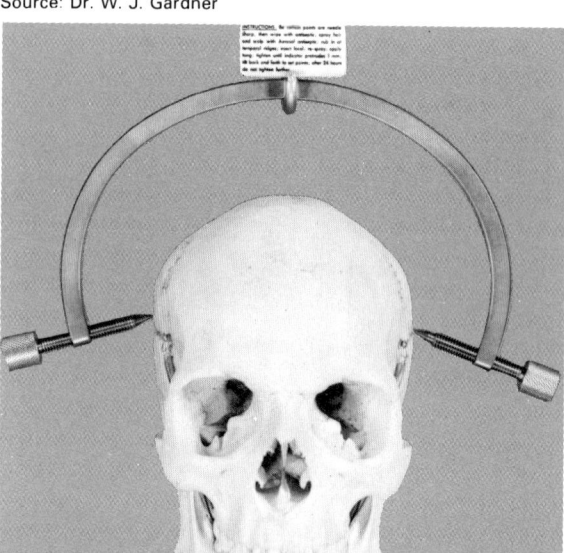

Source: Dr. W. J. Gardner

3. The traction should be applied directly above the ears. The desired degree of

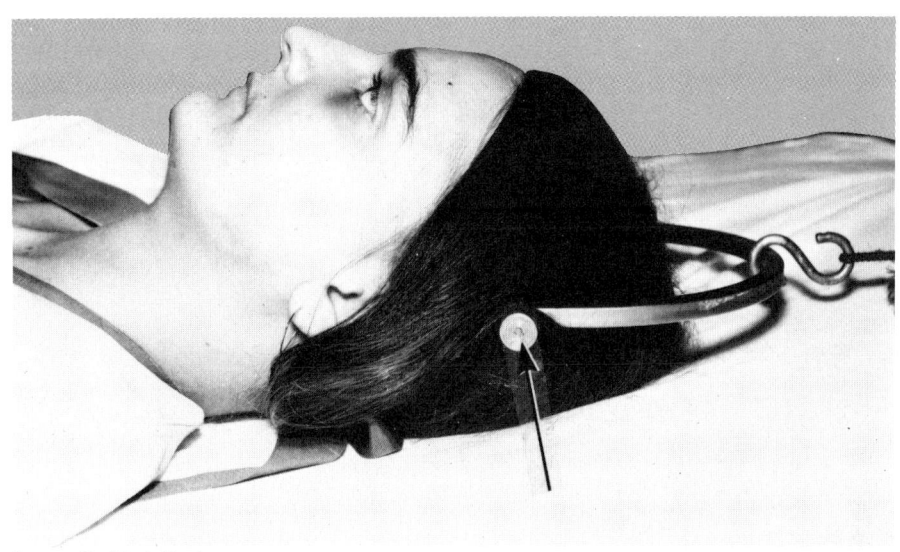

Source: Dr. W. J. Gardner

cervical flexion can be obtained by adjusting the height of the pulley.

PROCEDURE

1. It is <u>not</u> necessary to shave the scalp.
2. Prep the skin of the scalp by spraying with a solution of povidone-iodine. Spray the scalp at the temporal ridges, rub the agent into the scalp, and apply a second layer of spray.
3. Infiltrate the scalp with lidocaine at the site of application of the tongs, deepening the anesthetic to the periosteum.
4. Wipe the points of the tongs with antiseptic.
5. Apply the tongs to the scalp, screwing the points into position until the tension on the spring-loaded clamp indicates a squeezing pressure of 30 pounds. The amount of squeezing pressure is adequate when the indicator protrudes 1 mm from the knob of the screw.

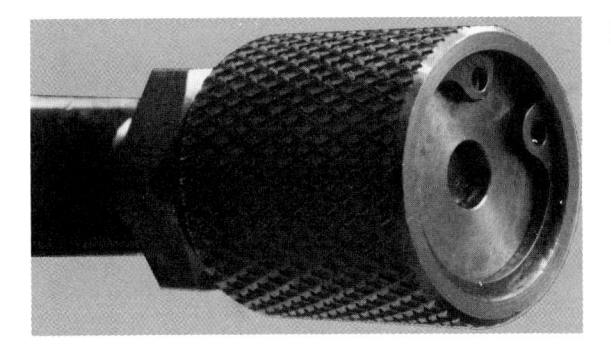

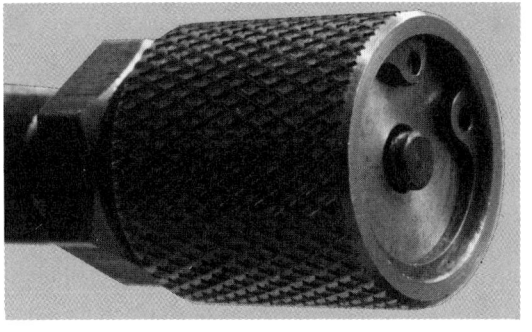

6. Tilt the tongs back and forth to be sure the pins are properly seated and readjust the pressure as necessary.
7. Attach the rope, pulley, and desired amount of weight.
8. Restrict rotation of the neck by placing sandbags on either side of the head, supporting the projecting knurled end of each screw.

NOTE: Be certain the points of the tongs are <u>needle-sharp</u> for better penetration.

BIBLIOGRAPHY

Gardner, W. J. The principle of spring-loaded points for cervical traction. J. Neurosurg. 39:543, 1973.

——— Personal communication.

Janese, W. W. Personal communication.

64 CYSTOGRAPHY AND STRESS CYSTOGRAPHY

INDICATIONS

1. Suspected injury to the bladder.
2. Following a normal urethrogram when lower urinary tract injury is suspected.
3. Presence of perineal hematoma.

EQUIPMENT

1. 16 or 18 Fr. Foley catheter (8 to 10 Fr. for pediatric patient)
2. Asepto syringe or Toomey syringe.

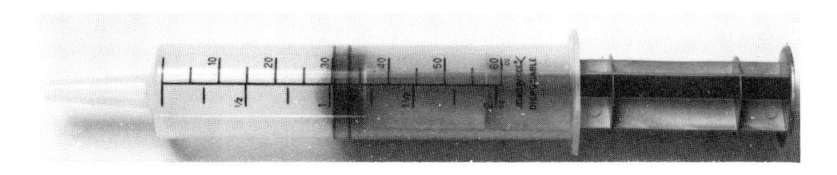

3. 14% Cystografin or a mixture of the following: ¼ Renografin, ¾ water (500 cc total)
4. Four towels
5. K-Y jelly
6. 500 cc metal pitcher

ANATOMICAL CONSIDERATIONS

1. The bladder is located in the midline of the pelvis, posterior to the symphysis pubis.
2. Injury to the bladder may involve any portion of its wall. Rupture may allow extravasation into extraperitoneal tissues or free rupture into the peritoneal cavity.

3. On occasion, the point of rupture may be occluded by omentum, a loop of bowel, or a blood clot. For this reason, filling of the bladder must be done under pressure in order to extravasate through the rupture (stress cystogram).

PROCEDURE

1. Place the patient supine on the x-ray table with one hip slightly elevated on a folded sheet.
2. Insert the Foley catheter into the bladder and allow all the urine to drain. Save samples for analysis, culture, and sensitivity.
3. Attach the barrel of the Asepto or the Toomey syringe to the open end of the catheter and allow the bladder to be filled with the radiopaque medium by gravity until the patient notes slight discomfort.

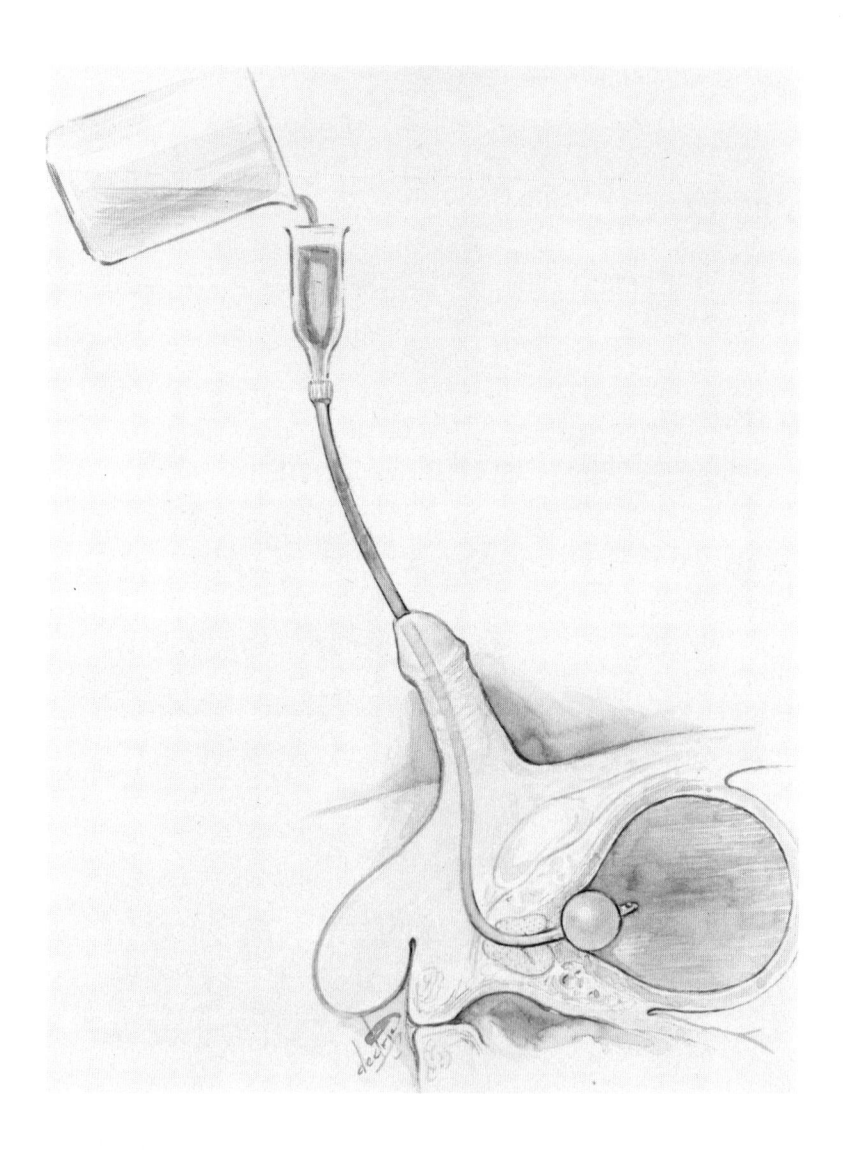

4. Clamp the catheter.
5. Call for the x-ray film.

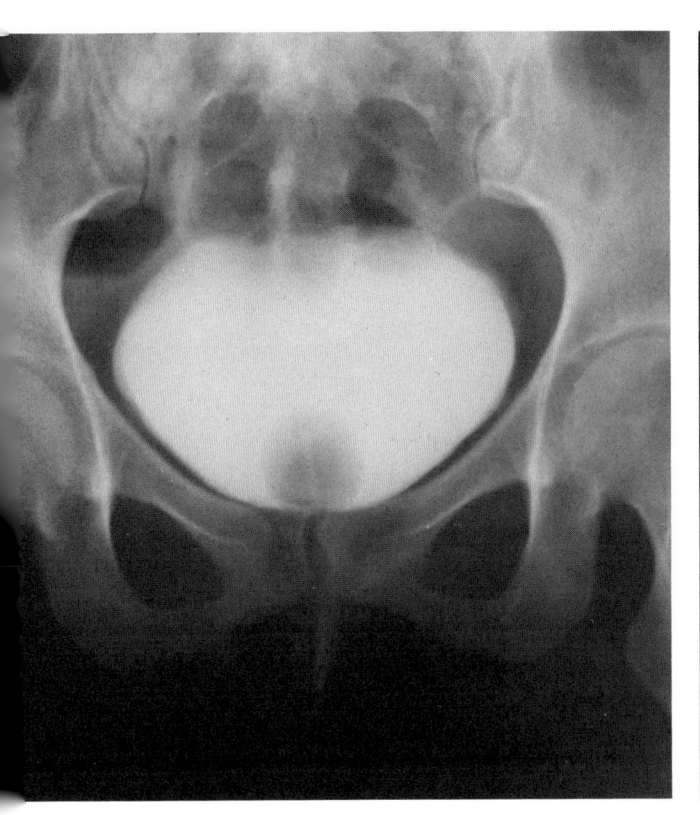

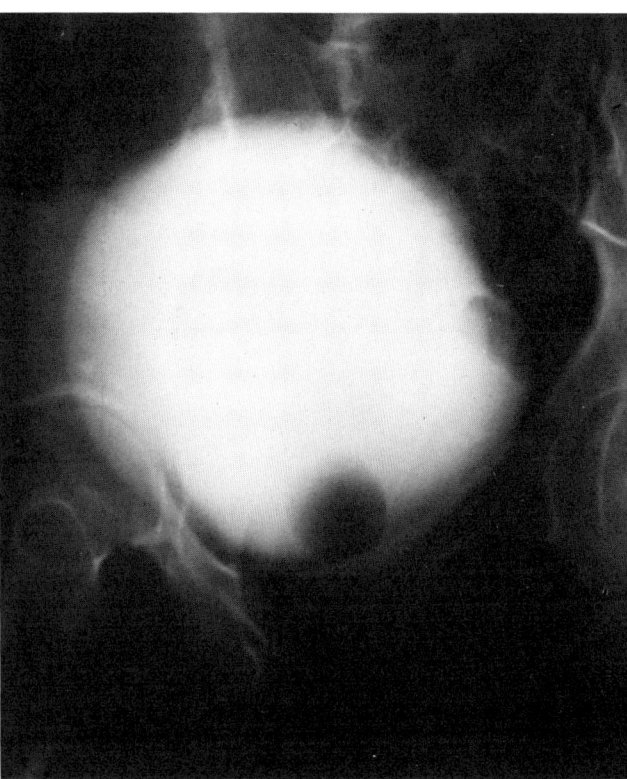

6. Place 30 cc of contrast material in the syringe with the plunger or bulb in place and inject this into the bladder under pressure. This is a "stress" cystogram.

BIBLIOGRAPHY

Carlton, C. E., Jr. Treatment of Urologic Injuries. In W. W. Oaks and S. Spitzer, eds., 23rd. Hahnemann Symposium. New York: Grune & Stratton, 1972, pp. 233-240.

65 TROCAR SUPRAPUBIC CYSTOTOMY

INDICATIONS
1. Acute urinary retention due to obstruction of the bladder outlet.
2. Acute urinary retention which cannot be relieved by transurethral catheterization.

EQUIPMENT
1. Local set
2. #3 knife handle with #10 blade
3. 0.5% lidocaine
4. 26 Fr. Campbell fenestrated trocar to allow passage of an 18 Fr. balloon catheter. In pediatric patients a 21 Fr. trocar is used, which will accept a 14 to 16 Fr. balloon catheter.
5. Foley catheter (18 Fr. for an adult, 14 to 16 Fr. for a child)

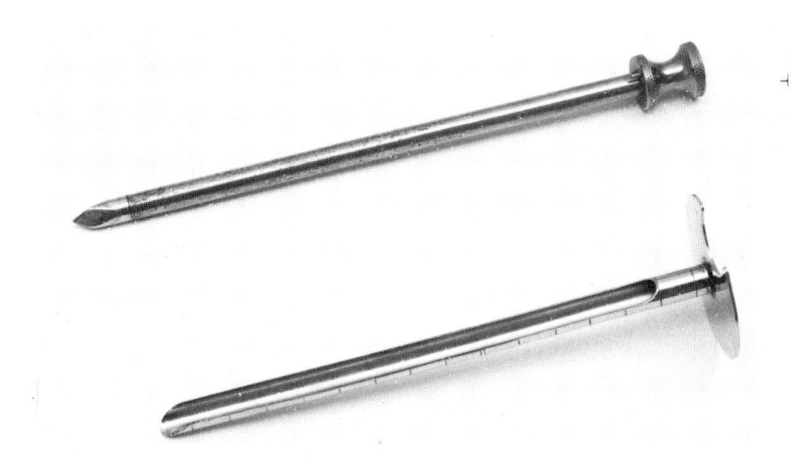

Campbell trocar

6. Catheter stylet or straight probe
7. Four towels
8. 000 silk suture on cutting edge needle
9. Twelve 4 × 4-inch gauze pads

NOTE: A number of disposable suprapubic drainage devices are available commercially.

ANATOMICAL CONSIDERATIONS

1. The urinary bladder is located in the midline of the pelvic area deep to the symphysis pubis. It is covered by peritoneum over its dome but is an extraperitoneal organ. As the obstructed bladder becomes distended, it rises out of the pelvis, much as a gravid uterus does, thus elevating the peritoneal reflection well above the symphysis.
2. The prevesical space of Retzius is located between the bladder and the posterior wall of the pubis. This space contains loose areolar tissue and small blood vessels. As the obstructed bladder rises out of the pelvis, the space of Retzius thins out and the anterior bladder wall lies in close proximity to the posterior margin of the rectus abdominis muscles. At this level, the posterior rectus sheath is absent.
3. The linea alba is located in the midline of the anterior abdominal wall and extends from the xiphoid to the symphysis pubis. This is the structure which should be incised to allow introduction of the trocar.

NOTE: It is extremely important to avoid entry into either rectus sheath where major blood vessels may be damaged, with resultant bleeding and/or hematoma formation.

4. The dome of the bladder should be palpated or percussed at least to a point midway between the umbilicus and the symphysis pubis.

PROCEDURE

1. Percuss or palpate the distended bladder to be certain its dome lies at the midpoint or above an imaginary vertical line drawn between the umbilicus and the pubis. A flat film of the abdomen may be taken to confirm this when physical findings are equivocal.
2. Place the patient in a supine position, prep the lower half of the abdomen with povidone-iodine, and drape.
3. Identify the point for insertion of the trocar 3 cm above the superior border of the symphysis.
4. Raise a skin wheal with 0.5% lidocaine, using a 25-gauge needle attached to a 10 cc syringe.
5. Change the needle to a 22-gauge 1½-inch size, introduce this into the skin wheal, and infiltrate full thickness of the abdominal wall, penetrating the linea alba and injecting the anterior wall of the distended bladder.
6. Make a 1 to 1.5 cm incision through the skin wheal and deepen this through the linea alba. Do not incise the bladder wall.
7. Insert the assembled trocar into the incision, and with the heel of the hand firmly push the trocar through the linea alba into the bladder in a slightly caudad direction toward the sacrococcygeal joint. The trocar should be inserted well into the bladder cavity.

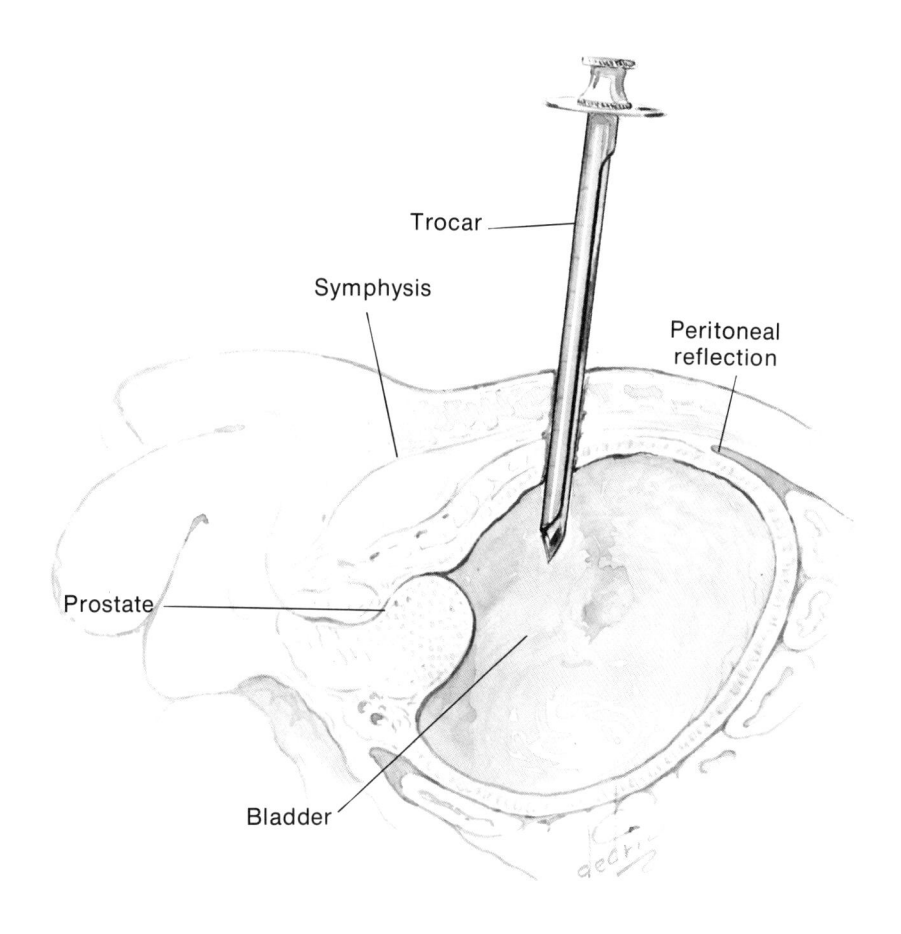

8. Holding the device in position, withdraw the pointed obturator, leaving the fenestrated cannula in the bladder. Insert the Foley catheter through the cannula into the bladder.

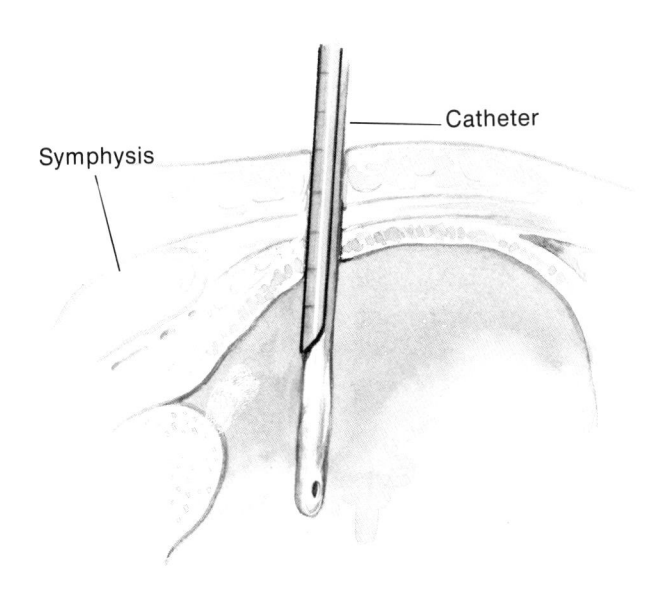

10. Inflate the catheter balloon with at least 5 cc of sterile water or saline.
11. Gently withdraw the cannula. The catheter will be kept in position by the balloon.
12. Withdraw the catheter until resistance is felt to snug the bladder against the abdominal wall.

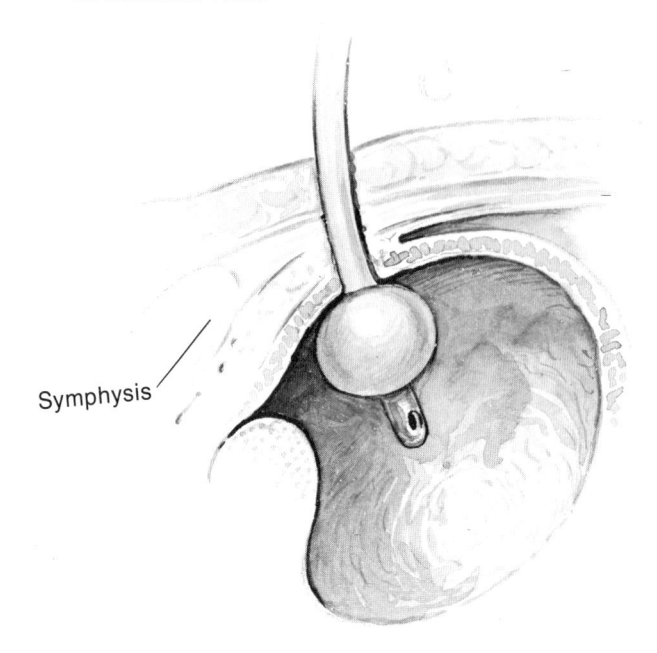

Symphysis

13. Attach the catheter to gravity drainage and measure and record the amount of urine obtained. An aliquot of urine should be set aside for routine analysis and another for bacteriologic studies, including culture and sensitivity.
14. Secure the catheter to the skin with a single silk suture placed through both margins of the incision and wrapped about the catheter.
15. Apply a dry sterile dressing.
NOTE: If difficulty is encountered passing the catheter through the cannula, insert a stylet into the catheter to give it some rigidity. The 18 Fr. catheter is considered too small for long-standing suprapubic drainage. Once the drainage tract is created, the catheter can be changed at weekly intervals and a larger catheter placed until the desired size (24 Fr.) is inserted.

66 URETHRAL CATHETERIZATION

The urethral catheters generally used in the emergency department are made of rubber, latex, or synthetic material. They are hollow tubes which are available in a variety of sizes, measured in the French scale, which indicates the external diameter. One unit on the French scale equals 0.3 mm; thus, three French units equals 1 mm; an 18 Fr. catheter has an external diameter of 6 mm.

There are several types of urethral catheters available which are generally straight or retention types. The straight catheter may have from one to six openings. Perhaps the one in most common usage is the Robinson catheter with two openings in the tip which is inserted into the bladder. Other varieties include the conical tip, whistle tip, or coudé olive-tip catheter. These catheters are most

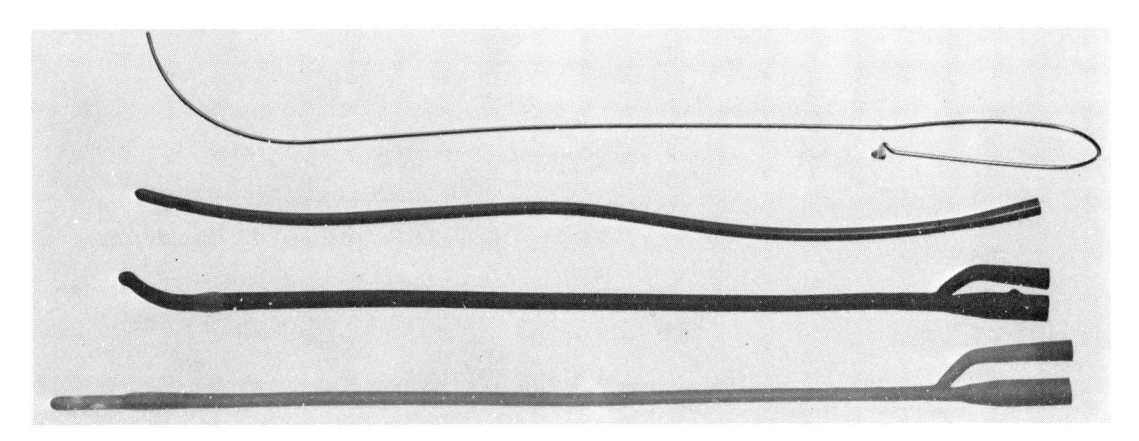

(top) Stylet (Center) Robinson catheter (Bottom) Retention catheter

often used for single insertion and withdrawal and may have a solid or hollow tip. The solid-tip catheter has a solid, rounded tip beyond the lateral opening. The hollow-tip has the lumen extending beyond the lateral opening and permits the use of a stylet.

Retention catheters are designed with an inflatable balloon near the tip which holds the catheter indwelling in the bladder. The balloons vary in capacity from 5 to 30 cc and are inflated with sterile water or saline.

Catheterization of the urethra and bladder requires the utmost caution and sterile technique. Catheterization of the female rarely presents any problems. However, male catheterization may be difficult, and sometimes impossible, without special sounds, or dilators, the use of which is best left to urologic surgeons who are familiar with them.

Assuming adherence to the technique of asepsis, the next most important principle of urethral catheterization is gentleness—DO NOT FORCE THE PASSAGE OF THE CATHETER. Inappropriate force may result in perforation or other damage to the urethra.

INDICATIONS

1. Need to establish bladder drainage to relieve urinary retention.
2. Need to obtain urine for diagnostic purposes in diabetes, urinary tract infections, and so on.
3. Need to perform diagnostic x-ray studies of the bladder in lower urinary tract trauma.
4. Need to obtain a sterile urine specimen, particularly in a female.

NOTE: If it is expected that multiple catheterizations may be needed, a retention catheter should be placed initially.

EQUIPMENT

1. Straight or indwelling catheter 16 or 18 Fr. (Sizes 4 Fr. to 24 Fr. should be available.) For infants and children the smaller sizes are used.
2. Lubricating jelly
3. Povidone-iodine prep
4. Curved hemostat
5. Cotton balls
6. Four towels
7. Collection bottles
8. 5 cc syringe
9. Sterile saline

NOTE: A variety of prepackaged sterile disposable catheterization trays are available commercially.

ANATOMICAL CONSIDERATIONS

1. In the male, the urethra has four parts named for their location:
   The penile urethra in the shaft of the penis. The posterior, or bulbous, urethra at the proximal end of the penis. It is a soft dilated portion of the urethra near the external sphincter. These portions of the urethra are flexible.

As the urethra passes through the muscular pelvic diaphragm, it becomes fixed and somewhat rigid and is called the membranous urethra. It then continues through the prostate gland as the prostatic urethra and enters the bladder.
2. It is at the fixed portion of the urethra (the membranous urethra) that iatrogenic injury may occur during rough instrumentation, especially if a stylet is used. This portion of the urethra may be damaged in certain fractures of the pelvis or the perineum.

PROCEDURE

The technique to be described is for the male patient.
1. Place the patient in the supine position.
2. Prep the external genitalia, including the glans and urethral meatus, with povidone-iodine.
3. Drape the entire area including the lower abdomen and upper thighs.
4. Stand on the right side of the patient and grasp the penis drawing it upward until it is perpendicular to the symphysis. If the patient is uncircumcised, retract the foreskin to expose the glans and urethral meatus.
5. Lubricate the catheter with sterile jelly.
6. Introduce the tip of the catheter into the urethral meatus and advance it gently into the urethra.
7. As the membranous portion of the urethra is reached it is found to be fixed in position. Do not force the catheter at this point, but maintain gentle pressure.
8. With continued pressure, pass the tip of the catheter through the sphincter into the bladder lumen. At this point, urine should escape from the end of the catheter.
9. Collect the specimens required for analysis or culture as necessary.
10. Measure the amount recovered and record this along with a gross description of the urine in the patient's hospital chart.
11. If the straight catheter is used, withdraw it after the bladder is completely empty.
12. If a retention catheter is used, inflate the balloon with sterile saline. Usually 5 cc is sufficient.

ALTERNATE PROCEDURE

As the operator gains experience, this variation of the classic method described above may be used. Aseptic technique is essential.
1. Stand to the right of the patient and grasp the penis in the left hand as described in step 4 above.
2. Prep the glans penis with povidone-iodine.
3. Take the curved hemostat in the right hand, keeping the ring and small fingers free. Place the jaws of the hemostat on the shaft of the catheter about 2 inches from its tip. Lift the catheter from the sterile tray, taking care not to touch the shaft of the catheter, thus contaminating it. Grasp the free end

between the ring and small fingers.
4. Dip the catheter tip in lubricating jelly and insert into the urethral meatus.
5. Follow steps 7 through 12 above.

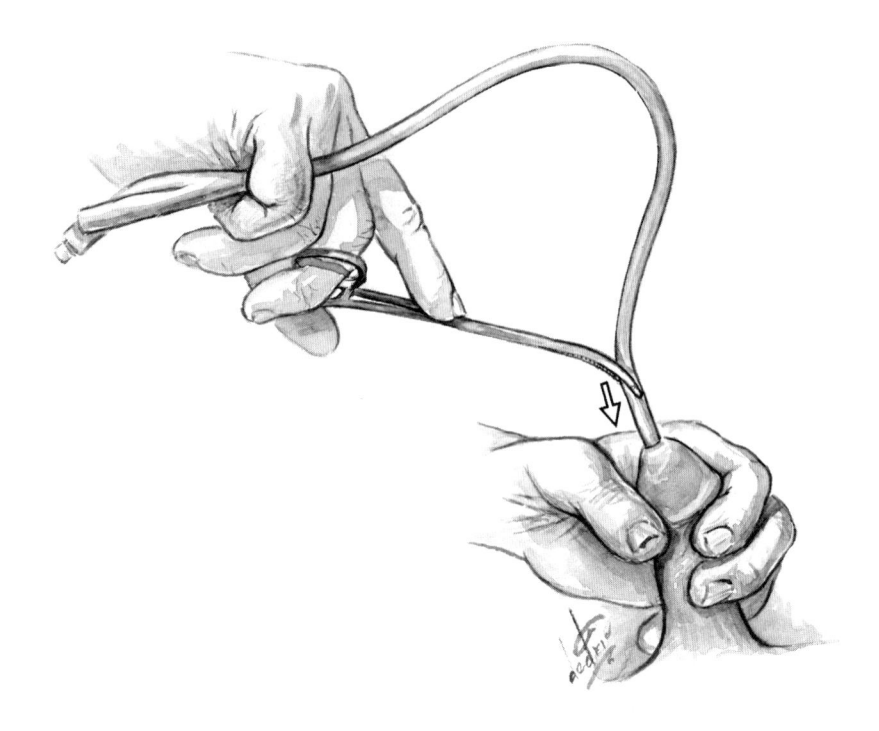

67 URETHROGRAM

INDICATIONS

1. Suspected injury to the urinary bladder.
2. Suspected injury to the posterior or prostatic urethra.
3. Evidence of perineal hematoma.
4. Traumatic hematuria.

EQUIPMENT

1. 50 cc Toomey syringe without Luer-Lok tip

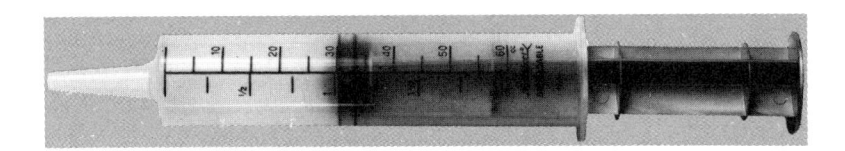

2. Cystograffin or mixture of the following: $1/3$ K-Y jelly, $1/3$ Renograffin, and $1/3$ water (500 cc)
3. Four towels
4. Povidone-iodine

ANATOMICAL CONSIDERATIONS

1. The urethra is normally located in the midline of the penis and extends behind the symphysis pubis.
2. To better visualize the urethra radiographically, the patient should be placed supine on the x-ray table with one hip elevated 2 to 3 inches by placing a folded sheet beneath it.

PROCEDURE

1. Prep the penis with povidone-iodine and drape the area.
2. Gently grasp the shaft of the penis behind the glans.
3. Carefully insert the tip of the syringe into the urethral meatus.

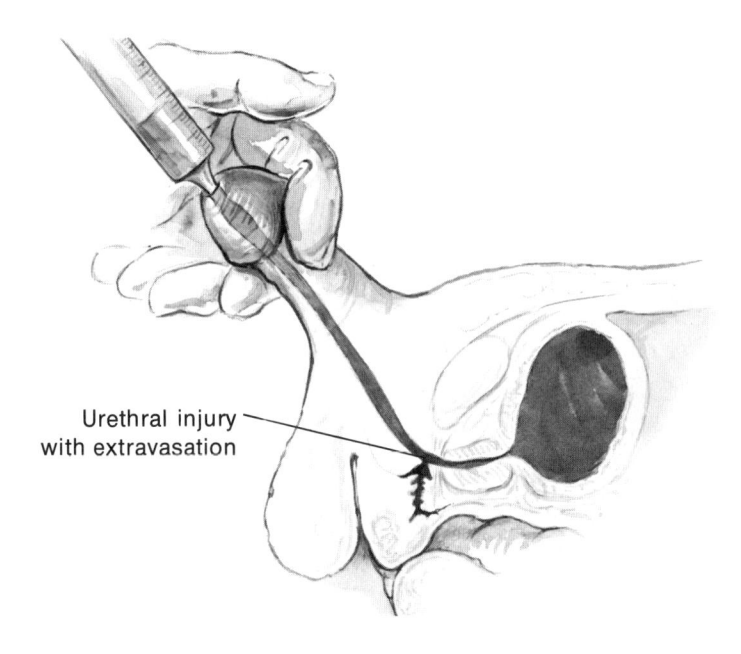

Urethral injury with extravasation

4. Gently inject 20 cc of contrast material into the urethra.
5. At the completion of the injection, maintain the syringe in position in the meatus and call for the x-ray exposure.

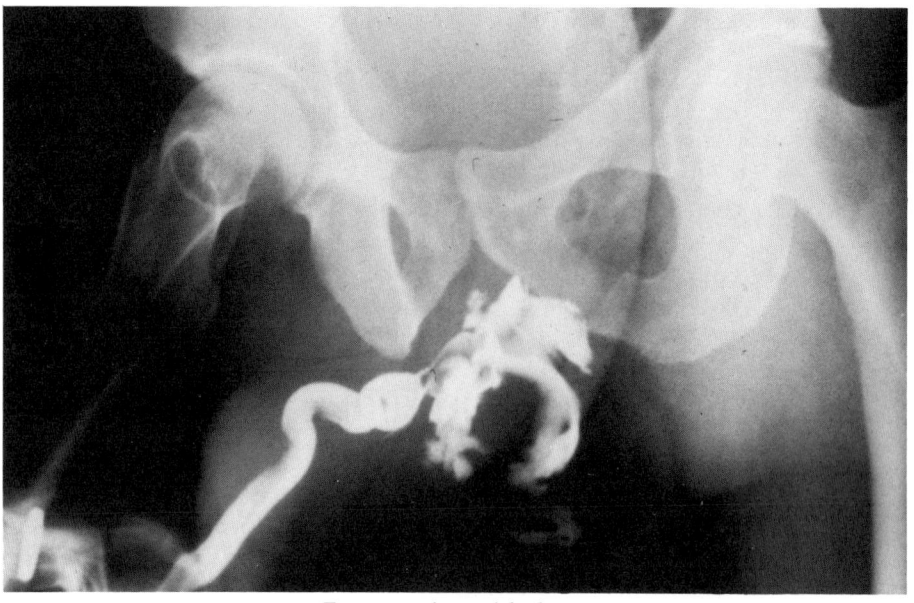

Extravasation with dye

NOTE: If the study reveals no damage to the urethra, prepare the patient for a cystogram.

BIBLIOGRAPHY

Baker, R. J. Newer techniques in evaluation of injured patients. Surg. Clin. N. Am. 55:31, 1975.

Brosman, S. A. and Fay, R. Diagnosis and management of bladder trauma. J. Trauma 13:687, 1973.

Clark, S. S. and Prudencio, R. R. Lower urinary tract injuries associated with pelvic fractures. Surg. Clin. N. Am. 52:183, 1972.

68 EMERGENCY MATERNITY CARE

Ambrose A. Macie, M.D.

BASIC PRINCIPLES

We deal here with what is usually a normal physiological process. For centuries women have been delivering infants spontaneously—many without benefit of assistance, much less professional help. The main objective is to deliver a healthy infant expeditiously with as little trauma as possible to the mother. Four considerations are of primary concern:

1. Delivery of the infant rapidly, but safely, without indulging in any unnecessary heroic manipulation.
2. Elimination of any extensive trauma to the mother.
3. Establishment of a free airway for the infant.
4. Close observation for excessive vaginal bleeding after delivery.

While it is agreed that human birth is a physiological process, experience has clearly demonstrated that the sterile environment of the hospital delivery room contributes to lower morbidity and mortality rates for both the newborn and the mother. Thus, when a patient in labor presents to the emergency setting and delivery appears imminent, care should be taken to maintain sterile precautions at all times. Before examining the patient, the perineal area should be washed with hexachlorophene soap and water, and sterile linens should be placed under the patient and draped about the perineum.

EQUIPMENT

1. Two hemostats
2. Scissors
3. Soft rubber bulb syringe
4. Sterile gloves
5. One dozen sterile gauze sponges
6. Sterile drapes or towels
7. 10 cc syringe
8. Two 5 cc syringes
9. 18-gauge 1½-inch needle
10. 25-gauge ⅝-inch needle
11. 22-gauge 1½-inch needle
12. 0.5% lidocaine for perineal anesthesia
13. Methylergonovine (0.2 mg dosage)
14. Oxytocin ampules (10 unit dosage)
15. 1,000 cc infusion liquid (dextrose in water or saline or Ringer's lactate)
16. Sterile linens
17. Povidone-iodine

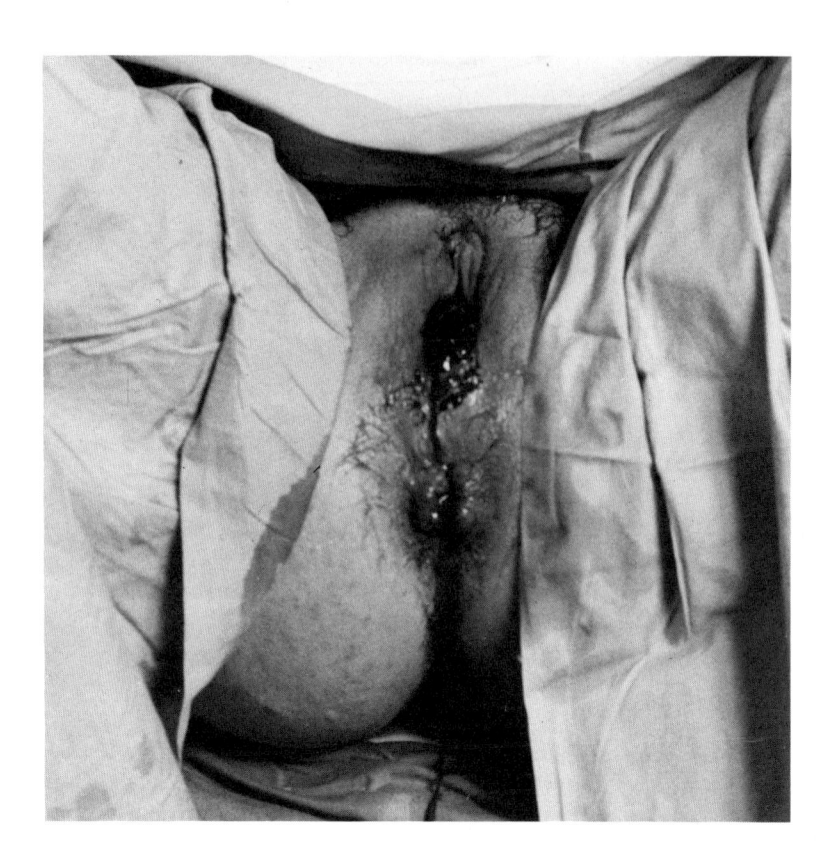

If an episiotomy is required, the perineum is prepped with povidone-iodine.

The examiner wears sterile gloves to assess the progress of the birth.

Good obstetric care includes attention to both the mother and the newborn infant.

THE STAGES OF LABOR

Labor is the process of the separation of the mature or nearly mature product of conception from the uterus of the mother.

There are three stages of labor. The first stage extends from the onset of labor pain until the cervix is fully dilated. It is usually during this stage that the membranes rupture. The second is the period of expulsion and extends from complete dilatation of the cervix to the birth of the child. The third is the placental stage and extends from the birth of the child to the extrusion of the placenta.

Generally, the duration of labor is longer in primiparous women (first pregnancy), averaging about 18 hours, than in multiparous women (second and later pregnancies), averaging 12 hours. With each succeeding pregnancy, the duration of labor shortens. The first stage is the longest, averaging 16 hours in primiparae and 10 hours in multiparae. This point should be kept in mind when managing a patient in labor in the emergency setting, for the physician may be faced with a less urgent situation when confronted with a primipara in the early or middle phase of the first stage of labor as opposed to a multipara in the same situation. Ideally, the birth should be accomplished in a delivery suite. Hence, accurate identification of the stage of labor will determine whether birth is imminent or the mother may safely be transported to an obstetrical unit.

Complications of infant malposition will be treated separately.

DIAGNOSIS OF THE PREGNANT PATIENT IN LABOR

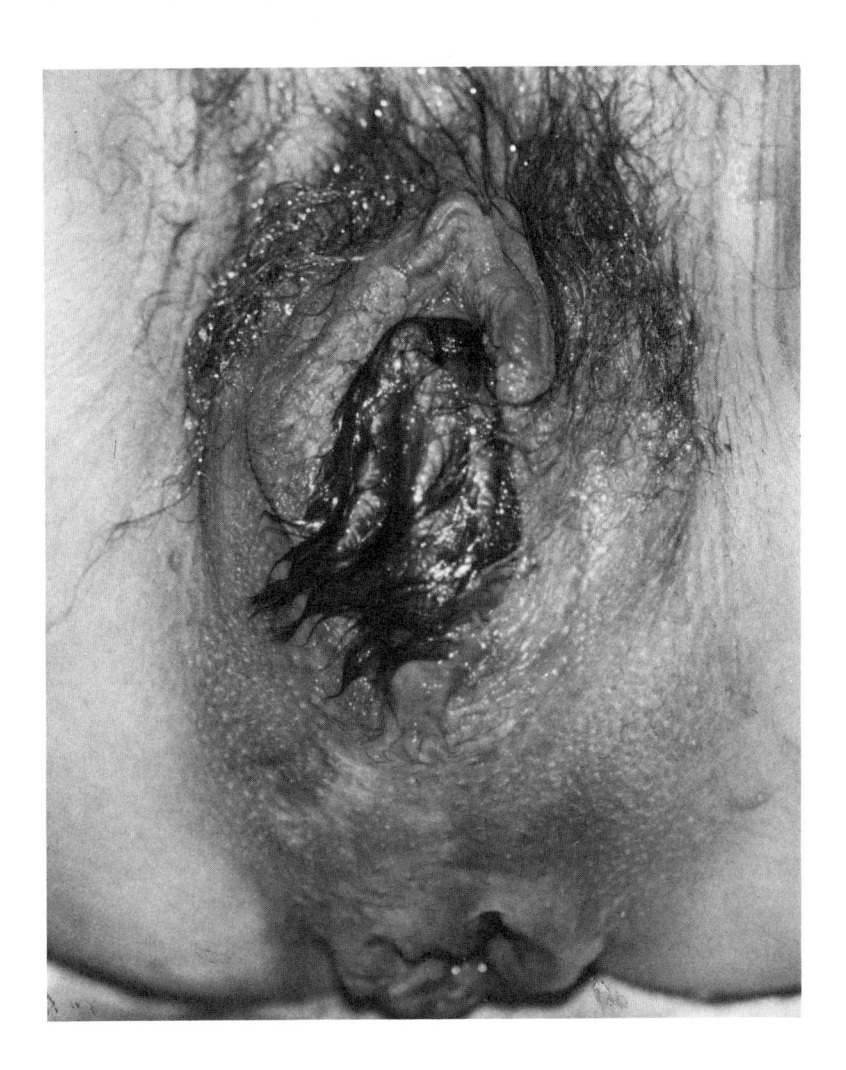

It would seem that the diagnosis of a pregnant woman should be self-evident. However, there are women who either through ignorance or emotional rejection may not realize that they are pregnant and in labor, despite the absence of menses for many months. Certainly the appearance in the emergency room of a woman of child-bearing age, with a prominent abdomen, who complains of intermittent abdominal pain should alert one to the probability of an intra-uterine pregnancy. An abdominal mass extending above the umbilicus must make one suspect such a diagnosis until proven otherwise. The application of a fetoscope to the abdomen, usually below the umbilicus, should allow one to hear fetal heart tones at a rate of 120 to 160 beats per minute, generally double the patient's pulse rate. Imminent delivery would be indicated by "bulging" of the perineum, particularly during one of the "pains." The presenting part of the infant may sometimes be seen when the labia are separated. Certainly a pelvic examination will confirm the suspicion. If the membranes have ruptured, the presenting part of the baby, generally the head, will be easily palpable. A hard firm mass (the head) that "pushes" toward the vaginal outlet with a pain is diagnostic. If the membranes of the amniotic sac are still intact, a soft bulging mass of fluid can be felt by the examining fingers. Should the cervix not be completely dilated, it can be felt as a ridge of tissue around the periphery of the vagina. If labor has not advanced to this stage, the patient should be transferred to an obstetrical delivery unit for further care. Let us assume that the patient arrives in the emergency room fully dilated and ready for delivery, and that the proper diagnosis has been established.

GENERAL CONSIDERATIONS

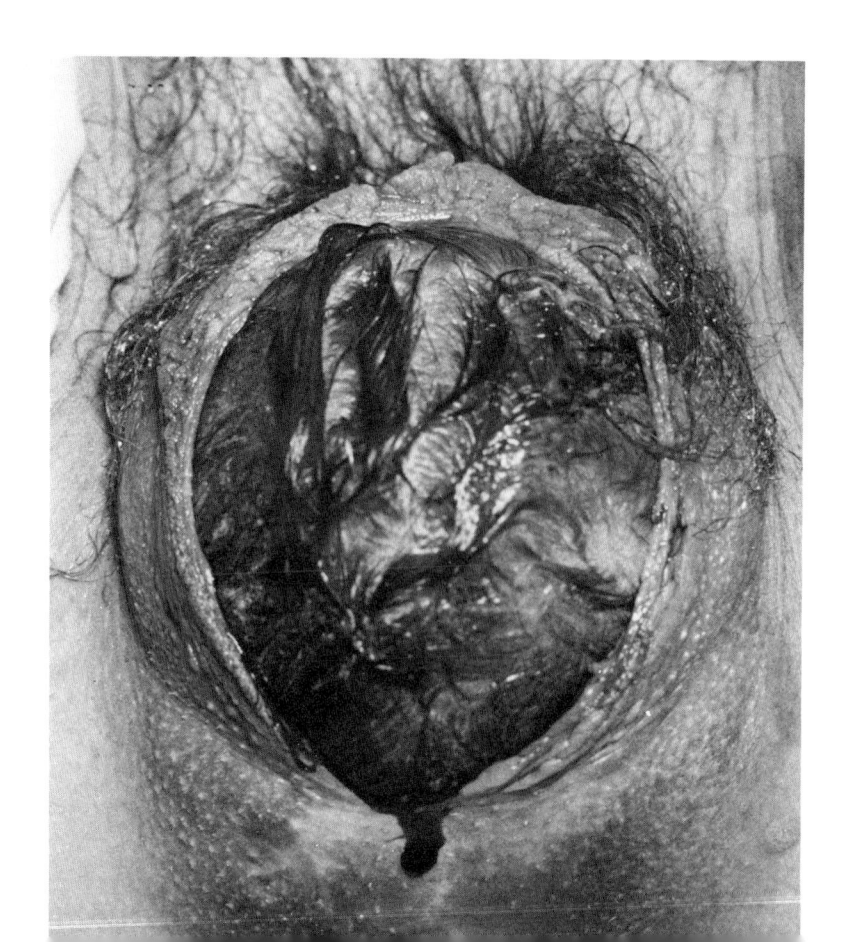

For the most part, a pregnant woman who presents in an emergency atmosphere with delivery imminent would have already accomplished most of the work. In most cases, such a rapid and apparently easy labor indicates that the presenting part of the fetus would be a vertex (a head presentation) and most likely in an occiput anterior position (with the face and chin pointing posteriorly toward the mother's rectum). The normal forces of labor should complete the delivery process. It remains for the delivering operator (accoucher) to "assist" the delivery. The patient should be placed in the lithotomy position (lateral Sims's or the supine position with the knees elevated and flexed on the abdomen. The operator should assist with the delivery of the head. Such assistance is initiated by the use of the Ritgen maneuver. Through a towel draped over the gloved hand, pressure is made posterior to the rectum in an effort to palpate the fetus' chin. A rocking motion of the fingers will thus extend the neck and help to deliver the head over the perineum. It is important to exert pressure on the baby's brow through the perineum with the opposite hand. The forces of labor can be quite explosive and a sudden surge of the head through the vaginal opening can cause extensive perineal lacerations. Thus this portion of the delivery should be controlled as carefully as possible. Once the head is delivered, the next essential step is to check for the umbilical cord which sometimes encircles the baby's neck. At this point, further progress of the birth with a tight cord around the neck

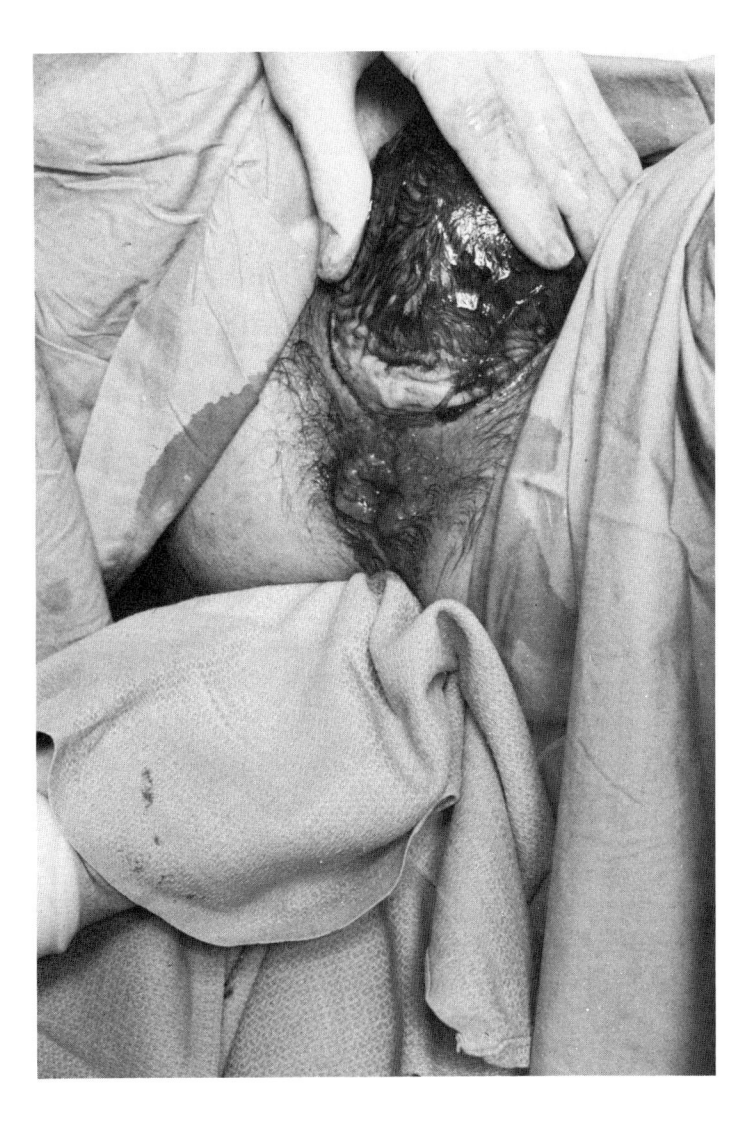

may tear the umbilical cord with significant blood loss to the infant, especially if the remainder of the delivery is prolonged. In this instance, place two hemostats in proximity to one another on the tight cord, cut the cord between the clamps with scissors, and unwind the loop or loops of cord from the infant's neck. The head will rotate toward one of the mother's thighs and lie transversely, placing the shoulders in an anteroposterior position. Gentle to moderate downward pressure on the infant's head toward the rectum of the mother will impinge the anterior shoulder of the infant under the mother's symphysis pubis. Remember, the mother's contractions are doing most of the work and undue pushing or pulling is unnecessary. As the anterior shoulder comes into view, lifting of the partially delivered infant upward (anteriorly) toward the symphysis pubis will complete delivery of the shoulders.

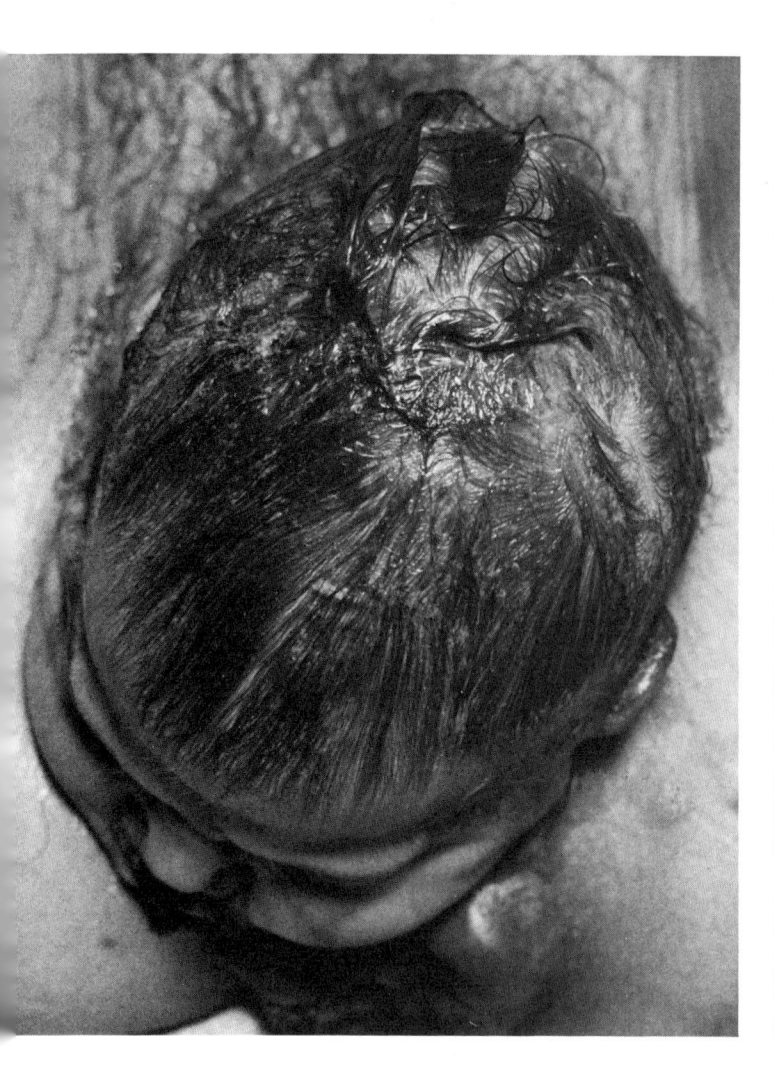

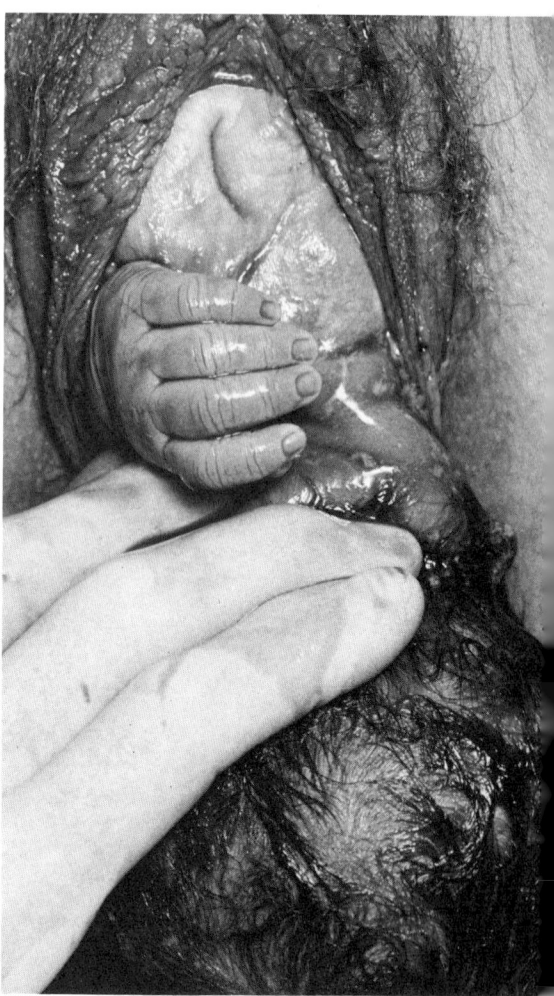

The remainder of the delivery will be accomplished by the forces of labor, with the operator providing a "guiding hand." The neck of the infant should be cradled in one hand and the remainder of the delivery effected by flexing the infant's body toward either the right or the left thigh of the mother — the direction depending on the direction the baby is facing.

After the delivery of the infant is complete, since it has been a "controlled" delivery, trauma to the mother should be minimal. This subject will be discussed separately. Of more import at this time is immediate care of the infant.

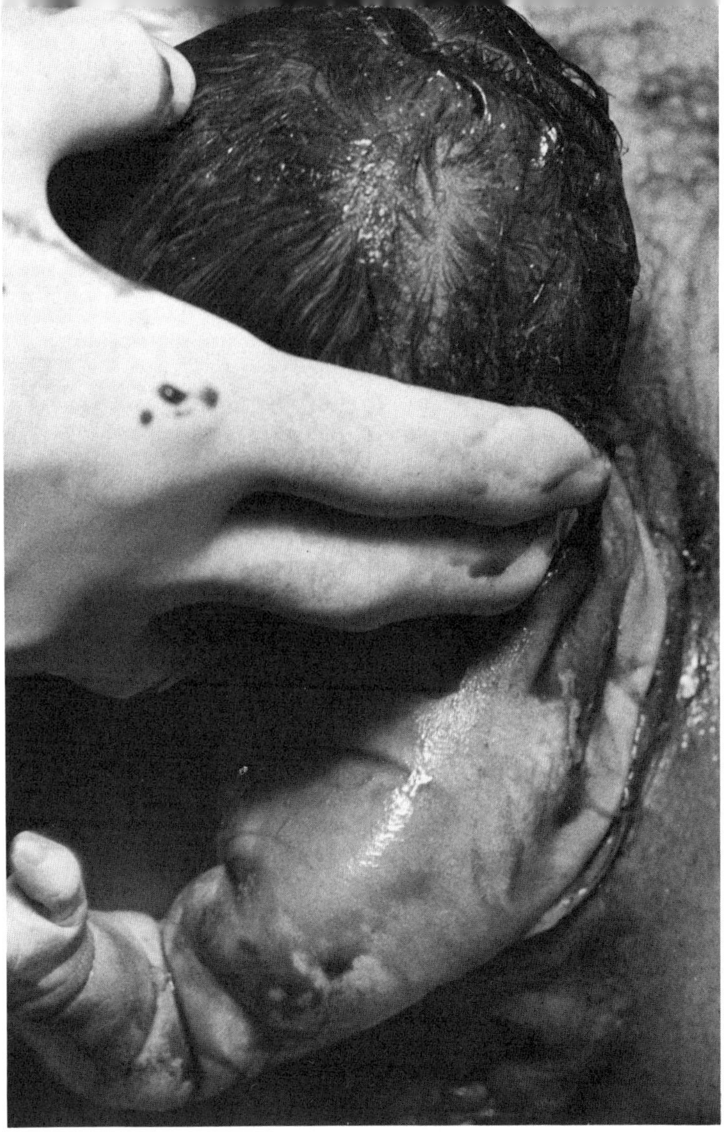

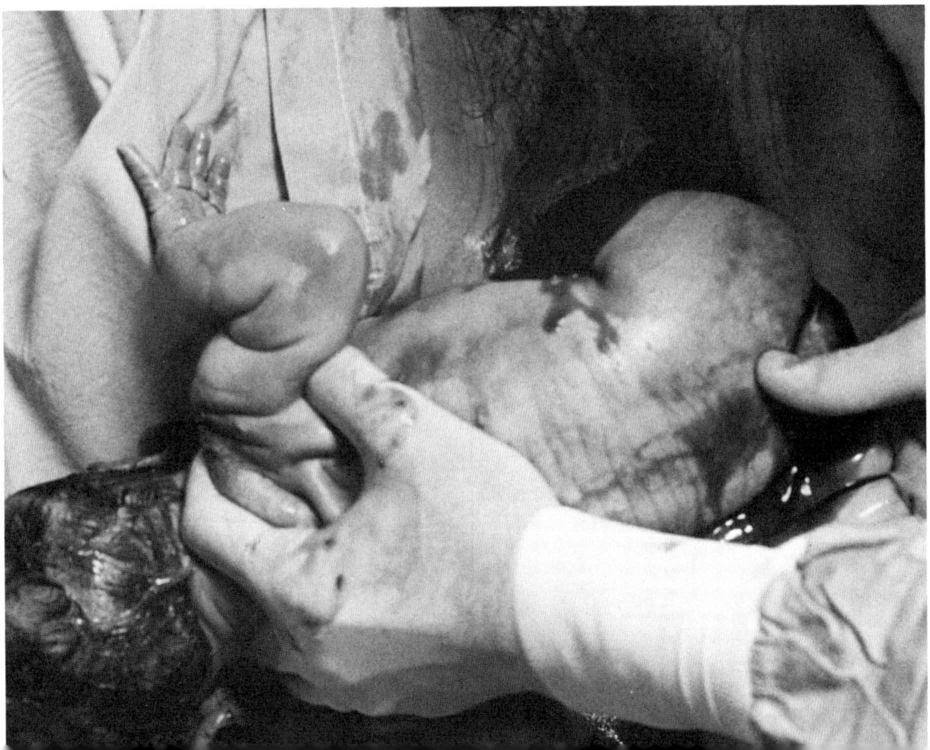

CARE OF THE NEWBORN

The baby should be held with the head in a dependent or downward position to facilitate drainage of mucus and/or aspirated amniotic fluid from the airway. The mouth, nostrils, and nasopharynx should be aspirated with a rubber bulb syringe. If one is not available, gentle "milking" of the trachea toward the mouth of the infant and wiping the baby's mouth out with gauze or even with a finger would be beneficial. Once a free airway is established and the infant is breathing spontaneously, the umbilical cord can be severed. An umbilical clamp and/or hemostats may be used for this purpose. Wrap the baby in a blanket as quickly as possible to eliminate excessive loss of body heat.

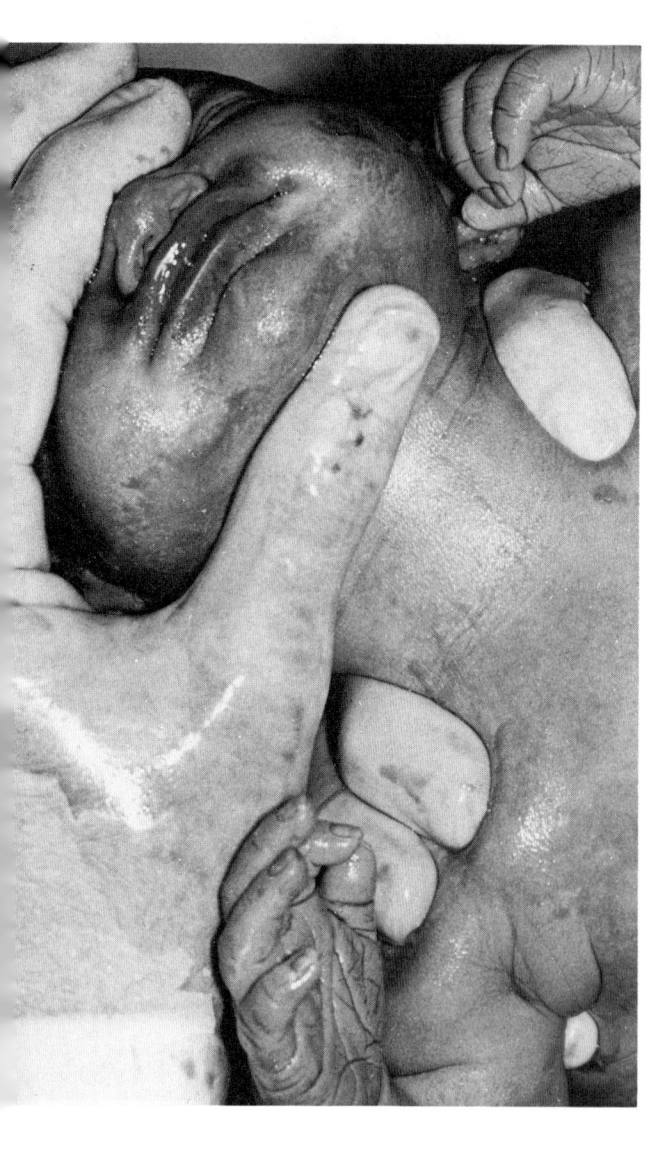

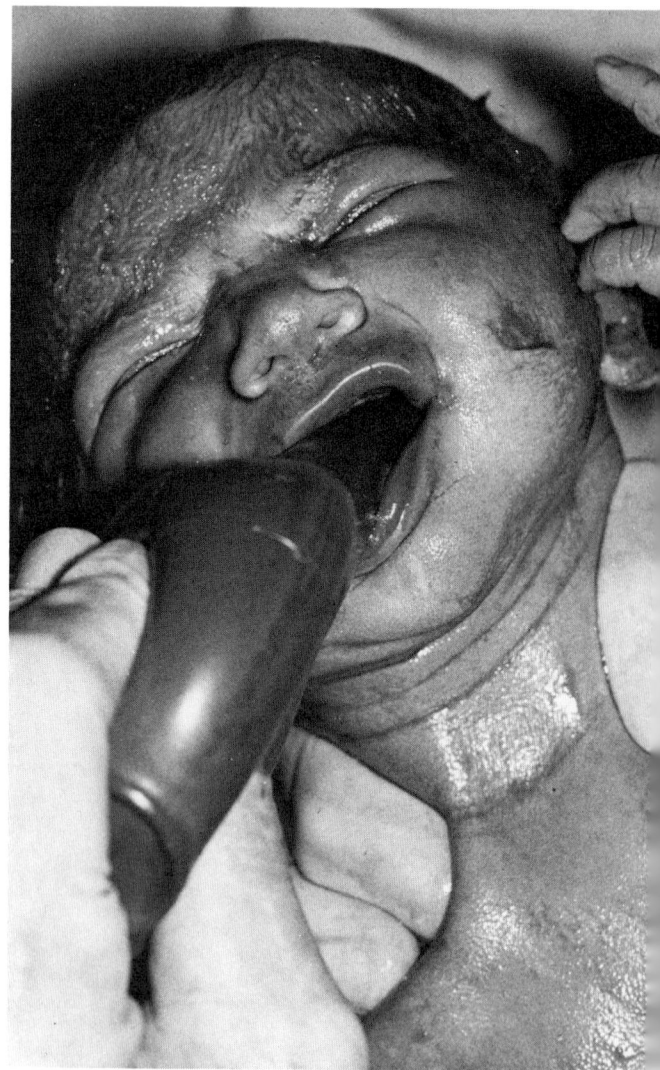

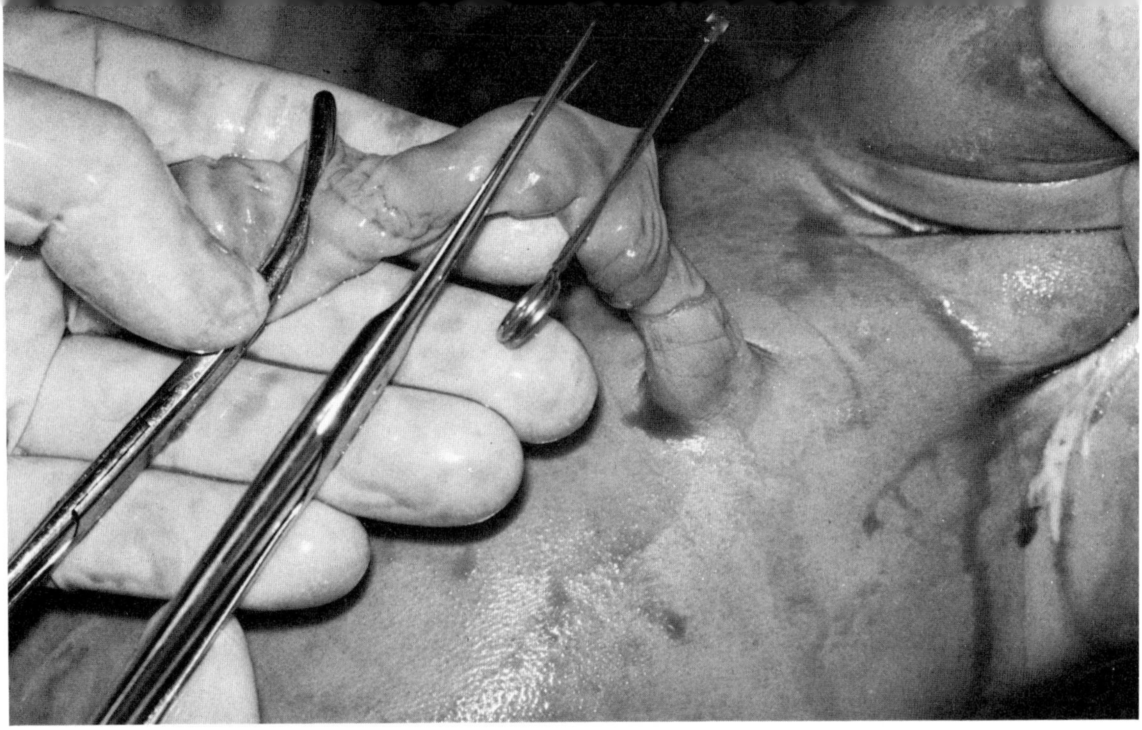

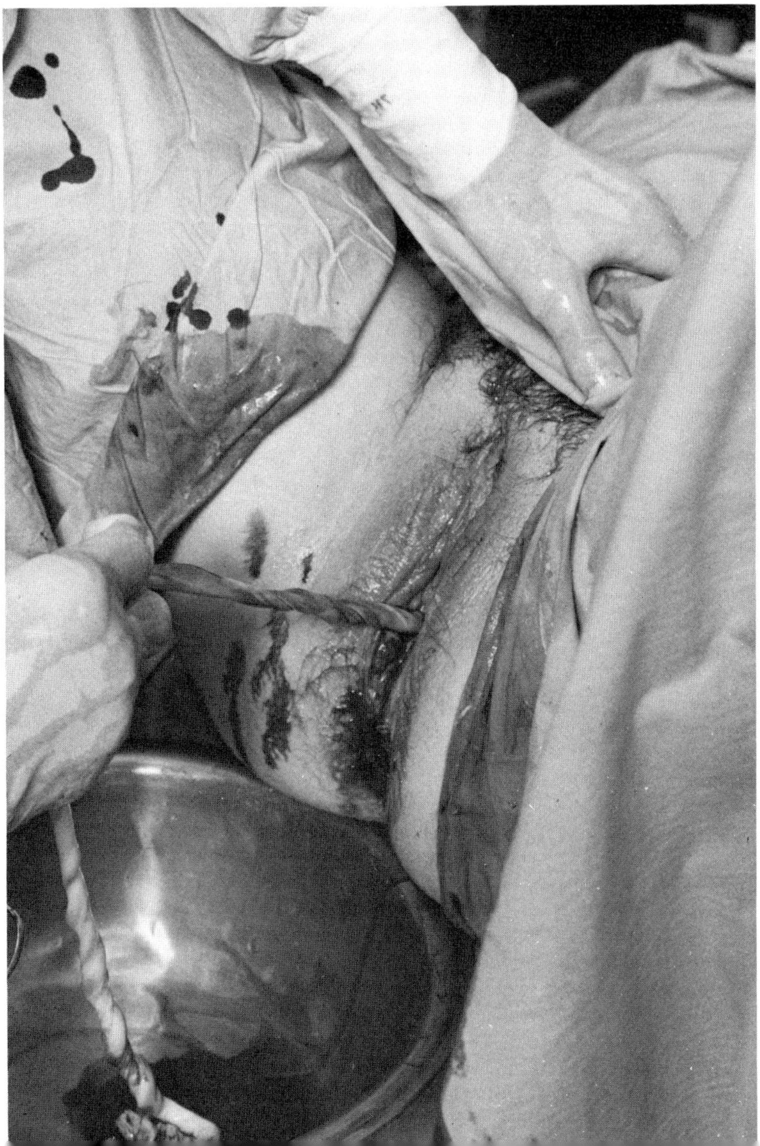

THE THIRD STAGE OF LABOR

Let us return to the delivered mother. Delivery of the placenta becomes the prime concern. Do not use excessive traction on the umbilical cord. Tearing of the cord at its placental insertion might necessitate manual removal of the placenta. Gentle traction on the cord combined with a gentle massaging action on the fundus of the uterus will usually accomplish the desired results. At this stage oxytoxic medication should be administered. Methylergonovine 0.2 mg IM and/or oxytocin 10 units IM or IV are the drugs of choice. This type of drug will help to stimulate the musculature of the uterus to contract. During this stage a moderate blood loss is expected, averaging 200 cc. Abnormal bleeding occurs when the loss exceeds 600 cc or 1 percent of body weight.

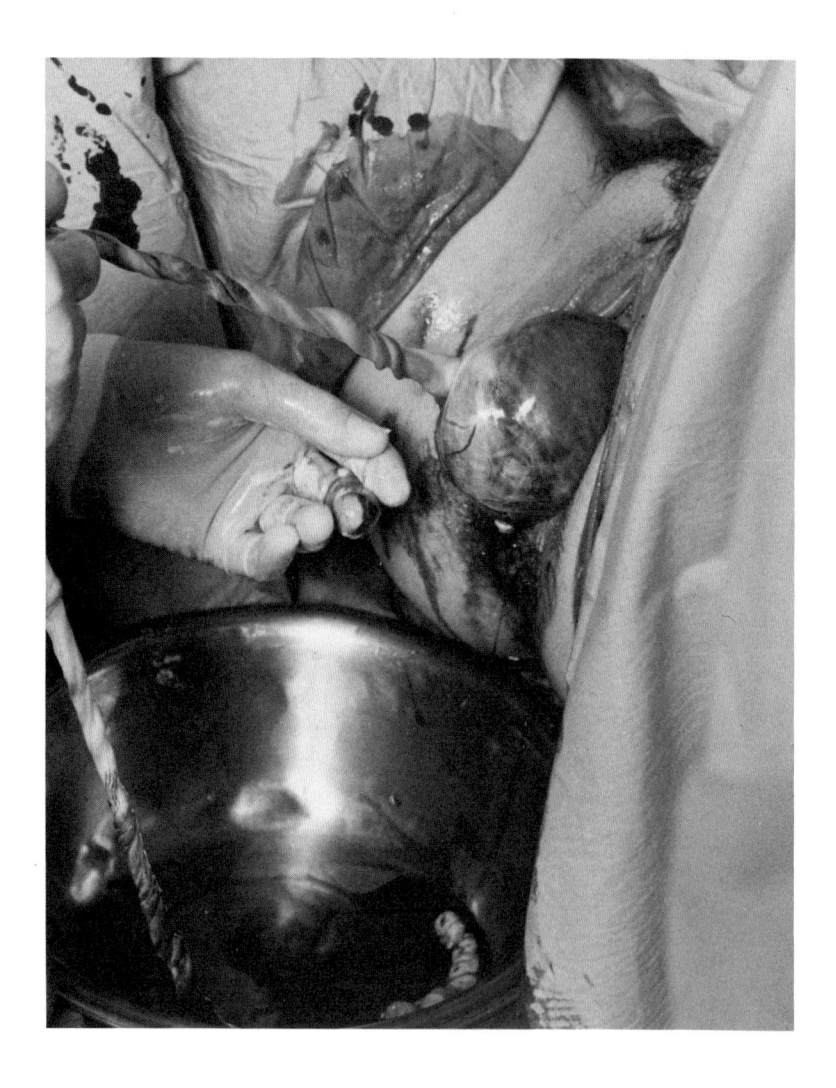

After the placenta is completely extruded, the mother should be examined for lacerations of the birth canal. The most common site for such trauma in a rapid delivery are in the peri-urethral area, that is, the lateral spaces anteriorly, immediately adjacent to the urethral orifice. The perineum must also be checked. The use of gauze sponges in either hand with lateral separation of the labia will easily expose these areas to visual examination. Minimal mucosal separation should be of little concern. More extensive lacerations with significant bleeding can temporarily be controlled by gauze-covered finger pressure until arrangements can be made for proper surgical repair.

POSTPARTUM CARE

One additional, but major, problem may be encountered at this time — postpartal bleeding. Patients delivering quickly enough to necessitate emergency care are usually multiparous women. Such women may be more likely to have excessive postpartal bleeding due to poor uterine muscle tone, so-called uterine atony. The uterus remains "boggy" and contracts poorly. An intravenous infusion containing 10 to 20 units of oxytocin in 1,000 cc. of fluid should be instituted immediately, preferably through an 18-gauge needle in case blood transfusion becomes necessary. In addition, bimanual uterine massage is indicated. One sterile gloved hand may be used vaginally to "lift" or push the uterus out of the bony pelvis. The contralateral hand is placed on the fundus of the uterus employing a gentle rotating massaging action. Should a sterile glove not be available, downward and upward pressure immediately above the symphysis pubis may accomplish the same objective.

Continued excessive vaginal bleeding after the above measures have been instituted necessitates movement of the patient to a surgical suite to better evaluate the perineum and external genitalia for more extensive lacerations which may be in the cervix or high in the vaginal vault and not readily recognized by previous visual examination. Again, such injury is more likely to occur in a rapid, precipitate delivery. Retained portions of placenta must also be considered as a possible cause of excessive bleeding. Treatment of all of the above problems can only be accomplished in a surgically sterile setting with benefit of some form of anesthesia.

COMPLICATIONS

We have discussed the diagnosis and delivery of a pregnant female with a normally presenting infant. This will accommodate 95 percent of all such women. Unfortunately there is one patient in twenty whose condition will not allow for the relatively simple procedures outlined above. Complications such as a prolapsed umbilical cord or malpresentations of the infant in relation to the maternal pelvis are most often encountered. Of extreme importance is the early diagnosis of such complications. Even minor problems may arise. Let us consider them individually.

THE NEED FOR EPISIOTOMY (PERINEAL INCISION)

The diagnosis of pregnancy, active labor, and imminent delivery has been established. If the patient's contractions, particularly a primipara, are strong and frequent (occurring every two minutes or less), and if a delivery room is not available, the need for an episiotomy should be considered. Such a procedure will facilitate delivery through an enlarged vaginal orifice with less trauma to the mother and the baby. A midline episiotomy may be considered. The perineal area between the posterior wall of the vagina and the rectum is prepped with povidone-iodine and local infiltration done with 0.5% lidocaine. An incision is made with scissors at the midpoint of the posterior vagina directed toward the rectum, and should extend down to, but not include, the anal sphincter fibers. With local anesthesia such an incision may be repaired in the emergency department utilizing 2-0 chromic catgut as a continuous suture. An inexperienced operator should call upon the services of an obstetrician or surgeon with more expertise in such a situation. Unless the episiotomy site bleeds excessively, closure may await the arrival of an experienced operator.

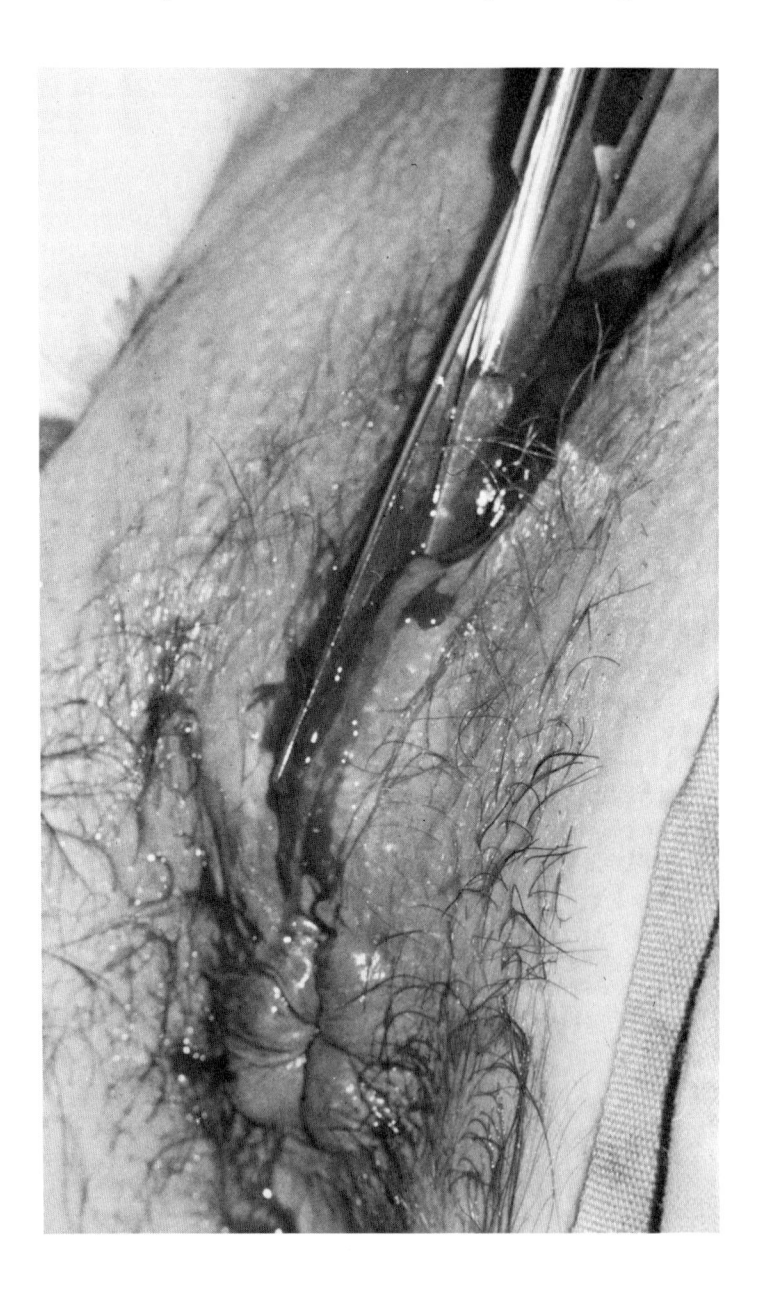

PROLAPSED UMBILICAL CORD

This is an absolute obstetrical emergency. Early diagnosis is imperative. If the membranes have ruptured, the cord may be visible at the introitus or lying outside of the vagina. If the membranes are intact the cord would be palpable through the "bag of waters." The diagnosis would be made by vaginal palpation of a pulsating soft loop or loops of cord. Such a patient should immediately be placed in Trendelenburg's position and be encouraged not to "push" with her pains. Oxygen is administered nasally and the loop or loops or cord cradled in the examining hand and replaced gently back into the vagina if prolapsed externally. Pressure should be exerted upward on the presenting part to prevent compression of the cord which causes fetal asphyxia and great danger to the fetus. In this situation, the degree of dilatation of the cervix is all important. If the cervix is completely dilated, delivery should be accomplished as quickly as possible. If the cervix is not completely dilated, the above measures must be continued while immediate preparations are made for cesarean section delivery.

BREECH PRESENTATION

Whereas a pelvic examination of a vertex presentation reveals a hard, convex "mass," a breech presentation will be much softer to the touch with prominences and depressions such as the gluteal crease and perhaps numerous small parts if the breech presents as a footling. Almost always the fetal heart tones are heard above the umbilicus of the mother—an important diagnostic point. Frank breech, where the fetus' legs are extended against the trunk and the feet lie against the face, is the most frequent type encountered.

Since fetal mortality and maternal morbidity are significantly higher in this type of presentation the attendance of an experienced accoucher would be most desirable. In the absence of such experience the best must be made of a dangerous situation. Hopefully, a spontaneous delivery may be accomplished and the most that can be expected in this circumstance is a so-called breech assist delivery. One of the major problems in a breech delivery is to attempt to deliver the infant through a cervix not completely dilated. Patience is essential. A midline episiotomy as described previously should always be done. Allow the mother to spontaneously deliver the infant. The desire to aid the mother by traction on the infant's legs must be restrained since undue haste at this point is not necessary and can cause injury to the baby. As the lower extremities and the pelvis of the baby are extruded, they should be wrapped in a towel or blanket. At the appearance of the baby's umbilicus, the rest of the delivery should be completed rapidly but not precipitately.

A loop of the umbilical cord should be pulled down to prevent tearing and the body of the infant guided with its back in a superior position. The mother is encouraged to push as hard as possible. If difficulty is encountered with the shoulder girdle, assistance may be necessary. A finger should be placed in the axillary fold of the infant and an attempt made to roll that shoulder anteriorly toward the symphysis of the mother. Do not press into the axilla. The arm may then be wiped out of the vagina along the baby's body. Further difficulty in delivery may necessitate repeating the maneuver with the opposite arm of the baby. After the shoulders are delivered, the body of the infant is cradled on the forearm and if possible one finger is placed in the baby's mouth to prevent the baby from making too many spontaneous gasps. The opposite hand steadies the baby's neck. Here, care must be exercised not to flex the baby's body too severely toward the symphysis of the mother. If the mother's expulsive effort is not sufficient to deliver the head, the accoucher may employ a pumping action — flexing the baby alternately toward the floor and then toward the ceiling. Excessive force must be avoided to decrease the possibility of intracranial injury, one of the more common causes of fetal damage in breech delivery.

TRANSVERSE LIE

In examining a pregnant women, if the normal, longitudinal ovoid of the uterus is replaced by a transverse one a problem should be immediately suspected. Upon pelvic examination, an empty vagina will confirm one's suspicion. The pelvic examination must be done with extreme care to avoid rupture of the membranes which would only compound the situation by increasing the likelihood of prolapse of the cord or an extremity of the baby. The patient should be placed in Trendelenburg's position and urged not "to bear down" with her pains. The delivery of a mother with a transverse lie is well beyond the scope of anyone but an experienced obstetrician, since cesarean section is indicated in all but the rarest of cases. All efforts must then be directed to prolonging the patient's labor and delaying delivery until such consultation can be obtained.

THIRD TRIMESTER HEMORRHAGE

Another of the more serious complications of pregnancy so often taken for granted is bleeding in the third trimester. Complete treatment of this problem is beyond the scope of emergency room personnel. Heavy vaginal bleeding in a pregnant woman in the third trimester is invariably due to placenta previa, in which the placenta lies between the baby and the cervix, or abruptio placenta, that is, premature separation of the placenta. Experience in delivery and treatment are of prime importance and delivery is not to be attempted except under a sterile double set-up where a cesarean section can be done immediately if a sterile examination shows this to be necessary. The diagnosis of pregnancy must be made by history and abdominal examination alone. All temptation to do a pelvic examination must be resisted since an inexperienced examiner can cause even more severe bleeding by being too enthusiastic when palpating. Of maximal importance is initiation of supportive measures. An intravenous line should be placed using a large bore needle (16 or 18 gauge), and Ringer's lactate infusion should be begun to initiate blood volume replacement. Venous blood samples are drawn for complete blood count and type and cross match. The patient's vital signs are monitored closely while the patient awaits obstetric consultation.

69 DENTAL EMERGENCIES

It is not unusual for a patient to be seen in the emergency setting with dental complaints. Invariably these result from a primary inflammatory disease process in the tooth or gum, or occur secondary to treatment recently given by a dentist.

The two most common symptoms are pain and/or bleeding. For the most part, emergency care of dental problems should be palliative; in other words, symptomatic relief is provided and the patient is referred back to his dentist.

Pain of dental origin is usually related to decayed teeth (dental caries). Pain due to caries is at first sharp and shooting and may later become more severe and throbbing. Often the patient can localize it to one tooth, or the examiner may identify the culprit by tapping the teeth with a dental mirror or hemostat. Poor oral hygiene may be noted in such a patient. If a cavity can be identified, it can be treated by the application of eugenol (oil of cloves) and zinc oxide.

Analgesics should be prescribed and the patient urged to take a light, preferably liquid, diet and to avoid fluids which are hot, cold, or sweet.

Pain following a dental surgical procedure, such as an extraction, is not uncommon. A patient with postextraction pain is most likely suffering from a "dry socket" or alveolar osteitis. It most often occurs after removal of a wisdom tooth and begins two to four days postoperatively. The patient may note a bad taste in his mouth. Careful and gentle examination of the operative site is necessary and may reveal a dry socket containing no blood clot, or a clot that is necrotic and foul-smelling. Management includes gentle irrigation of the socket with warm saline solution and loose packing of the defect with iodoform gauze to which has been added eugenol and benzocaine. Analgesics should be prescribed as needed.

Postoperative dental bleeding may follow an extraction. Though it is rarely, if ever, life-threatening, it can be most annoying. Inevitably, the patient has swallowed some of the blood and may complain of nausea and emesis. The patient should rinse his mouth with a warm saline or peroxide solution which should be spit out, NOT swallowed. The oral cavity, especially the operative site, should be examined to locate the bleeding point. A suction unit may be needed to remove the blood. Once the bleeding point has been localized, a 2 × 2-inch gauze pad is placed over the site and the patient is told to bite down on this, holding the gauze in position for 30 to 45 minutes. Then the patient is re-examined to determine whether the bleeding is controlled. If not, the socket may be sutured closed with one or two chromic or silk sutures after injection of a local anesthetic agent or application of a topical anesthetic agent to the mucosa. Invariably these methods will control further bleeding. If this is not the case, the patient should have immediate testing of his clotting mechanism, including complete blood count, platelet count, and partial thromboplastin time to uncover any blood dyscrasia.

SUMMARY

Patients with urgent problems of dental origin not uncommonly seek treatment in the emergency setting. The two most common symptoms are pain and bleeding. Unless a dentist is available, the preferred treatment is palliative — give symptomatic relief and refer the patient to his dentist promptly.

INDEX

Abruptio placenta, 308
Adam's apple, 21
Advanced life support, 94–108
  defined, 93
Airway management, 1–9. See also Cardiopulmonary resuscitation
  endotracheal intubation, 8, 15–20, 99
  esophageal obturator, 8, 11–13
  Heimlich maneuver, 39–43
  needle cricothyrotomy, 8, 21–23
  tracheostomy, 8, 25–37
Alveolar osteitis, 309
Ambu bag, 6–7, 20
Anatomical snuffbox, 208
Anesthesia, local. See Local anesthesia
Angiograms. See Arteriograms
Angle of Lewis, 242, 253
Antecubital vein, 71
Arterial blood gas values, 9
Arterial puncture, 59–62
Arteriograms
  axillary, 45–46
  femoral, 47–51
Artificial breathing. See Ventilation, artificial
Artificial circulation. See Circulation, artificial
Artificial ventilation. See Ventilation, artificial
Antishock suit, 115–119
Aspiration. See also Taps
  of bursa, 81–84
  of cul-de-sac, 269–270
  of ganglion cyst, 91–92
  gastrointestinal. See Gastrointestinal tubes
Atony, uterine, 305
Atropine sulfate, in cardiopulmonary resuscitation, 107
Axillary arteriogram, 45–46
Axillary artery, 46

Balloon flotation catheter, 121
Basic life support, 94–102
  defined, 93
Basilic vein, 126

Bicipital tendon sheaths, injection of, 77–80
Bicipital tenosynovitis, 77
Bladder drainage
  suprapubic, 283–286
  urethral, 287–290
Blakemore-Sengstaken tube, 157, 159–160, 175–177
Bleeding. See also Hematoma; Hemorrhage
  dental, 309–310
  from esophageal varices, 157, 159, 175
  nasal, 227–232
  urinary, 291
Blood gas values, arterial, 9
Blood pressure monitoring. See Central venous catheterization; Intra-arterial pressure monitoring
BLS. See Basic life support
Brachial artery, 60
Breathing
  artificial. See Ventilation, artificial
  assessment of, 94–96, 98–99
Breech presentation, 307–308
Bupivacaine, 180
Bursa
  aspiration of
    olecranon, 81–82
    patellar, 83–84
  injection of
    radiohumoral, 85–86
    subacromial, 87–89
Bursitis, 81, 83, 85
  tendinitis vs., 77, 87
Butterfly device, 54

Calcium chloride, in cardiopulmonary resuscitation, 108
Cannula, indwelling, 63–64, 65–69
Cantor tube, 158–159, 167–170
Cardiac arrest. See Cardiopulmonary resuscitation
Cardiac compression, external. See Closed chest compression
Cardiac monitor, with transvenous pacemaker, 112

311

Cardiac tamponade, 237
Cardiopulmonary resuscitation, 93–108
   airway management in, 94, 96–98. *See also* Airway management
   breathing assessment in, 94–95, 98–99
   circulation assistance in, 95–96, 100–102
   contraindications to, 108
   CVP line in, 105
   defibrillation in, 102–104
   drug therapy in, 104–108
   intravenous line in, 105
   termination of, 108
Carotid pulse, palpation of, 95
Catheters
   balloon flotation (Swan-Ganz), 121
   central venous, 122–123
   Foley. *See* Foley catheter
   intra-arterial, 121
   Robinson. *See* Robinson catheter
   urethral, 287–288
Catheterization
   central venous. *See* Central venous catheterization
   urethral, 287–290
Central venous catheterization, 57, 121–123
   antecubital approach, 125–126
   in cardiopulmonary resuscitation, 105
   external jugular approach, 127–131
   subclavian approach, 133–135
Cephalic vein, 126
Cervical traction, 275–278
Childbirth, 295–308
Circulation, artificial, 93, 95–96, 100–102
   with cardiac compression, 99, 101
Closed chest compression, 93, 95–96, 100–102
   with artificial breathing, 99, 101
   in infants and children, 101–102
Closed chest drainage, 251–258
   with needle drainage, 243
Closed thoracostomy, 251–258
Cocaine solution, in nasal pack, 228
Compression, cardiac. *See* Closed chest compression
Conical tip catheter, 287
Contact lens removal
   hard, 141–142
   soft, 143–145
Coracoid process, 77
Coudé olive-tip catheter, 287
Countershock, electrical, 102–104
CPR. *See* Cardiopulmonary resuscitation
Cricothyroid membrane, 21
Cricothyrotomy, needle, 8, 21–23
Cul-de-sac aspiration, 269–270
Cutdown, venous, 71–75
CVC. *See* Central venous catheterization
Cyanosis, signs of, 2
Cyst, ganglion, aspiration of, 91–92
Cystography, 279–281
Cystotomy, suprapubic, 283–286

Decompression, gastric, 157, 163
Defibrillation, 102–104
   with transvenous pacing, 112
Dental emergencies, 309–310
Digital nerve block, 215–218

Drainage
   of bladder. *See* Bladder drainage
   closed chest, 243, 251–258
   of felon, 147–148
   gastrointestinal. *See* Gastrointestinal tubes
   of hemopericardium, 237–239
   of hemothorax, 8, 245–249, 255–257
   needle, 241–243
   of pleural effusion, 245–249
   of pneumothorax, 8, 241–243, 252–255
   of subungual hematoma, 149–150
   by thoracentesis, 8, 245–249
   by thoracostomy, 8, 251–258
   underwater. *See* Underwater drainage
Drugs
   cardiac, 105–106
   local anesthetic, 180–181
Dry socket, 309

Ear
   irrigation of, 226
   removal of foreign body from, 223, 224–226
EKG
   with pericardiocentesis, 239
   with transvenous pacemaker, 112–113
Electrical countershock, 102–104
Electrocardiogram. *See* EKG
Endotracheal intubation, 8, 15–20, 99
Epicondylitis, 85
Epiglottis, 16
Epinephrine
   in cardiopulmonary resuscitation, 107
   with local anesthetic, 180–181
     avoidance of, 218
Episiotomy, 296, 305–306
Epistaxis *See* Nasal packing
Esophageal obturator airway, 8, 11–13
Esophageal varices, 157, 159, 175
Eyelid, eversion of, 137–139
Extensor pollicis brevis, 208
Extensor pollicis longus, 208
External cardiac compression. *See* Closed chest compression
External jugular vein, 127

Felon, drainage of, 147–148
Femoral arteriogram, 47–51
Femoral artery, 48, 59
Femoral vein puncture, 65
Fibrillation, ventricular, 102, 107
Field block anesthesia, 179, 185–187
Fish hook removal, 155–156
Flail chest, 1, 3
   endotracheal intubation in, 15–20
   tracheostomy in, 25–37
Flank tap, 259–260
Flexor carpi radialis, 205
Flexor carpi ulnaris, 212
Fluoroscopy, with transvenous pacemaker insertion, 112
Foley catheter
   in cystography, 280
   in cystotomy, 285
   in thoracostomy, 254, 257
Food bolus removal, by Heimlich maneuver, 39–43

Foreign body removal
  from airway, 94, 99
    Heimlich maneuver, 39–43
  from ear, 223, 224–226
  from eye, 137–139
  from nose, 223–224
Four-quadrant tap, 261–262
Fractures, spinal. *See* Traction

Gag reflex, 233, 235
Ganglion, aspiration of, 91–92
Gardner-Wells traction tongs, 275–278
Gastric aspiration. *See* Nasogastric tubes
Gastric decompression, 157, 163
Gastric lavage, 157, 163, 165, 172
Gastrointestinal tubes, 157–177
  Blakemore-Sengstaken, 157, 159–160, 175–177
  Cantor, 158–159, 167–170
  Levin, 157–158, 163–165
  Miller-Abbott, 158–159, 171–174
  nasogastric, 157–158, 163–165
    Blakemore-Sengstaken tube with, 177
    esophageal obturator airway with, 13
    Robinson catheter as, 157, 160, 163
    placement of, 160–161
  Salem-sump, 157–158, 163–165
Glottis, 16

Head-tilt maneuver, 4, 96
Heart block, transvenous pacemaker in, 111–113
Heimlich maneuver, 39–43
Heimlich valve, 254
Hematoma
  perineal, 279, 291
  subungual, drainage of, 149–150
Hematuria, 291
Hemopericardium, drainage of, 237–239
Hemorrhage. *See also* Bleeding
  antishock suit in, 115–119
  gastrointestinal, 163, 165
  intraperitoneal, 259–262, 265–268, 269–270
  pericardial, 237–239
  in pregnancy, 308
  thoracic. *See* Hemothorax
Hemothorax, 245, 251
  due to central venous catheterization, 123
  evacuation of, 8
    by thoracentesis, 245–249
    by thoracostomy, 255–257
Hypoxia, endotracheal intubation in, 15–20

Indirect laryngoscopy, 233–235
Indwelling cannula, 63–64, 65–69
Infiltration, local, 179, 185
Infraorbital canal, 194
Infraorbital foramen, 194
Infraorbital nerve block, 193–195
Infusion sets, for vascular puncture, 55
Intercostal nerve block, 201–202
Intercostal neurovascular bundle, 201, 242
Intestinal aspiration. *See* Gastrointestinal tubes

Intra-arterial catheter, 121
Intra-arterial pressure monitoring
  by arterial puncture, 59–62
  with central venous catheterization, 121
Intraperitoneal bleeding, 259–262, 265–268, 269–270
Intravenous line
  in cardiopulmonary resuscitation, 105
  in transvenous pacing, 112
Intubation, endotracheal, 8, 15–20, 99
Irrigation. *See also* Lavage
  of ear, 226

Jaw-pull maneuver, 97
Jaw-thrust maneuver, 97
Jugular vein, external, 127

Keisselbach's area, 227

Labor
  care of patient in, 295–308
  stages of, 296–297, 304–305
Laryngoscopy, indirect, 233–235
Lavage
  gastric, 157, 163, 165, 172
  peritoneal, 265–268
Levin tube, 157–158, 163–165
Lidocaine, 180
  in cardiopulmonary resuscitation, 107–108
Linea alba, 284
Local anesthesia, 179–218
  adverse reactions to, 183
  drugs used in, 180–181
  techniques used in, 182–183
  types of, 179–180
    field block, 179, 185–187
    local infiltration, 179, 185
    nerve block, 179–180, 189–218
      digital, 215–218
      infraorbital, 193–195
      intercostal, 201–202
      median, 203–205
      mental, 197–199
      radial, 207–209
      supraorbital, 189–191
      ulnar, 211–213
Local infiltration anesthesia, 179, 185
Lumbar puncture, 219–221

Maternity care, emergency, 295–298
Median basilic vein, 71
Median nerve block, 203–205
Mental foramen, 197
Mental nerve block, 197–199
Mepivacaine, 180
Miller-Abbott tube, 158–159, 171–174
Mirror laryngoscopy, 233–235
Monitor, cardiac, with transvenous pacemaker, 112
Morphine sulfate, in cardiopulmonary resuscitation, 108
Mouth-to-nose technique, 95
Mouth-to-mouth ventilation, 95, 98–99

Myocardial infarction, transvenous pacemaker in, 111–113

Nasal packing
  anterior, 227–228
  posterior, 229–232
Nasogastric tubes, 157–158, 163–165
  Blakemore-Sengstaken tube with, 177
  esophageal obturator airway with, 13
  Robinson catheter as, 157, 160, 163
Nasopharyngeal airway insertion, 6
Needle cricothyrotomy, 8, 21–23
Needle drainage, 241–243
Nerve block anesthesia. See under Local anesthesia
Neurogenic airway problems, 1–2
Newborn care, 302
Nose
  packing of. See Nasal packing
  removal of foreign body from, 223–224

Obstructive airway problems, 1–2
Obturator, esophageal, 8, 11–13
Olecranon bursa, aspiration of, 81–82
Oropharyngeal airway
  endotracheal intubation with, 20
  insertion of, 6

Pacemaker, transvenous, 111–113
Packing, nasal. See Nasal packing
Palmaris longus tendon, 204
Papoose Board, 72, 182, 224
Paradoxical respiration, 2
Parenchymal airway problems, 1–2
Patellar bursa, aspiration of, 83–84
Pericardiocentesis, 237–239
Peritoneal flank tap, 259–260
Peritoneal four-quadrant tap, 261–262
Peritoneal lavage, 265–268
pH, of tissue, and local anesthesia, 180
Placenta
  delivery of, 304
  premature separation of, 308
  retained, 305
Placenta previa, 308
Pleural cavity, needle drainage of, 241–243
Pleural effusion, 245–249
Pneumothorax, 1, 3, 251
  due to central venous catheterization, 123, 135
  due to thoracentesis, 249
  evacuation of, 8
    by needle drainage, 241–243
    by thoracostomy, 252–255
Pouch of Douglas, 269
Precordial thump, 100
Procaine, 180
Pulmonary pressure measurement, 121
Punctures. See also Aspiration; Taps
  bladder, 283–286
  cricothyroid membrane, 8, 21–23
  lumbar, 219–221
  pleural cavity, 241–243, 245–249, 251–257
  vascular. See Vascular punctures

Queckenstedt's test, 221

Radial artery, 60
Radial nerve block, 207–209
Radiohumeral bursa, injection of, 85–86
Regional anesthesia, 185–187
Respiration
  artificial. See Ventilation, artificial
  paradoxical, 2
Respiratory arrest. See also Cardiopulmonary resuscitation
  esophageal obturator airway in, 11–13
Respiratory insufficiency
  endotracheal intubation in, 15–20
  esophageal obturator airway in, 11–13
  tracheostomy in, 25–37
Retention catheters, 287, 288
Ring, removal of, 151–153
Ritgen maneuver, 298
Robinson catheter, 287
  as nasogastric tube, 157, 160, 163

Salem-sump tube, 157–158, 163–165
Saphenous vein, 71
Shock, antishock suit in, 115–119
Skeletal airway problems, 1–2
Sodium bicarbonate, in cardiopulmonary resuscitation, 103, 106–107, 108
Space of Retzius, 284
Spinal tap, 219–221
Steinman pin insertion, 271–273
Stokes-Adams disease, transvenous pacemaker in, 111–113
Straight catheters, 287
Stress cystography, 279–281
Subacromial bursa, injection of, 87–89
Subclavian vein, 133
Subungual hematoma, drainage of, 149–150
Sucking wounds, 1
  defined, 3
Suction
  with Blakemore-Sengstaken tube, 177
  with Cantor tube, 170
  with Miller-Abbott tube, 173
  with Salem-sump tube, 165
Supraorbital nerve block, 189–191
Suture method (ring removal), 153
Swan-Ganz catheter, 121

Tamponade, cardiac, 237
Taps. See also Aspiration; Punctures
  pericardial, 237–239
  peritoneal
    flank, 259–260
    four-quadrant, 261–262
    with lavage, 265–268
  spinal, 219–221
  thoracic, 8, 245–249
Tendinitis, 77
  bursitis vs., 77, 87
Tendon sheaths, injection of, 77–80
Tennis elbow, 85
Thoracentesis, 8, 245–249
Thoracostomy, 8, 241, 251–258
Thoracotomy, 239
Thyroid isthmus, 31
Thyroid notch, 21

Trachea, 16–17, 22, 27
Tracheostomy, 8, 25–37
Traction
 cervical, 275–278
 with Steinman pin, 271–273
Transvenous pacemaker, 111–113
Transverse lie, 308
Trocar suprapubic cystotomy, 283–286
Trocar thoracostomy, 257–258
Tubes, gastrointestinal. *See* Gastrointestinal tubes

Ulnar nerve block, 211–213
Umbilical cord
 in breech presentation, 307
 prolapsed, 307
 tight, 299
Underwater drainage, 8
 with needle drainage, 241, 243
 with thoracostomy, 241, 254, 257
Urethra, male, 288–289
Urethral catheterization, 287–290
Urethrogram, 291–293
Uterine atony, 305
Uvula, 16

Valsalva's maneuver
 with central venous catheterization, 130
 with lumbar puncture, 220
Varices, esophageal, 157, 159, 175
Vascular punctures, 53–57. *See also* Arteriograms; Central venous catheterization
 arterial, 59–62
 venipuncture, 56–57, 63–69
  femoral, 65
  site selection for, 56–57
 venous cutdown, 71–75
Venipuncture, 56–57, 63–69
Venous cutdown, 71–75
Ventilation, artificial, 4, 6–7. *See also* Airway management
 with cardiopulmonary resuscitation, 94–95, 98–99, 101
 with sodium bicarbonate administration, 107
Ventricular fibrillation, 102, 107
Vocal cords, 235

Whistle tip catheter, 287

X-ray studies
 arteriograms
  axillary, 45–46
  femoral, 47–51
 of Cantor tube placement, 170
 of central venous catheter placement, 126, 128, 131, 135
 cystogram, 281
 fluoroscopy, with transvenous pacemaker, 112–113
 of Miller-Abbott tube placement, 174
 with thoracentesis, 245, 249
 with thoracostomy, 255, 257, 258
 urethrogram, 291–293